Deb McClung

MAGNETIC RESONANCE IMAGING
Physical and Biological Principles

MAGNETIC RESONANCE IMAGING
Physical and Biological Principles

Stewart C. Bushong, Sc.D.

Professor, Department of Radiology,
Baylor College of Medicine,
Houston, Texas

With 547 illustrations

The C. V. Mosby Company

St. Louis • Washington, D.C. • Toronto 1988

MOSBY

A TRADITION OF PUBLISHING EXCELLENCE

Editor: David T. Culverwell
Editing and Design: Editing, Design, & Production, Inc.

The C. V. Mosby Company
11830 Westline Industrial Drive, St. Louis, Missouri 63146

Library of Congress Cataloging-in-Publication Data

Bushong, Stewart C.
    Magnetic resonance imaging: physical and biological principles /
Stewart C. Bushong.
        p.   cm.
    Includes index.
    ISBN 0-8016-1820-7
    1. Magnetic resonance imaging.   I. Title.
    [DNLM: 1. Nuclear Magnetic Resonance.   2. Nuclear Magnetic
Resonance—diagnostic use.   WN 445 B979m]
    RC78.7.N83B87   1989
    616.07'54—dc 19
    DNLM/DLC
    for Library of Congress

C/VH/VH   9 8 7 6 5 4 3 2   01/C/077

To
Bettie,
Leslie,
Stephen,
Andrew,
Butterscotch,†
Jemimah,†
Geraldine,†
Casper,†
Ginger,†
Sebastian,†
Buffy,†
and Eboney

†R.I.P.

Preface

Magnetic resonance imaging has burst onto the scene as a diagnostic imaging tool with even more intensity than did computed tomography some 15 years ago. Its similarities to computed tomography are somewhat obvious, but the underlying physical principles are new to imaging physicians and technologists and are considerably more difficult to understand. Whereas computed tomography is an extension of x-ray imaging, whose basic physics has been well integrated into radiology training programs, the physical basis for MRI is totally different. MRI is confounding because much of the terminology and most of the mathematics are foreign to those involved in medical imaging.

In 1982, we at Baylor College of Medicine installed our first MR imager. Following the experience we gained with that initial system, we began to offer a week-long program combining lectures and laboratory sessions for physicians, scientists, and engineers getting started in MRI. Fully 80% of the week's activities was devoted to the physics of MRI, and the remainder to image appearance and interpretation.

This week-long program was later supplemented by a 2-day course for radiologic technologists. This course did not go nearly as deeply into the physics and mathematics of MRI, and there was no laboratory work. Still, it has been shown to meet the needs of radiologic technologists very effectively.

This volume is an outgrowth of these courses. It represents the combined efforts of many members of the faculty of the Department of Radiology at Baylor College of Medicine, whose contributions are evident throughout the text. Listed below are the faculty members who made this volume possible:

Susan E. Blair, B.S., Administrative Coordinator of MRI
R. Nick Bryan, M.D., Ph.D., Professor of Radiology
Marvin H. Chasen, M.D., Associate Professor of Clinical Radiology
Joseph J. Ford, Ph.D., Research Assistant Professor of Radiology
Michele A. Gable, R.T., Technical Director of MRI
John E. Madewell, M.D., Vice Chairman and Professor of Radiology
Marilyn H. Sackett, R.T., Technical Director of Radiology
Steven L. Sax, M.D., Fellow in MRI
Nicholas Schneiders, M.S., Research Assistant Professor of Radiology
Paul T. Weatherall, M.D., Fellow in MRI
Susan W. Weathers, M.D., Research Assistant Professor of Radiology
Richard E. Wendt III, Ph.D., Research Assistant Professor of Radiology
Robert L. Willcott, Ph.D., Adjunct Professor of Radiology

Chapters 13 through 16 are the result of efforts by Drs. Weatherall and Madewell, who assembled the images and prepared the discussions of planar anatomy.

I am also deeply indebted to Elaine Casey, Judy Matteau, Gina Foster, and Jo Ann Dinnean for their patient help in assembling and processing the manuscript. The text illustrations for this volume are by Ann Sparks, Spencer Phippen, and Kraig Emmert. Their talent and clever ideas added sense where concepts were sometimes hard to express. The cover was designed by Angie Dinnean, who once again demonstrated exceptional skill.

The goal of this text is to present the fundamentals of MRI in such a way that they are easily understood by physicians and technologists with little or no background in physics and mathematics. Abundant use has been made of illustrations, but only the most basic mathematics has been included. Interested readers will find a more complex mathematical development in Appendix A.

I would like to encourage readers of this book to inform me of any sections that they find difficult to understand. Such comments will be taken into account in the development of future editions. By the way, I have purposefully inserted a significant error in this book to see how closely it is read. The first person to discover the error and let me know will receive a very special award as well as recognition in subsequent editions.

I trust that this volume continues my efforts to make medical imaging understandable and **medical physics fun**.

Stewart C. Bushong

Contents

Chapter
ONE

An Overview of Magnetic Resonance Imaging

HISTORICAL TRAIL

One hundred years ago, if one wanted to make an image of a patient, what could be done? Actually not much of anything. At that time only photography or hand-drawn images were available. Both types of images use the narrow band of the electromagnetic spectrum, called the **visible light** region, as shown in Figure 1-1. This figure representing the electromagnetic spectrum shows that electromagnetic radiation can be characterized by any one of three parameters: wavelength, energy, and frequency. Although we can only sense electromagnetic radiation in the visible light region, we know that the range of such radiation extends over many orders of magnitude.

How does photography work? Visible light reflects off an object, and the photons of light are captured by something that is sensitive to that kind of radiation, such as a photographic emulsion. Therefore, a photograph is made with reflected electromagnetic radiation and a suitable receptor. Nineteenth-century physicists studying visible light detailed its wavelike properties accord-

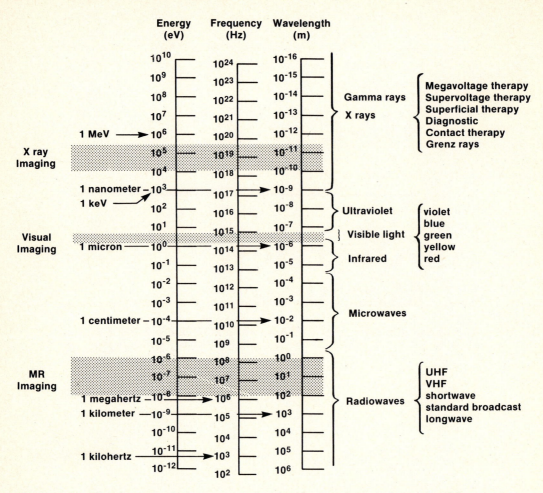

Figure 1-1. The electromagnetic spectrum showing the imaging windows of visible light, x-rays, and radiowaves.

ing to how it interacted with matter—reflection, diffraction, and refraction. Consequently, visible light has always been characterized by its wavelength.

When Roentgen discovered x-rays in 1895, suddenly there was another, equally narrow region of the electromagnetic spectrum from which medical images could be made. For that discovery, he received the first Nobel Prize in Physics in 1901. One reason for that award was that within about 6 months Roentgen conducted numerous cleverly designed experiments that allowed him to describe x-rays pretty much as we know them today. Some of the experiments indicated to him that this "x-light" interacted not as a wave but as a particle. Therefore, x-ray emissions are identified according to their energy. One refers to **kVp,**—kilovolt peak—but in fact it is more accurate to use **keV**—kilo electron volt—to identify x-radiation.

How is an x-ray image made? A source of electromagnetic radiation—x-rays—is shone on a patient. Some of the radiation is absorbed, and some of it is transmitted through the patient to an image receptor. Therefore, one obtains a shadowgram, like one children make with their hands. The x-ray shadowgram, however, results from partial absorption of electromagnetic radiation, not reflection.

During the latter nineteenth century, following Edison's early work, engineers and physicists were working to develop radio communications. To create a radio emission, one must in some way cause electrons to oscillate in a conductor. This requires the construction of an electronic circuit called an **oscillator.** The oscillator is the basis for radio electronics. The electromagnetic radiation emitted is called a **radio frequency (RF)** emission. Physicists identify this radiation according to the frequency of oscillation.

Commercial broadcast, both AM and FM, is similarly identified. The AM RF band ranges from 540 to 1640 KHz and the FM RF band from 88 to 108 MHz. Magnetic resonance images are made with RF in the range from about 1 MHz to 80 MHz. One could just as easily identify these various RF emissions by their energy or wavelength as seen in Figure 1-1.

What is really spectacular about contemporary medical imaging is the use of the RF region of the electromagnetic spectrum to produce an image. This is **nuclear magnetic resonance (NMR),** or as we have settled on, **magnetic resonance imaging (MRI),** or **magnetic resonance imaging and spectroscopy (MR).** Some of the leaders in radiology were concerned about the use of the word *nuclear* around patients, and so *nuclear* was dropped from the term.

How does one make an MR image? For a visible image, radiation is reflected from the body. For an x-ray image, radiation is partially transmitted through the body. For an MR image, the body is stimulated to emit electromagnetic radiation, which by some very clever methods is detected, interpreted, and used to produce an image, as illustrated in Figure 1-2.

Felix Bloch

A 1946 Nobel Prize–winning paper by **Felix Bloch** (1905–1984) started it all. Bloch, therefore, is to MR imaging what Roentgen is to x-ray imaging. Bloch was a theoretical physicist who proposed some rather novel properties for the atomic nucleus. One of Bloch's proposals was that the nucleus behaves like a small magnet. He described this nuclear magnetism by what is now called the **Bloch equations.** These equations are covered in simplistic form in Appendix A for the interested reader.

Bloch's equations explain that a nucleus, because it spins on an imaginary axis, has an associated magnetic field. This field is called a **magnetic moment.** Nucleons that have charge such as a proton and that spin have an even stronger magnetic field.

The experimental verification for the Bloch equations did not come until the early 1950s. By 1960 several companies were producing analytical instruments called **NMR spectrometers.** During the sixties and seventies, NMR spec-

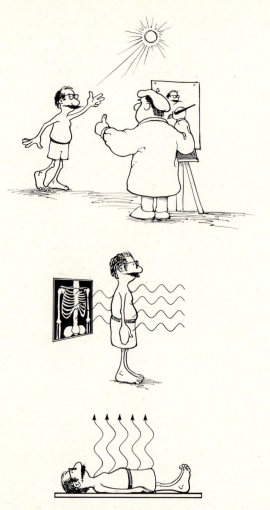

Figure 1-2.   Illustrating how images are made using the three regions of the electromagnetic spectrum.

trometry became very widely used in academic and industrial research. Such use of NMR allows the investigator to determine the molecular configuration of a material from analysis of its NMR spectrum.

Damadian and Lauterbur

In the late 1960s, engineer-physician Raymond Damadian, was doing NMR spectroscopy. He first showed that malignant tissue has a different spectrum from that of normal tissue. Furthermore, he showed the parameters associated with NMR—spin density, T1, and T2—differ between normal and malignant tissue. Because of his unique academic background, in 1974 Damadian produced a crude NMR image of a rat tumor, which appeared on the cover of

TABLE 1-1. **Spatial and contrast resolution characteristics of several medical imaging procedures**

	Radioisotope Imaging	Ultrasound	Radiography	Computed Tomography	Magnetic Resonance Imaging
Spatial resolution (mm)	5	2	0.1	0.5	0.5
Contrast resolution (mm at 0.5%)	20	10	10	4	2

Science magazine. His first body image was accomplished in 1976, and it took almost 4 hours to produce.

During this same period Paul Lauterbur was engaged in similar research. There is considerable discussion as to which of these two should be recognized for bringing us MRI. In all likelihood both will ultimately share this recognition.

WHY DO MRI?

When a plain radiograph of the abdomen is placed on a view box for interpretation, what does one see? Not very much! The image is gray and flat, with very little detail. To enhance the detail of such an image, one could do a conventional tomogram or an angiogram. These two radiographic examinations have one thing in common: they enhance the contrast of the image and thereby improve the visualization of structures.

Contrast Resolution

If such an image is not satisfactory, what else can be done? A computed tomography (CT) scan could be requested. The advantage of CT imaging over radiographic imaging is superior **contrast resolution.** The **spatial resolution** of CT scanning is worse than that of screen-film imaging. Likewise, the spatial resolution of MRI is considerably worse than that of radiography. But the contrast resolution or the resolution of low-contrast objects is even better with MRI than with CT. **Contrast resolution is the principal advantage of MRI.**

Spatial resolution refers to the ability of a process to identify very small but dense objects such as metal fragments or microcalcifications. Contrast resolution allows visualization of low-density objects with similar soft tissue characteristics such as liver-spleen or white matter–gray matter. Table 1-1 shows representative values of spatial resolution and contrast resolution for various medical imaging devices.

In x-ray imaging, spatial resolution is principally a function of the geometry of the system. Focal spot size and source to image receptor distance (SID) are two important geometric considerations. In x-ray imaging, contrast resolution in principally limited by the amount of scatter radiation present. X-ray beam collimation and use of radiographic grids reduce scatter radiation and therefore improve contrast resolution.

In x-ray imaging, differential x-ray absorption in body tissues is determined by the x-ray attenuation coefficient. The x-ray attenuation coefficient in turn is dependent on the energy of the x-ray beam and the atomic number of the tissue being imaged. The basis for the MR image, however, is far different. It is a function of several intrinsic properties of the tissue being imaged. The three most important properties are **spin density (SD), spin lattice relaxation time (T1),** and **spin-spin relaxation time (T2).** There are also secondary properties such as motion, paramagnetism, and chemical shift.

To produce a radiographic image, two principal controls cover technique selection—kVp and mAs (milliampere-second). By carefully selecting kVp and mAs, one can optimize the contrast resolution of an image without compromise of the spatial resolution.

In MRI it is not that way at all. There are many combinations of how one sequences the RF emissions, called **RF pulses,** to maximize contrast resolution. There are three principal RF pulse sequences—**partial saturation, inversion recovery,** and **spin echo**—each of which has a large selection of timing patterns for the RF pulses. How one times the RF pulses will determine the appearance of the image. Furthermore, it is becoming clear that precise RF pulse sequencing may be associated with optimum visualization of various disease states.

Multiplanar Imaging

A second advantage to MRI is the ability to obtain direct sagittal, coronal, and oblique plane images. Conventional radiographs show superimposed anatomy regardless of the plane of the image. In CT imaging one reconstructs sagittal and coronal images from a set of contiguous transaxial images. With MR images one can obtain a very large data set, all acquired during a single imaging sequence, and with proper data processing reconstruct any particular anatomic plane for display.

Viewing images obtained from various anatomic planes requires a different kind of knowledge on the part of the physician and the technologist. During residency training, radiologists spend 4 years studying image recognition. Except for CT images nearly all of the images are parallel with the axis of the body. The MR image interpreter now views anatomic planes that have not been imaged before. The required interpretive skills will come with experience.

When students are enrolled in a program of radiologic technology, the emphasis of the curriculum is **technique selection** and **positioning.** Patient positioning in radiography is important to ensure that the structure being imaged is parallel and close to the image receptor. MR images are directly available as high-contrast projections in any plane, without attention to patient positioning. The operator may need to know a little trigonometry, but all planes are easily acquired because of the design of the operating console and software.

MR Spectroscopy

Another advantage to MRI is the possibility of doing in vivo spectroscopy. This subject is dealt with only superficially here. It is possible that one could make an MR image, see a suspicious lesion, put the cursor on that lesion, and encompass it within a **region of interest (ROI).** One could then retrieve the NMR spectrum from the lesion for analysis. An interpretation of the NMR spectrum then would tell whether the tissue is normal or abnormal, and if it is abnormal, it would reveal the molecular nature of the abnormality.

This ability may come to pass, although it is being developed much, much slower that was initially anticipated. Furthermore, unless they become organic chemists, physicians are not going to read these spectra. If in vivo NMR spectroscopy becomes a clinical reality, an organic chemist will probably be needed in the reading room with the radiologist.

No Radiation

MRI's advantage over x-ray imaging of having no radiation has been well publicized. No radiation, or precisely no ionizing radiation, has been used very effectively to promote MRI to the medical community and the public. MRI uses RF electromagnetic radiation and magnetic fields, which do not cause ionization and therefore do not have the associated potential harmful effects of ionizing radiation. There are some known bioeffects of RF and magnetic fields, but they do not occur at the low intensities of MRI and they are not associated with induction of malignant disease. This advantage is probably overstated since the radiation doses employed in x-ray imaging are so low.

MRI HARDWARE

Just as a radiographic system can be identified by its three main components—x-ray tube, high-voltage generator, and operating console—so are there three main components of an MR imager. These are the **gantry,** the **computer,** and the **operating console.**

The gantry is the large, usually cylindrical device that accommodates the patient during imaging. Unlike a CT gantry, the MRI gantry has no moving parts. Everything is controlled electronically. The patient aperture is usually 50 to 60 cm in diameter. Surrounding the patient in this aperture are the RF coils, or **RF probe.** Surrounding the RF probe are **gradient coils, shim coils,** and in the case of an electromagnet **primary coils** to produce the main magnetic field.

The computer required for MRI is similar to that for CT, only faster and bigger. During an MR scan more data are collected, and the computations required are longer and more difficult than with CT.

The MRI operating console is similar to that for CT. It has the same controls for windowing and data analysis through an ROI. Whereas CT employs mechanical incrementation for patient localization, there is no movement of the patient in MRI. An MRI console has RF controls rather than kVp, mA, and scan time controls.

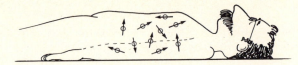

Figure 1-3.   Under normal conditions nuclear magnetic dipoles in the body are randomly distributed, resulting in zero net magnetization.

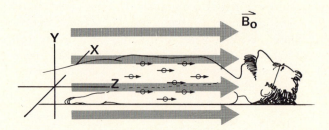

Figure 1-4.   When a strong external magnetic field, B_0, is applied, the patient becomes polarized and net magnetization, M, appears.

MRI BRIEFLY

Figure 1-3 shows a patient on an imaging couch. The hydrogen nuclei in the patient, protons, behave like tiny magnets. Hydrogen is abundant in the human body, constituting 80% of all atoms, which makes it very useful for MRI. Furthermore, because it is a single charged spinning nucleon, the hydrogen nucleus exhibits relatively strong magnetism. The little arrows in Figure 1-3 represent these individual proton magnets. Under normal circumstances, these magnetic dipoles are randomly distributed in space. Consequently, if you attempt to measure the net magnetic field of a patient, it would be zero, because all of the individual magnets will cancel out.

Net Magnetization

When the patient is placed in the presence of a strong external magnetic field, the individual nuclear magnetic moments, or **dipoles,** align with the external magnetic field, as shown in Figure 1-4. A mathematician will always show the cartesian coordinate axis, X, Y, and Z, with the Z axis as the vertical axis. To develop the physics of MRI, vector diagrams will be employed using the mathematician's rendering of the coordinate system.

A vector is a quantity that has not only magnitude but also direction. In Figure 1-4 the Z axis is drawn along the long axis of the patient. By convention, in MRI the Z axis coincides with the axis of the main magnetic field. In the most popular electromagnetic imagers, the main magnetic field is horizontal and therefore the Z axis is also. In a permanent magnet imager the Z axis is vertical as in the vector diagrams to follow.

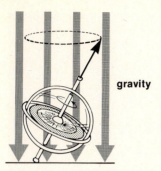

gravity

Figure 1-5. A gyroscope, when spinning in outer space, just spins. On the Earth it precesses as it spins.

The symbol for the main magnetic field is B_0. It has an intensity expressed in **tesla (T).** An often asked question about MRI is, how many rads are equal to 1 tesla? The answer is none. There is no relationship between ionizing radiation and magnetic field strength. Nothing about MRI can be measured in rads because **MRI employs no ionizing radiation.**

With a patient positioned in an external magnetic field, the proton dipoles align with the field, as shown in Figure 1-4. Actually this is an oversimplification and is not exactly true. Only about one out of each million dipoles becomes so aligned. When individual magnetic dipoles are so aligned, the patient is said to be polarized, and **net magnetization** of the patient has been created. The patient now has a north pole and a south pole.

Precession

In addition to polarization, a second phenomenon occurs when a patient is placed in a strong magnetic field. To understand this phenomenon, consider the gyroscope shown in Figure 1-5. A gyroscope has an annulus of heavy metal attached by spokes to an axis. Early space station designs were like saucers, spinning to produce an artificial gravity. Figure 1-6 shows the current design. Hand and foot clips will provide moorings for space station inhabitants. If one takes the gyroscope onto a space station and spins it, the gyroscope will spin and that is all. But if one spins the gyroscope on Earth in the presence of a gravitational field, not only will gyroscope spin, but as it slows it will begin to wobble. Physicists call this wobble **precession.** The gyroscope is said to precess.

Precession is the interaction between the spinning mass of the gyroscope and the mass of the Earth that is manifest through the gravitational field. By spinning, the gyroscope creates angular momentum, which interacts with the angular momentum of the spinning Earth and causes the precessional motion.

Similarly, if a spinning magnetic field, such as the magnetic moment of the proton in Figure 1-7, is in the presence of an external magnetic field, it will not only spin but will also precess.

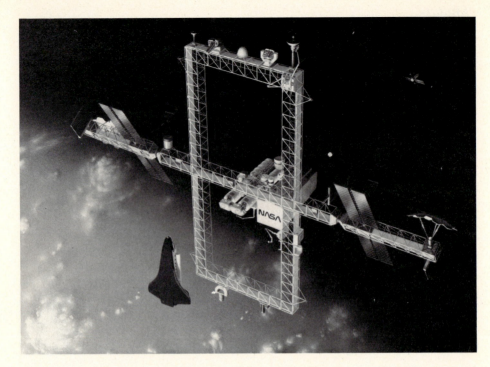

Figure 1-6. A proposed space station of the twenty-first century. (Courtesy National Aeronautics and Space Administration.)

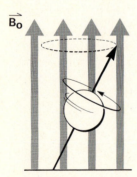

Figure 1-7. In the presence of an external magnetic field a spinning proton will precess.

The fundamental equation for MRI is the **Larmor equation,** which identifies the frequency of this precession:

$$\omega = \gamma\, B \qquad\qquad \textbf{(1-1)}$$

where ω is the frequency of precession, and
γ represents the gyromagnetic ratio.

TABLE 1-2.   Nuclei of medical interest and their gyromagnetic ratios

Nucleus	Gyromagnetic Ratio (MHz/T)
^{1}H	42.6
^{19}F	40.1
^{31}P	17.2
^{23}Na	11.3
^{13}C	10.7
^{2}H	6.5
^{17}O	5.8
^{39}K	2.0

The Larmor equation relates B, the strength of the magnetic field, to the precessional frequency omega (ω) through gamma (γ), which has a precise value that is characteristic of each nuclear species.

Gamma is to MRI what lambda (λ), the disintegration constant, is to radioactive decay. Each radionuclide has its own characteristic disintegration constant, and each nuclear species has its own characteristic gyromagnetic ratio. The units of the gyromagnetic ratio are MHz/T. For instance, hydrogen has a gyromagnetic ratio equal to 42.6 MHz/T. Omega is the frequency at which that nuclear species precesses in a magnetic field. For instance, if the external magnetic field is 1 tesla and the gyromagnetic ratio is 42.6 MHz/T, then the precessional frequency would be 42.6 MHz. The precessional frequency is also called the **Larmor frequency.**

Table 1-2 shows the principal nuclei that are of biologic interest in MRI. Medical applications of MRI concentrate on hydrogen because of its relative abundance and high gyromagnetic ratio. Compared with other nuclei in the body, hydrogen has the highest sensitivity for producing an NMR signal.

Free Induction Decay

Having placed the patient in the strong magnetic field, we have polarized the patient as in Figure 1-4. The proton magnetic dipoles have aligned with the main magnetic field. We therefore summarize the action of all of these individual proton dipoles with one large arrow as in Figure 1-8. This arrow represents a vector quantity called **net magnetization.**

Now begins the NMR experiment. Figure 1-8 includes a coil or wire, which represents a radio transmitter. Using this antenna, one transmits into the patient a pulse of RF at the Larmor frequency. For hydrogen imaging with a magnetic field of 1 tesla, the RF would be tuned to 42.6 MHz.

Figure 1-9 shows a country-and-western star plucking the G string of a guitar. If a harp were nearby, one of its strings might begin to vibrate. But only one string would vibrate—the G string; the other strings would remain unaffected. Just the harp string that has the same fundamental resonance as the plucked guitar string would vibrate. The *R* in MRI stands for **resonance.** The

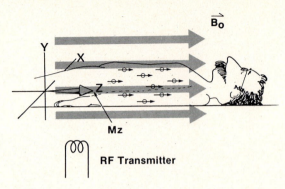

Figure 1-8. Net magnetization along the Z axis is represented by M_z and the large arrow.

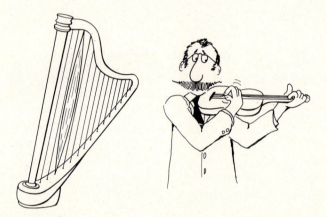

Figure 1-9. Plucking the string of G on a guitar will cause only the G string of a nearby harp to vibrate.

RF pulse transmitted into the body must be at the resonant frequency of the precessing hydrogen nuclei in order for energy to be absorbed.

Most objects in nature have a **fundamental resonance.** Energy transfer is always most efficient at resonance. For example, at a large hotel in Kansas City a few years ago people were dancing on a suspended bridgelike walkway. They hit a resonance that was fundamental to the walkway and it collapsed. Marching military personnel are instructed to break cadence when crossing a bridge for the same reason. Figure 1-10 shows the collapsing Tacoma Narrows suspension bridge that was subjected to harmonic buffeting winds.

With net magnetization in the Z direction as shown Figure 1-11, not only are the proton magnetic dipoles aligned, but each individual proton is precessing at the Larmor frequency. When one pulses the RF signal at resonance into the patient, the individual energy states of each proton may be changed. This causes enough protons to flip into the negative Z direction while still precessing

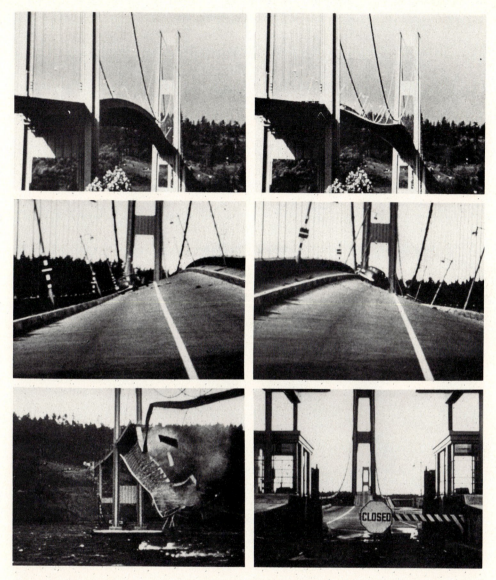

Figure 1-10. The Tacoma Narrows suspension bridge collapsed in buffeting gale force winds that set up a resonant oscillation. (Courtesy Civil Engineering Department, Rice University, Houston, Texas.)

as shown in Figure 1-12. Net magnetization is now in the negative Z direction and precessing.

When RF is pulsed into the patient, the protons individually flip over into the negative Z direction while continuing to precess, and then one by one these protons start flipping back to their normal state in the positive Z direction. The

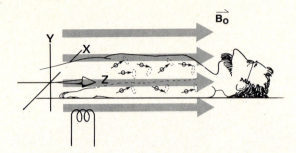

Figure 1-11.   Placing a patient in a strong magnetic field polarizes the patient and causes each proton dipole to precess randomly.

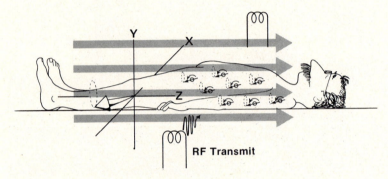

Figure 1-12.   Net magnetization is changed to the negative Z direction, and the protons precess in phase when a proper RF pulse is transmitted into the patient.

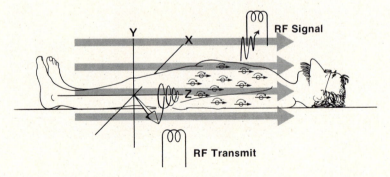

Figure 1-13.   Precessing net magnetization induces an RF signal in a receiving antenna. That RF signal is called a free induction decay (FID).

normal state is called the **equilibrium** state because the protons are at equilibrium in the main magnetic field. As the individual protons return to equilibrium, the net magnetization precesses around the Z axis and slowly returns, **relaxes,** to equilibrium, as in Figure 1-13.

   To a disinterested observer, such as the RF receiving antenna in Figure 1-13, such precession will not be obvious. All that is observed is a magnetic

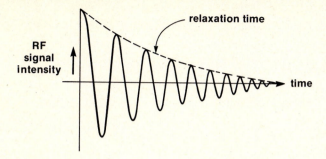

Figure 1-14. The FID is a decreasing harmonic oscillation of the Larmor frequency.

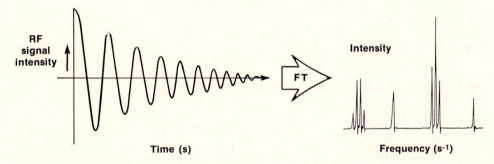

Figure 1-15. When a Fourier transformation (FT) is performed on the FID, an NMR spectrum results.

field first approaching and then receding harmonically. Any time there is a moving magnetic field, an electric current can be **induced** in a properly designed antenna. The induced current represents a radio signal emitted by the patient. This signal is the **free induction decay (FID).** The signal received by the RF antenna surrounding the patient is an oscillating signal that decreases with time, as shown in Figure 1-14. It decreases as each individual proton flips back until the signal gets back to equilibrium magnetization. The time that is required for that signal to "relax" back to equilibrium is a **relaxation time.** There are two such relaxation times. T1 and T2 are independent, but both can be obtained from the FID.

Fourier Transformation

The free induction decay is a plot of NMR signal intensity as a function of time as shown in Figure 1-14. This FID can be expressed mathematically as a sinusoidal variation in signal intensity. If a mathematical operation called a **Fourier transformation (FT)** is performed on the FID, the result appears as in Figure 1-15.

The result of this Fourier transformation is an NMR spectrum. Whereas the FID is a plot of signal intensity versus time, the NMR spectrum is a plot of signal intensity versus inverse time, s^{-1}, or hertz (Hz). Therefore, the NMR spectrum is a plot of signal intensity as a function of frequency. Each of the

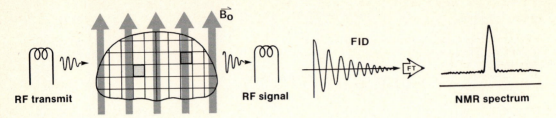

Figure 1-16.   If the same tissue were in the two highlighted voxels, both voxels would be represented by the same peak in the NMR spectrum.

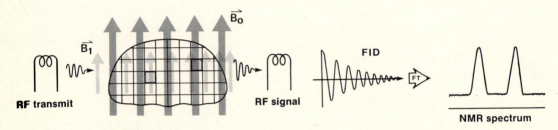

Figure 1-17.   In the presence of a gradient magnetic field, B_1, the NMR spectrum provides information on pixel location.

peaks in the NMR spectrum represents some characteristic of the tissue under investigation.

How is an image obtained from an NMR spectrum? The following explanation is simplistic and will be developed in detail throughout this volume. Figure 1-16 presents a transaxial cross-section through the trunk. Two pixels in the patient are highlighted, and the patient is in a uniform magnetic field. If both voxels contain the same tissue, the peak in the NMR spectrum will represent both voxels. Therefore, one can tell from the spectrum what is in both voxels but cannot tell where each is located.

If instead of a uniform magnetic field we impress across the patient a **gradient magnetic field, B_1,** the result is shown in Figure 1-17. A gradient field is a nonuniform, continuously varying magnetic field. The tissue in the voxel at the lower magnetic field strength has a lower Larmor frequency than that at the higher magnetic field even though it is the same tissue. The free induction decay in this situation is considerably more complicated. Following Fourier transformation, instead of having one peak the spectrum has two peaks. **A uniform magnetic field is required for spectroscopy. Gradient magnetic fields are required for spatial information.**

Those two peaks carry spatial information, one representing the voxel at the lower magnetic field and the other signifying the voxel at the higher magnetic field. Such a spectrum could be considered a projection as in CT.

Multiple projections could be obtained as in CT by electronically rotating the gradient magnetic fields around the patient to produce a set of projections

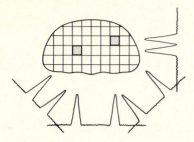

Figure 1-18. By rotating the gradient magnetic field around a patient, projections (spectra) can be obtained, from which an image could be reconstructed by back projection.

as shown in Figure 1-18. Back projection reconstruction could then be implemented to produce an image. The earliest MR images were made this way.

This is not the way MR images are now constructed. The spatial information still comes from the application of magnetic gradients superimposed on the main magnetic field, but the reconstruction of an image is through a process termed **two-dimensional Fourier transformation (2DFT).** Although this is a special application of higher mathematics, it will be developed schematically later in this volume.

SUMMARY

Magnetic resonance imaging had its beginnings in the work of Felix Bloch, who described nuclear magnetic resonance in the late 1940s. During the 1960s and 1970s nuclear magnetic resonance spectroscopy developed into an effective and widely used tool in chemical research and development. In 1972 Raymond Damadian demonstrated the first magnetic resonance image.

The advantages of magnetic resonance imaging over other medical imaging modalities include superior contrast resolution, direct multiplanar imaging, and absence of ionizing radiation. The process employs the magnetism of the hydrogen nucleus, the proton, and its interaction with external magnetic and electromagnetic fields.

First a patient is placed in a strong magnetic field, which causes the nuclear magnetism of protons to become aligned and precessing. Then a radio frequency pulse at the resonant frequency is transmitted into the patient under very controlled and prescribed conditions. Finally the patient responds to this stimulation by emitting a radio frequency signal that is computer processed to produce an image.

Chapter
TWO

Electricity and Magnetism

Both electric and magnetic fields and electromagnetic radiation are employed in MR imaging to produce an image. These are not unlike the physical agents used in x-ray imaging, although their method of use is vastly different. Electricity is used to produce the main and the gradient magnetic fields. These magnetic fields interact with the intrinsic nuclear magnetism of tissue, which is then stimulated to emit electromagnetic radiation. This stimulation is accomplished with electromagnetic radiation in the form of a radio frequency (RF) wave produced by an electrically stimulated antenna. This antenna also receives RF information emitted from the body.

A modest understanding of these fundamental physical concepts of electricity and magnetism is necessary for an understanding of MRI. A logical sequence for dealing with such subjects is to discuss electrostatics and electrodynamics to develop an understanding of electricity. This is followed by a discussion of the phenomenon of magnetism, which leads into electromagnetism and electromagnetic radiation.

ELECTROSTATICS

Electrostatics deals with stationary electric charges. The smallest unit of electric charge is contained in the electron. The proton likewise contains one unit of

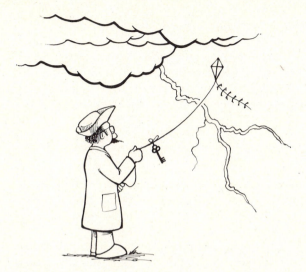

Figure 2-1.   Benjamin Franklin described electricity as the flow of positive electrification rather than electrons.

positive electric charge. Electric charge, unlike other fundamental properties of matter such as mass, cannot be subdivided. Furthermore, larger quantities of charge can only be multiples of the unit charge. Although the magnitude of the electric charge of an electron and proton is the same, the mass is approximately 1840 times the mass of the electron. Protons are relatively fixed by virtue of their position in the nucleus of an atom, whereas electrons are free to migrate from atom to atom under some circumstances.

This was not always thought to be the case. Although the electron was hypothesized by Dalton in 1688, it was not until the 1750s that Benjamin Franklin first scientifically described the nature of the electric charge. As illustrated in Figure 2-1, Franklin's experiments have been popularly associated with flying kites, which is indeed true. However, he was and is credited with also being a laboratory scientist. Nevertheless, Franklin erroneously assumed that it was positive charges that migrated down his kite string. He called this migration of charge electricity, and therein lies the origin of our confusing convention: that electric current (I) in a conductor flows opposite to electron movement. It was not until the work of J.J. Thompson in the 1890s that the electron was identified as the fundamental charged particle responsible for electricity.

The Coulomb

The fundamental unit of electric charge is the **coulomb (C).** One coulomb consists of 6.24×10^{18} electronic charges; therefore, it is a sizable number of electrons. This definition, adopted at an international congress in 1910, is such a strange number because the system for electrical measurement had already been established before the discovery of the electron. Ideally, the electron should be the smallest unit of electric charge. Instead, the charge on an electron is 1.6×10^{-19} coulombs.

The coulomb is an unfamiliar quantity to most of us, although we experience electric charges daily. The lightning associated with a thunderstorm ranges from perhaps 10 to 50 coulombs. The shock one experiences when grasping a doorknob in the dry air of winter is measured in microcoulombs (μC) a mere 10^{12} electrons!

Electrification

Whenever electrons are added to or removed from material, the material is said to be **electrified**. Electrification can occur by contact, friction, or induction.

Electrification by **contact** always occurs when an object having an excess number of electrons contacts a neutrally charged object or an object with a deficiency of electrons. Scuffing across a wool carpet and rubbing a balloon on your hair to make it stick to the wall are examples of electrification by **friction.** The loosely bound electrons of wool and one's hair are mechanically transferred so that one's body and the balloon become electrified.

Electrification by **induction** occurs when a highly electrified object comes close to a neutral object so that electrons are transferred by spark. Lightning bolts jump from cloud to cloud or cloud to earth in order to shed themselves of excess electrons. The earth is the ultimate sink for excess electrons and is called an earth ground, or just **ground** in engineering terms. This phenomenon is correctly termed **electrostatic induction,** and as we shall see, it is closely related to **magnetic induction** and **electromagnetic induction. Induction refers to the transfer of a physical property between objects without actual contact between the objects.**

The Electric Field

Unlike mass, charge cannot be destroyed by conversion to another form. In the universe, the total number of negative charges equals the total number of positive charges, and the net charge is always the same—zero. Furthermore, charge is quantized; it comes in discrete bundles rather than in a continuum of values. Why this is so is unknown; however, there is an imaginery field associated with each charge that is a continuum.

This imaginary field is called the **electric field.** We know it exists for much the same reason we know a gravitational field exists—because a force is exerted. The gravitational field produces a force that causes one mass to be attracted to another. Similarly, the electric field creates a force between one charge and another. However, whereas the gravitational force is always attractive, the force of the electric field can be attractive or repulsive, depending on the nature of the charges involved.

The electric field is most easily visualized as imaginary lines radiating from an electric charge, as shown in Figure 2-2. The strength of the electric field is proportional to the concentration of lines, and therefore, the electric field strength decreases as the square of the distance from the charge. The

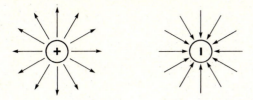

Figure 2-2.   The electric field, E, radiates from a positive charge and into a negative charge.

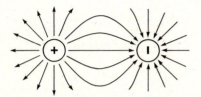

Figure 2-3.   The electric field is continuous, beginning on positive charges and ending on negative charges.

strength of the electric field is termed the **electric field intensity,** or simply the electric field, and it is symbolized by **E.**

E is a vector quantity; that is, it not only has magnitude but also has direction. The direction of the electric field is determined by the movement of a positive **search charge** or **test charge** in the electric field. In the presence of an electron, the search charge would be attracted, and therefore the imaginary lines of the electric field are directed in toward the electron. Alternately, if the search charge is in the field of a proton, it will be repelled and the imaginary lines will radiate from the proton. In any electric field the lines of force begin on positive charges and end on negative charges, as shown in Figure 2-3.

The magnitude of the electric field is defined as the force on a unit charge in the field as follows:

$$E = F/Q \qquad\qquad (2\text{-}1)$$

where E is the electric field intensity (newtons/coulomb),
F is the force on the charge (newtons), and
Q is the electric charge (coulombs).

The strength of the electric field produced by a charge, Q, at a distance, d, from that charge is given by:

$$E = k\, Q/d^2 \qquad\qquad (2\text{-}2)$$

where k is a constant that equals 9.0×10^9 N m^2/c^2.

Although electric charges are discrete quantities, their associated electric fields are continuous, and this is the fundamental basis for **field theory.** Particles add in a quantized fashion; fields add in a continuum by **superposition.** Consider a home television antenna. The force on an electric charge in that antenna is determined not only by the movement of charges in the broadcast antenna but also by the electric fields produced by all other electric charges near and far. Such is **field superposition.** The subject of antennae as related to MRI will be addressed more completely later.

Electrostatic Laws

The nature and intensity of the electric field form the basis for the four principal laws of electrostatics.

UNLIKE VERSUS LIKE CHARGES.   Because of the vector nature of the electric field, **like electric charges repel, and unlike electric charges attract.** Particles having no net electric charge such as neutrons are not influenced by an electric field.

COULOMB'S LAW.   The force of attraction or repulsion between electrostatic charges was first described by Charles Coulomb in the 1780s. Coulomb noted that the force was proportional to the product of the two charges and inversely proportional to the distance separating them. From the equivalent expressions of equations 2-1 and 2-2 describing the strength of the electric field, Coulomb's law can be stated:

$$E = F/q = k\ Q/d^2 \qquad\qquad \textbf{(2-3)}$$

or

$$F = k\ q\ Q/d^2 \qquad\qquad \textbf{(2-4)}$$

where F is the force (newtons),
      q and Q are the charges (coulombs),
      d is the distance between them (meters), and
      k is the proportionally constant of equation 2-2.

The electrostatic force is one of the five fundamental forces in nature. It is 10^{37} times stronger than the **gravitation force,** 100 times as strong as the **weak interaction,** about equal to the **magnetic force,** and about one one-hundredth of the **strong nuclear force.** An electrified balloon will attract paper or repel a small stream of water. The electrostatic force of attraction holds electrons in orbit in an atom. The electrostatic force of repulsion among protons limits the size of the nucleus.

CHARGE DISTRIBUTION.   Because protons are fixed whereas electrons are free to move, the remaining discussion of electrostatic phenomenon concerns electrons. Because of the radial nature of the electric field associated with each electron, electrons on any electrified object tend to be separated uniformly and to the maximum dimensions possible, as shown in Figure 2-4. Therefore, free electrons are distributed on the surface of the object, not inside it.

CHARGE CONCENTRATION.   If the electrified object is regularly shaped, such as a sphere or wire, the distribution of electrons on the surface will be uniform.

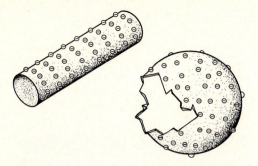

Figure 2-4.   Electrons are distributed on the surface of electrified objects.

On the other hand, if the surface is irregularly shaped—for instance, has a point as in an electrified cattle prod or a microfocus field emission x-ray tube, electrons will be concentrated at the sharpest region of curvature.

Electric Potential Energy

When two like charges are pushed together or two unlike charges are pulled apart, work is required. The resulting system will have the ability to do work and therefore will have potential energy or electric potential energy. Electric potential energy is also called **electromotive force (emf).** The work done to create electric potential energy comes from an **energy source,** and the work obtained from the potential energy is deposited in an **energy sink.** A hydro generator and steam generator are common energy sources that convert mechanical energy into electric potential energy. Energy sinks, such as motors, lamps, and heaters, abound.

The electric potential energy of a charge, q, is converted to kinetic energy when the charge is in motion and work is done. The electric potential energy of a charge influenced by the electric field of other charges is given by:

$$E = QV \qquad \qquad \text{(2-5)}$$

where E is the potential energy (joules),
   Q is the electric charge (coulombs), and
   V is a function of the position of the charge called the **electric potential.**

Because the potential energy of any system is created to do work, equation 2-5 is usually written:

$$W = QV \qquad \qquad \text{(2-6)}$$

where W is the work done (joules).

When the electric potential (V) is expressed as a measure of the work done per unit charge:

$$V = W/Q \qquad \qquad \text{(2-7)}$$

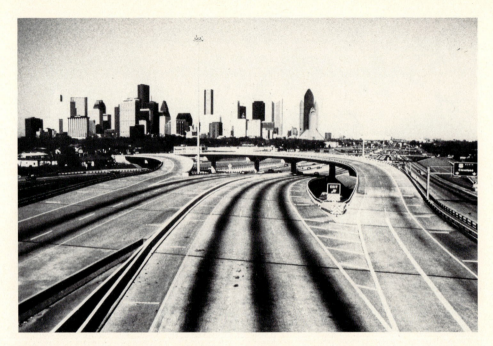

Figure 2-5. This Houston freeway at rush hour is analogous to an electric current, with the cars serving as electrons.

it is called an emf. Because it has units of joules/coulomb, it is not a force at all but rather a force used to do work. Therefore, emf is given a special name, **volt,** and is commonly called voltage.

ELECTRODYNAMICS

The investigation of electric charges in motion is **electrodynamics.** Basically electrodynamics has to do with what is commonly called an electric current, or **electricity.** We know that electricity deals with the flow of electrons in a conductor.

A Houston freeway at rush hour as seen in Figure 2-5 is analogous to an electric current. Normally, about 10,000 cars each hour will pass any given point on a six-lane freeway. If there is a wreck or construction, the speed of each car will be reduced at that point and the flow of traffic restricted. At an interchange, some cars may exit onto alternate routes. This allows those cars remaining on the main freeway and those that exited to travel faster. The traffic flow in each branch will be reduced because there are fewer cars in each route but the total flow will remain constant.

Electric Current

The electrons flowing in a conductor behave not unlike the automobiles on the freeway. For an electric current to exist, a closed circuit is necessary. Each

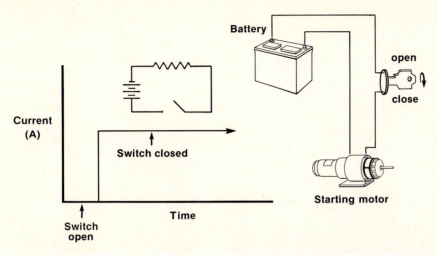

Figure 2-6.   The electric circuit in an automobile is an example of direct current.

electron must have a place to go. If there is a barricade in a conductor, such as an open switch, electron flow ceases. The reason for investigating electricity is that work can be extracted from the kinetic energy of electrons moving in a conductor.

To determine the work done by an electric current, we need to know not only the number of electrons involved but also the energy given up by each. The number of electrons involved is given a special name, the **ampere (A)**, which is equal to the flow of 1 coulomb each second (**1** A **= 1** C/s**).**

An ampere is a rather large electron flow, 6.24×10^{18} electrons. We cannot count electrons that fast, so we quantitate electric current by devices that measure the associated magnetic field. Electric currents range from thousands of amps in lightning volts to picoamps in electronic equipment. Household current can be up to about 30 A on any circuit. A current of only 100 mA at 110 volts is almost always fatal, and that is why grounded circuits and ground fault interrupters are necessary elements in home wiring.

DIRECT CURRENT.   If the energy source propels electrons in only one direction, as with an automobile battery, the form of electricity is **direct current (DC).** This is diagrammed in Figure 2-6. At time zero, when the switch is open, no current flows. The instant the switch is closed electrons will flow, but only in one direction.

ALTERNATING CURRENT.   On the other hand, if the energy source is of the alternating form, as in Figure 2-7, **alternating current (AC)** will be produced. At time zero with the switch open, again no current flows. When the switch is closed, electrons will first flow in one direction and then reverse direction and flow oppositely.

When electrons begin flowing in the positive direction, they begin very slowly at first and speed up to a maximum, represented by the first peak of the current waveform. Then they begin to slow down, still traveling in the same

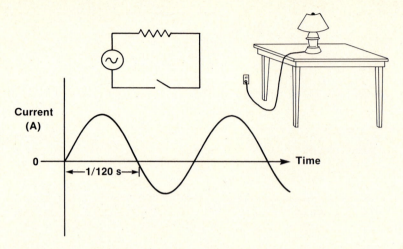

Figure 2-7.   Normal household current is provided as an alternating current.

direction, until they momentarily come to rest. This moment of rest occurs 120 times each second and is represented by the zero crossing of the waveform. Then the electrons reverse direction, first speeding up to a maximum, then slowing down to zero again. The number of electrons in the circuit remains constant, and their net movement is zero. Their velocity determines the intensity of the current and their direction—the direction of the current. Remember that by convention electron flow is opposite to current flow. Both AC and DC are used to great advantage in MRI.

PHASE.   The current waveform shown in Figure 2-7 illustrates that at any instant all electrons are moving in the same direction with the same velocity. They are said to be in **phase,** and the electricity is commonly called single-phase current. Actually, commercial electric power is generated and transmitted as three-phase current. A three-phase waveform is shown in Figure 2-8. At any instant, not all electrons are moving in the same direction, and those that are have different velocities. They are out of phase with one another. The concept of phase is important to the understanding of how an MR image is produced, and that will be addressed later.

Ohm's Law

Electrons do not flow in a circuit unimpeded. They behave much like an individual walking along a crowded sidewalk, bumping into people. Electrons bump into other electrons of the conductor. This property of any electric device is called **impedance,** and it is a function of the size, shape, and composition of the conductor or circuit element. There are three types of electric impedances—capacitive, inductive, and resistive. If the work done on the device changes the electric energy into heat, the impedance is called a **resistance** to current flow, and it is equal to the electric potential divided by the current.

Such heating may be a problem with a resistive-type MRI magnet. The

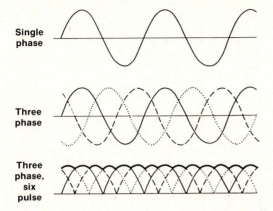

Figure 2-8. Electric power is generated and transmitted in three-phase form.

heating can require a closed cooling system incorporating a high-efficiency heat exchanger. Superconducting MRI magnets do not have this difficulty because the resistance to electron flow is near zero. The electrons are walking along empty sidewalks, as it were.

The resistance of a conductor or circuit element is usually a fixed quantity and follows a simple relationship first enunciated by George Ohm in the 1840s, known as Ohm's Law:

$$R = V/I \qquad\qquad \textbf{(2-8)}$$

where R is the resistance in ohms (Ω)

V is the electric potential in volts (v), and

I is the electric current in amperes (A).

Although Ohm's Law is fundamental to electronics, many electric devices are employed because they do not obey Ohm's Law. Vacuum tubes, transistors, and integrated circuits are prime examples.

Materials used in electric circuits are sometimes classified by their resistance. Those with low resistance, such as copper, aluminum, and seawater, are called **conductors.** Those with high resistance, such as quartz, rubber, and glass, are called **insulators.** Some materials that lie in between are called **semiconductors.** Silicon and germanium are semiconductors used extensively in fabricating diodes and integrated circuits. If the resistance is very low or even zero, they are called **superconductors.** However, to behave as a superconductor, such as niobium and titanium, material must be in an extremely cold or cryogenic environment. This electric classification of material is summarized in Table 2-1.

Electric Power

When an electric current flows, it will do so because of an electric potential or voltage. Because of the impedance of circuit elements to electron flow, energy must be supplied. Such energy was expressed in equation 2-5 as E = QV. This

TABLE 2-1.   The four electrical classifications of matter

Class	Property	Material
Insulator	Resists the flow of electrons	Rubber, glass, plastic
Semiconductor	Can behave as an insulator or a conductor	Silicon, germanium
Conductor	Allows the flow of electrons with difficulty	Copper, aluminum
Superconductor	Freely allows the flow of electrons	Titanium, niobium

equation relates the energy required to move a charge, Q, through an electric potential, V, sometimes called a voltage drop or usually a voltage. Power **(P)** is the rate at which energy **(E)** is used or work **(W)** is performed; that is:

$$P = E/t = W/t \text{ (joules/second)} \qquad \text{(2-9)}$$

therefore:

$$P = QV/t = IV \qquad \text{(2-10)}$$

Alternately, applying Ohm's Law, one can express power as:

$$P = I^2R = V^2/R \qquad \text{(2-11)}$$

The quantity for power, the joule per second, is given a special name in physics, the **watt (W).** The watt, therefore, is the unit of electric power.

In terms of human activity, the watt is very large. A construction worker might be able to work sufficiently hard to power a few 100-W light bulbs. In terms of human consumption, the watt is a small quantity. In the United States, we require about 6 kW per person continuously. In many of the developing nations, the figure is less than 500 W.

Resistive-type MRI magnets require considerable amounts of power. Some may require as much as 100 kW, and with the cost of electric power now running close to 10 cents per kilowatt per hour, one can see that this portion of the operating expense could be substantial.

MAGNETISM

Like mass and charge, magnetism is a fundamental property of matter. All matter is magnetic to some degree. We know that an iron magnet will pick up a steel paper clip but not a copper penny. We commonly call steel **magnetic** and copper **nonmagnetic.** Actually, copper is also magnetic but to a very small degree. Even subatomic particles, such as protons, have magnetic properties. Basically, magnetism is an imaginary field associated with certain types of ma-

A
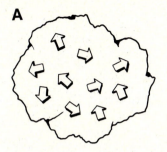

B
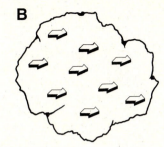

Figure 2-9.   **A,** In most matter magnetic domains are randomly oriented. **B,** Magnets exist when magnetic domains are aligned.

terial that are said to be magnetic. The magnetic field is similar in many ways to the electric field, but its manifestation is different.

The earliest magnets were described several thousand years ago as naturally occurring black stones that would attract iron. These "leading stones," or **lodestones,** were thought to be magic by the natives in a region of present-day western Turkey, then known as Magnesia. The term magnetism was adopted and persists.

Magnetic Domains

The smallest region of magnetism is called a **magnetic domain.** Most materials have their magnetic domains randomly oriented as in Figure 2-9, *A,* and therefore exhibit no magnetism. Material such as that in Figure 2-9, *B,* however, that has its magnetic domains aligned becomes a magnet.

The strength and number of magnetic domains in a material are associated with its electric configuration. As we shall discuss, an electric charge in motion creates a magnetic field. In the case of common magnetic materials and electromagnetism, the magnetism is related to moving electrons. In the case of nuclei, the magnetism is related to the much weaker magnetic properties of the spinning, electrically positive nucleus. The magnetic field of paired electrons cancel; therefore, atoms with closed electron shells exhibit little magnetism, whereas those with unpaired electrons produce strong magnetic domains. Atoms with nearly half-filled shells have the strongest magnetism because electrons generally will not begin pairing spins until a shell is half full.

Because of the various electron configurations, there are basically three types of magnetism—**ferromagnetism, paramagnetism,** and **diamagnetism.** Materials with such properties are distinguished from each other according to the strength and alignment of their magnetic domains in the presence of an external magnetic field.

Ferromagnetic materials are easily magnetized and have a **magnetic susceptibility** greater than 1. Such materials include iron, cobalt, nickel, and gadolinium. These materials make the strongest magnets and are used singly and

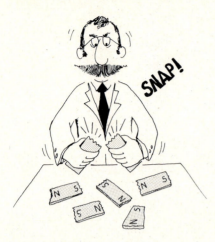

Figure 2-10.   If a magnet is broken into smaller and smaller pieces, baby magnets result.

in combination with the many MRI magnets. Perhaps the most common permanent magnet is one made of an alloy of aluminum, nickel, and cobalt—**alnico.**

Paramagnetic materials include platinum, oxygen, tungsten, manganese, and aluminum. These materials have a magnetic susceptibility less than 1. They are weakly influenced by an external magnetic field but do not exhibit measurable magnetic properties of their own.

Diamagnetic materials have negative magnetic susceptibilities and, in fact, are slightly repelled by magnets. Such materials include mercury, silver, copper, carbon, and hydrogen.

The Laws of Magnetism

DIPOLES.   Unlike the situation that exists with electricity, there is no smallest unit of magnetism. Because each magnetic domain exists with two poles—a north pole and a south pole—it is commonly called a **dipole.** A large magnet also has two poles, but the intensity of each cannot be subdivided until there is a single magnetic pole. Unlike electric charge, a magnet cannot exist with a single pole, only as a dipole. Dividing a magnet simply creates two smaller magnets, as illustrated in Figure 2-10.

ATTRACTION/REPULSION.   As with electric charges, like magnetic poles repel, unlike magnetic poles attract. Also, by convention the imaginary lines of the magnetic field leave the north pole of a magnet, as shown in Figure 2-11, and return to the south pole. How do we know that these imaginary lines exist? They can be demonstrated by the action of iron filings near a magnet, as shown in Figure 2-12.

The polar convention of magnetism actually has its origin in the compass. The end of a compass needle that points to the earth's North Pole (actually, its magnetic South Pole) is the north pole of the compass. As shown in Fig-

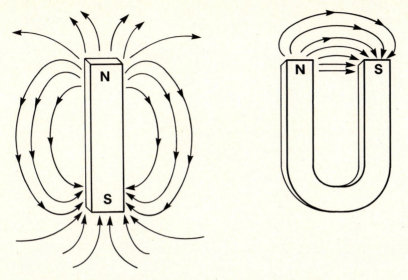

Figure 2-11. The imaginary lines of the magnetic field leave the north pole and enter the south pole.

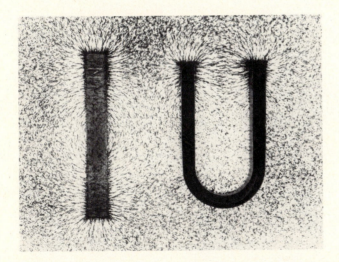

Figure 2-12. Demonstration of magnetic lines of force with iron filings. (Courtesy Robert Waggener, University of Texas Health Science Center, San Antonio, Texas.)

ure 2-13, if a compass were taken to the North Pole, it would point into the earth. At the South Pole, it would point to the sky.

MAGNETIC INDUCTION. Just as an electrostatic charge can be induced from one material to another, so nonmagnetic material can be made magnetic by induction. The imaginary magnetic field lines just described are called magnetic **lines of induction,** and the density of lines is proportional to the intensity of the magnetic field.

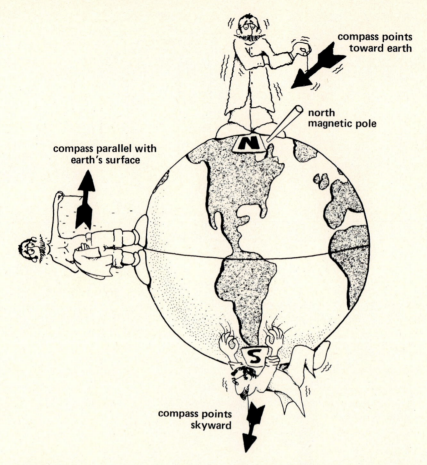

Figure 2-13.   A free-swinging compass reacts with the earth as though it were a bar magnet.

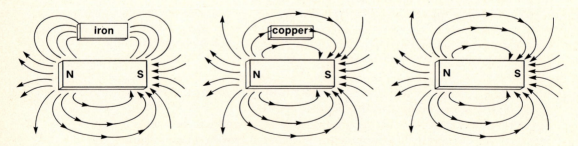

Figure 2-14.   Ferromagnetic material such as iron attracts magnetic lines of induction, whereas nonmagnetic material such as copper does not.

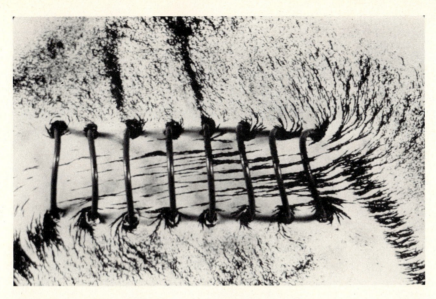

Figure 2-15.   Iron filings show the magnetic field lines of an electromagnet. (Courtesy Murray A. Solomon, San Jose, California.)

When ferromagnetic material such as a piece of soft iron is brought into the vicinity of an intense magnetic field, the lines of induction will be altered by attraction to the soft iron, as seen in Figure 2-14, and the iron will be made temporarily magnetic. If copper, a diamagnetic material, were to replace the soft iron, there would be no such effect.

This principle is employed with many MR imagers that utilize an iron magnetic shield to reduce the level of the fringe magnetic field. Ferromagnetic material acts as a magnetic sink by drawing the lines of induction into it. This is also the basis of antimagnetic watches, but don't believe it if you work near the strong field of an MR imager.

When ferromagnetic material is removed from the magnetic field, it usually does not retain its strong magnetic property. Soft iron, therefore, makes an excellent **temporary magnet.** It is a magnet only while its magnetism is being induced. If properly tempered by heat or exposed to an external field for a long period, however, some ferromagnetic materials will retain their magnetism when removed from the external magnetic field and become **permanent magnets.**

Another type of magnet is the **electromagnet.** It owes its magnetism to an electric current, which induces magnetism, as shown in Figure 2-15, but only while the current is flowing. MR imagers employ permanent magnets, resistive electromagnets, or superconductive electromagnets.

MAGNETIC FORCE.   The force created by a magnetic field behaves similarly to that of the electric field. The electric and magnetic forces were joined by Maxwell's field theory of electromagnetic radiation.

TABLE 2-2.   Three fundamental forces

	Gravitational	Electric	Magnetic
The force is:	Attractive only	Attractive and repulsive	Attractive and repulsive
Acts in:	Mass, m	Charge, q	Pole, p
Through an associated field:	Gravitational field, g	Electric field, E	Magnetic field, B
With intensity:	$F = mg$	$F = qE$	$F = pB$
The source of the field is:	Mass, M	Charge, Q	Pole, P
The intensity of the field at a distance from the source is:	$g = \dfrac{GM}{d^2}$	$E = \dfrac{kQ}{d^2}$	$B = \dfrac{kP}{d^2}$
The force between fields is given by:	Newton's Law $F = -G\dfrac{Mm}{d^2}$	Coulomb's Law $F = k\dfrac{Qq}{d^2}$	Gauss' Law $F = k\dfrac{Pp}{d^2}$
where:	$G = 6.678 \times 10^{-11}\,\dfrac{Nm^2}{kg^2}$	$k = 9.0 \times 10^9\,\dfrac{Nm^2}{C^2}$	$k = 10^{-7}\,\dfrac{W}{A^2}$

Table 2-2 summarizes some of the similarities of three fundamental forces. Note that the defining equation is precisely the same among the three. The magnitudes are different, however. The gravitational force is a long-range force, and if it is assigned a relative value of 1, the electric and magnetic forces would have a value of 10^{37} times its magnitude in newtons.

The equation of interacting magnetic fields is named for Karl Gauss, who in the 1840s used Coulomb's Law to explain magnetism. The magnetic force obeys the inverse square law principle, and its magnitude is proportional to the product of the two interacting magnetic poles. Its formulation is:

$$F = k\, pP/d^2 \qquad\qquad (2\text{-}12)$$

where F is the force in newtons (N),
P and p are the relative pole strengths in ampere meters (AM),
d is the separation distance in meters (m), and
K is a proportionality constant with a value of 10^{-7} W/A^2

As with the gravitational force and the electric force, the magnetic force does not need a conducting medium. It acts through space.

The Magnetic Field

The imaginary lines of magnetic induction create a field effect. We define the strength of the magnetic field by placing an imaginary north pole in it and measuring the force on the pole. This is similar to our definition of the electric field by its force acting on a positive search charge. Therefore, the magnetic field **B** is given by:

$$B = F/p \tag{2-13}$$

where   B is the field strength in tesla (T),
          F is the force in newtons (N), and
          p is the pole strength in ampere meters (AM).

The tesla (T) is the SI unit for the magnetic field. The older unit, but still very much in use, is the gauss (G). One tesla equals 10,000 G. As with other types of fields, the strength of magnetic fields ranges over many orders of magnitude.

ELECTROMAGNETISM

A motionless electron has an electric field associated with it. An electron in motion has both an electric and a magnetic field. The interaction between the electric field and the magnetic field is the basis for **electromagnetism.**

Oersted's Experiment

Until the 1820s, electricity and magnetism were considered two separate, unrelated, and independent manifestations. As with many great discoveries, Hans Christian Oersted accidentally noted that a compass was deflected by a DC current, as shown in Figure 2-16. When no current exists in the circuit, the compass needle placed close to the conductor will point to the earth's North Pole. Once the switch is closed and current flows, the compass will immediately align itself perpendicular to the current-carrying wire. If the electron flow is as illustrated in Figure 2-15, the north pole of the compass will be attracted to the wire as shown. Reversing the current would cause the south pole of the compass to point to the wire.

Oersted's observation demonstrated that **a magnetic field is always associated with a moving charged particle.** Furthermore, if either the electric field or the magnetic field is time variant—that is, changing in intensity with time—profound interactions can occur. Figure 2-17 illustrates the magnetic field induced by a moving electron. Note that the magnetic field lines exist radially from the axis of motion. How do we know that moving charged particles create a magnetic field? This cannot be shown in an isolated frame of reference. Such a demonstration requires another magnetic field, so that one observes the interaction between the two magnetic fields.

Study the situation shown in Figure 2-18. An electron is moving out of the page between the poles of a magnet. We know the electron is coming out of the page because of the ⊙. The ⊙ represents the head of an arrow. If the

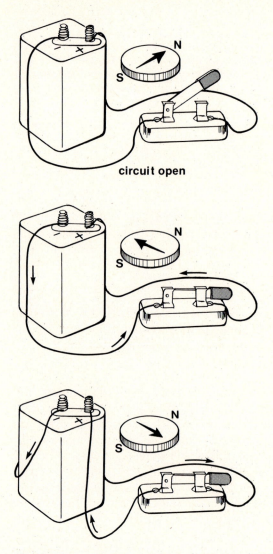

circuit open

Figure 2-16. A compass will be deflected by a DC current, and the direction of deflection depends on the direction of the electric current.

electron were moving into the page, one would see ⊗, representing the tail of an arrow. This convention holds not only for charged particles but also for electric and magnetic field lines.

The electron moving in the magnetic field experiences a force that is at right angles to both its velocity and the external magnetic field. This force tends to deviate the electron in its motion, causing it to follow a curved path. The direction of the force is given by the left-hand rule, as shown in Figure 2-19. Applying the left-hand rule, one would conclude that the electron in Fig-

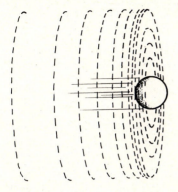

Figure 2-17.   A moving charged particle will induce a magnetic field in a plane perpendicular to its motion.

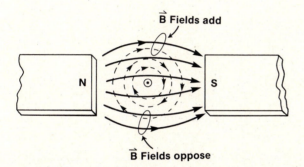

Figure 2-18.   An electron moving in a magnetic field experiences a force tending to cause it to curve. The force results from the interaction between the electron's magnetic field and the external magnetic field.

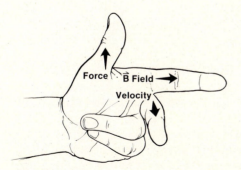

Figure 2-19.   The left-hand rule demonstrates the directional relationships between force, velocity, and external magnetic field.

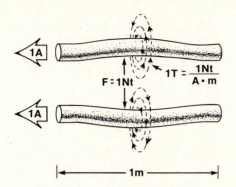

Figure 2-20. Parallel current-carrying wires will repel each other. This forms the basis for the definition of the tesla.

ure 2-18 should move down the page. This is so because the external magnetic field and that of the electron reinforce one another above the path of the electron and oppose one another below that path.

The magnitude of this force is given by:

$$F = qvB \tag{2-14}$$

where   F is the force in newtons (N),
     q is the charge in coulombs (C),
     v is the electron velocity in meters per second (m/s), and
     B is the magnetic field in tesla (T).

This expression is yet another approach to the definition of the magnetic field. **A magnetic field of 1 T** N/Am exists where 1 coulomb traveling at 1 meter per second is acted on by a force of 1 newton.

The total force on a moving electron is the sum of the forces owing to external electric and magnetic fields as follows:

$$F = qE + qvB \tag{2-15}$$

This is called the **lorentzian force,** and it is the basis for such diverse yet readily recognizable phenomena as the **aurora borealis** (northern lights), the cathode-ray tube, and the operation of a cyclotron for positron-emission tomography (PET) scanning.

When electrons move in a conductor, the Lorentzian force determines their use in electromechanical devices such as motors and generators. In an MR imager, this force can be used to explain the operation of the main magnet, the gradient coils, and the RF antenna.

THE SOLENOID.   Still another method for defining a magnetic field is based on the force on a very long section of current-carrying wire as shown in Figure 2-20. The external magnetic field B could be created by a permanent magnet or an adjacent current-carrying wire. The defining equation for the strength of the magnetic field is:

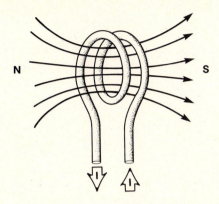

Figure 2-21.   A magnetic dipole is produced by a current-carrying loop of wire.

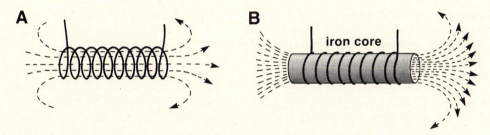

Figure 2-22.   A, A coil of current-carrying wire will produce a magnetic field and is called a solenoid. **B,** With an iron core, it is called an electromagnet.

$$B = \frac{F}{Idl}$$ **(2-16)**

where F is force in newtons (N),

I is the current in amperes (A), and

dl is an incremental length (m) of a long wire.

If the force on a 1-meter section of wire conducting 1 ampere is 1 newton, then the magnetic field has a strength of 1 T.

If the straight length of wire is shaped to form a loop, a **magnetic dipole** will be produced, as shown in Figure 2-21. Reverse the current, and the polarity of the dipole will be reversed.

If, instead of one loop, a series of loops is formed from a current-carrying wire, a more intense magnetic field will be produced, as in Figure 2-22, *A.* Such a helically wound coil of wire is called a **solenoid,** and it is the first step in making an electromagnet.

THE ELECTROMAGNET.   If one inserts a rod of ferromagnetic material inside the solenoid, as in Figure 2-22, *B,* the intensity of the induced magnetic field will be greatly strengthened because of the concentration of magnetic field

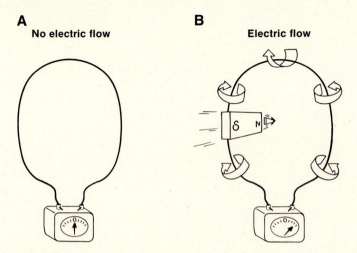

A
No electric flow

B
Electric flow

Figure 2-23.   A, There is no electric current in a closed circuit having no source of electric potential. **B,** When a magnetic field is moved through a closed loop of wire, an electric potential is created and an electric current will be induced.

lines. Such a device is an **electromagnet,** and it is the basis for switches, large industrial magnets, and one type of MRI magnet. It is also the foundation for more complicated electromagnetic devices such as motors, generators, and transformers. All of these devices function because coils of current-carrying wire are wrapped around ferromagnetic cores and magnetic fields are induced.

A motor is a device that converts electric energy into mechanical energy. A generator does quite the opposite; it converts mechanical energy into electric energy. The intermediate step in each of these devices is the **induced magnetic field.** Mechanical motion can be extracted from electric power or supplied to produce electric power because of the force on a current-carrying wire in the presence of a magnetic field.

Faraday's Law—Induction

Recall that a force is exerted on a length of current-carrying wire when a magnetic field is present. The force is perpendicular to both the magnetic field and the direction of electron flow.

Now consider the situation depicted in Figure 2-23, *A.* A loop of wire is connected to an ammeter to produce a closed circuit, but there is no current in the loop because there is no source of emf or voltage. If one now moves a permanent magnet toward the loop as in Figure 2-23, *B,* a current will flow. The changing magnetic field **induces** a voltage in the circuit, causing electrons to flow. This phenomenon was demonstrated by Michael Faraday in the 1830s and is stated as Faraday's Law of electromagnetic induction:

$$V = -\frac{\triangle B}{\triangle t}$$

(2-17)

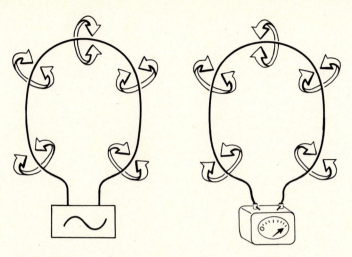

Figure 2-24. An alternating current in one coil creates an alternating magnetic field that can induce an alternating current in a nearby second coil.

where V is the induced voltage (V),

$\triangle$B represents the changing magnetic field, and

t is the time taken for that change.

The negative sign in Faraday's Law is a consequence of **Lenz's law.** The direction of the induced electron flow, and therefore the induced voltage, is such that it opposes the agent that induced the flow. Note that in Figure 2-23, *B,* the electron flow induced by moving the north pole of the magnet toward the loop is in such a direction that the north pole of the induced magnetic field opposes a further push of the magnet. Were the permanent magnet pulled away from the loop, or the south pole of the magnet pushed toward the loop, the induced electron flow would be reversed and the polarity of the induced magnetic field reversed. Regardless of whether the magnetic field or the loop of wire is moved, a current will be induced, which in turn will induce a secondary magnetic field to oppose the inducing field.

If one used an opposing loop of wire instead of a permanent magnet as the inducing agent, as in Figure 2-24, one would have a simple transformer. If the first coil is energized by a source of AC power, the magnetic field associated with the first coil will alternate in polarity. This primary alternating magnetic field will interact with the second coil as though one alternately pushed, then pulled, a permanent magnet along the axis of the second coil. The induced electron flow in the secondary coil will be AC, and the induced magnetic field will always oppose the action of the primary field.

THE TRANSFORMER. This principle is the basis for the **transformer.** A transformer incorporates hundreds of loops of wire coiled on a ferromagnetic core. The core concentrates and intensifies the magnetic field. Because a moving magnetic field is required, a transformer will not work on DC, only AC.

THE ANTENNA.   Return for a moment to the situation illustrated in Figure 2-24. The current in the primary coil induces a current in the secondary coil through magnetic induction, but only when the primary current varies in intensity, not if it is constant. However, one must carry the phenomenon of Faraday induction one step further. If the electrons are not only varying in intensity but also being accelerated and decelerated alternately, **electromagnetic radiation** will be emitted. If the frequency of emission is appropriate, the electromagnetic radiation emitted by a transmitting antenna will induce a similar movement of electrons in a receiving antenna.

ELECTROMAGNETIC RADIATION

We have seen that a resting electric charge radiates an electric field. When the charge is in motion, a magnetic field is generated as well as an electric field. When the moving electric charge is joined by others and confined to a conductor to produce an electric current, the associated magnetic field results in a force being applied to the conductor. If the conductor is properly fashioned, as in a coil, and current is supplied as AC, the varying magnetic field may be used to induce an electric current in a secondary coil.

　　When a moving electric charge undergoes acceleration or deceleration, a photon of electomagnetic radiation is emitted. Radiologists know that bremsstrahlung x-rays are produced by a deceleration of the projectile electron in the vicinity of the nucleus of a tungsten atom in the anode of an x-ray tube. Acceleration of excited electrons dropping back into an outer electron shell can produce a photon of visible light. Electrons accelerated within the conducting element of a radio antenna will emit a photon of radio emission. This phenomenon was described mathematically in the 1860s by James Clerk Maxwell.

Maxwell's Wave Equations

Maxwell synthesized the then-known laws of electricity and magnetism into what is now known as Maxwell's wave equations of electromagnetic fields. At that time, the only electromagnetic radiation recognized was visible light. Maxwell described light mathematically in terms of oscillating electric and magnetic fields and showed that the interaction of these fields caused a wave to be propagated in free space at a direction 90 degrees to the fields. Furthermore, the velocity of propagation was shown to be 3×10^8 m/s by these equations.

　　Maxwell's mathematical equations describe a photon of electromagnetic radiation that can be illustrated as in Figure 2-25. Note that the electric and magnetic fields are at right angles to one another and are also at right angles to the propagation vector of the photon. Because the field disturbance is perpendicular to the direction of propagation, such a photon is known as a **transverse wave.** Compare this with an ultrasound wave, in which the molecules oscillate in the direction of the propagation vector. Consequently, ultrasound is known as a **longitudinal wave.** The terms *transverse* and *longitudinal* will be used again to describe the two MRI relaxation times.

　　The intensity of each photon begins at zero and increases rapidly to a maximum, decreasing to zero again. It is only during acceleration of a charged

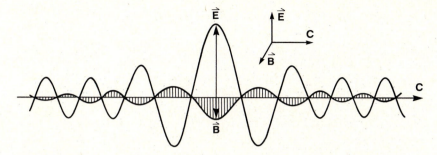

Figure 2-25.   An electromagnetic photon consists of electric and magnetic fields oscillating at right angles to one another and traveling at the speed of light.

particle that such an electromagnetic disturbance is possible. Consequently, each photon does have an origin and a termination. The energy of the electromagnetic photon is determined by the amount of kinetic energy gained or lost by the charged particle.

Maxwell's equations also demonstrated that an electromagnetic photon obeyed the classical wave equation:

$$c = \lambda \nu \qquad \text{(2-18)}$$

where λ is the photon wavelength (m),
ν is the photon frequency (Hz), and
c is the constant photon velocity (m/s).

A decade later, the velocity of light was measured by Albert Michelson and Edward Morley, who showed that Maxwell's theoretically determined value was correct.

The Electromagnetic Spectrum

A mention of Albert Einstein's 1905 theory of relativity and Max Planck's 1915 formulation of quantum mechanics is required to complete our current understanding of electromagnetic radiation. Einstein showed that electromagnetic photons behaved relativistically; that is, if two electrons are accelerated together, a stationary observer would observe the emission of two photons. However, if the observer were on one of the electrons, he or she would be able to verify that the neighboring electron had only an electric field; no electromagnetic radiation would be detected. Furthermore, Einstein showed not only that energy was conserved by the conversion of kinetic energy into electromagnetic energy but also that electromagnetic energy could represent the conversion of matter into energy according to his famous equation:

$$E = mc^2 \qquad \text{(2-19)}$$

where E is the energy in joules (J),
m is the particle mass (kg), and
c is the photon velocity (m/s).

By the time of Max Planck, the various forms of electromagnetic energy were recognized as being different manifestations of a similar fundamental disturbance. The great body of physical measurements, resulting from the previous 100 years' experience with light and optics, held that the interaction of electromagnetic radiation with matter was wavelike in nature. Planck's quantum theory quantized electromagnetic radiation into photons and showed how such radiation could behave as a particle during its interaction with matter. The proof of this is the photoelectric effect and the fundamental equation underlying Planck's theory:

$$E = h\nu = \frac{hc}{\lambda} \qquad \textbf{(2-20)}$$

where E is the energy of the photon (J),

h is Planck's constant, 6.63×10^{-34} J $\cdot$ s and

c, ν, and λ are as in the wave equation.

Planck further showed that electromagnetic radiation indeed actually possessed a duality of nature insofar as its interaction with matter was concerned. Electromagnetic radiation does interact as a photon or as a wave, depending basically on the photon energy.

Electromagnetic radiation extends over an enormously wide range, as was shown in Figure 1-1. This span of electromagnetic radiation is known as the **electromagnetic spectrum,** and it extends from radio emissions on the low-energy side through microwaves, infrared, visible light, and ultraviolet light to high-energy x- and gamma-radiation.

This representation of the electromagnetic spectrum contains three scales, E, λ, and ν, each of which is equivalent according to the Planck equation (2-20). Also, each scale has some historical interest, reflecting the manner in which the photons are produced and interact with matter. Light was the earliest electromagnetic radiation to be studied. It was shown to interact primarily as a wave and therefore was usually characterized by its wavelength. Radio emissions are produced by oscillating electric circuits. This was first demonstrated by Heinrich Hertz in the 1880s. Because the oscillation of emission was the principal design parameter, these waves are identified by their frequency. Roentgen discovered x-rays in 1895, and they were characterized by the voltage of production. When Einstein and Planck explained their interaction with matter as particles, it became convention to identify such photons by their energy.

Our interest in radiologic imaging lies in the three distinct regions of the electromagnetic spectrum called **imaging windows.** Each of the three windows is described by one of the three scales.

THE VISIBLE WINDOW. Visible light interacts with matter more like a wave than a particle. Diffraction, refraction, reflection, and interference are all properties of wavelike interactions, and they all apply to visible light. Visible light photons range from approximately 400 to 700 nm, and this corresponds to a

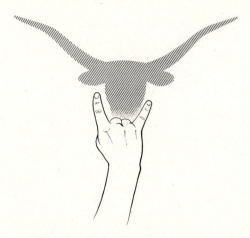

Figure 2-26. X-ray images are similar to a shadowgram except that they provide outlines of internal structures as well as the surface. (Dedicated to Xie Nan Zhu, Guangzhou, People's Republic of China.)

frequency of 4.32×10^{14} to 7.5×10^{14} Hz and a photon energy of 1.8 to 3.1 eV, respectively. Visible light is produced essentially by electron shifts from an excited energy state to the ground state of the outermost shell of an atom. Its wavelength allows it to interact with the receptor cells of the eye, but its quantum energy is too low to ionize matter.

Imaging with visible light occurs by sensing the reflection of light from a patient. The image of the patient is therefore a surface image and not an image of interior structures. Individual light photons are detected by specially evolved optical light sensors—the rods and the cones—of the human eye or by the special molecules in the emulsion of a photographic film.

THE X-RAY WINDOW. The radiologist is most familiar with the x-ray imaging window, which encompasses high-energy imaging. X-rays are produced by changes in the kinetic energy of very fast moving electrons. Bremsstrahlung photons can simplistically be viewed as being created by the deceleration of a high-velocity electron in the vicinity of the nucleus of a target atom. Characteristic x-rays are produced when the outer-shell electrons are accelerated to an inner shell. The energy of photons used for x-ray imaging ranges from about 30 to 150 keV. This corresponds to frequencies of 0.7×10^{18} to 3.6×10^{18} Hz and wavelengths of 400 to 80 pm, respectively.

X-rays are used to image the body in much the same way a shadowgram is produced with a beam of light, as in Figure 2-26. Of course, in a shadowgram one images only the outline of the figure. During x-ray examination, one images not only the outline but also the internal structures.

X-ray imaging is possible because of the particle-like interactions between x-ray photons and tissue atoms. These interactions occur principally by way of photoelectric effect and Compton scattering, although at low energies coherent scattering may also contribute to the attenuation of the x-ray beam. A radiograph, therefore, represents the pattern of x-ray attenuation while passing through the patient. The resulting image is a function of the x-ray linear attenuation coefficient.

THE MRI WINDOW.   Electromagnetic radiation having frequencies of approximately 5 to 200 MHz (6 to 60 m and 21 to 210 meV) is used in MRI and NMR spectroscopy. These photons lie in the **RF** portion of the electromagnetic spectrum. RF photons are used extensively in communications—television, radio, and microwaves. Standard commercial AM broadcast operates from about 540 to 1640 kHz. FM radio and television occupy a band of frequencies from about 50 to 100 MHz. This range overlaps with the range employed in MRI.

There are many sources of RF radiation in this frequency range, all of which can interfere with an NMR signal. Measures must usually be taken to ensure that these extraneous sources of RF are attenuated or entirely excluded from the antenna used to receive the NMR signals. This can present a problem similar to that encountered in x-ray imaging. An x-ray examination room is shielded to ensure that x-radiation does not escape from the room and create a radiation hazard to persons nearby. An MRI room may require shielding to exclude extraneous RF from the imager. Such a shielded room, called a **Faraday cage,** is discussed in Chapter 8.

SUMMARY

An understanding of the production of a magnetic resonance image requires some knowledge of the basic physics of electricity and magnetism. Electrostatics is the study of resting electric charges, and the nucleus of a hydrogen atom represents such a resting charge. When electric charges move in a conductor, electricity is produced. Also produced will be a magnetic field, and this phenomenon is the basis for most magnetic resonance imagers.

Electrons moving in a conductor produce the magnetic field that creates the environment for most MR imagers. The induction of an electric current by a moving magnetic field is the fundamental step in the NMR experiment. In MRI, electromagnetic radiation stimulates patient tissues to induce a changing magnetic field, which in turn results in the RF signal basic to MRI.

Chapter
THREE

Nuclear Magnetism

As the name *nuclear magnetic resonance* indicates, the MRI signal originates from the nuclei of atoms resonating in a patient in the presence of a magnetic field. Because this is a nuclear phenomenon, an accurate and complete description requires the use of **quantum mechanics.** Quantum mechanics is that branch of physics that describes the behavior of very small particles such as protons, neutrons, and electrons. This branch of physics has evolved since the turn of the century and is the basis for contemporary investigations into the structure of matter. Quantum mechanics, though, is rather complex and does not provide an intuitive understanding of what is really happening at the subatomic level. It is highly mathematical and abstract, and although it most accurately describes NMR, it will be avoided here.

Much of what we need to understand can be described in terms of **classical mechanics.** Classical mechanics is the branch of physics that describes the behavior of large objects like rockets and ping pong balls. It has its origins in the seventeenth-century ideas of Sir Isaac Newton. These differences are demonstrated in Figure 3-1. For many cases, the statistical averaging that occurs over a normal patient reduces the quantum mechanical description to a classical mechanical description. One quantum mechanical concept, however, that cannot be overlooked or avoided, is **nuclear spin.**

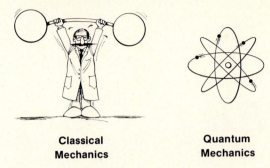

Classical Mechanics   **Quantum Mechanics**

Figure 3-1. The motion of large objects is described by classical mechanics and that of subatomic particles by quantum mechanics.

TABLE 3-1.   NMR properties of medically important nuclei

Isotope	Spin Quantum Number	Gyromagnetic Ratio (MHz/T)	Percent Abundance
^{1}H	½	42.6	99
^{12}C	0	0	98
^{13}C	½	10.7	1.1
^{16}O	0	0	99
^{17}O	5/2	5.8	0.1
^{19}F	½	40.0	100
^{23}Na	3/2	11.3	100
^{25}Mg	5/2	2.6	10
^{31}P	½	17.2	100
^{33}S	3/2	3.3	0.7
^{57}Fe	½	1.4	2.2

QUANTUM MECHANICAL DESCRIPTION

According to quantum mechanics, every nucleus has an associated quantity called **spin.** This quantity is not exactly what we normally think of as spin, but it's close enough for our purposes. There is one anomaly, though, in that this spin is **quantized** into units of half-integer values, which are called the **spin quantum number.** That is, there are only certain precisely allowed states of spin. The allowed values are 0, ½, 1, 3/2, and so on. Each nucleus has its own characteristic spin quantum number. For instance all hydrogen atoms of atomic mass 1 have a spin quantum number of ½. All carbon atoms of atomic mass 12 have a spin quantum number of 0. All carbon atoms of atomic mass 13 have a spin quantum number of ½.

The spin quantum number dictates many of the magnetic resonance properties of a given isotope and produces the term *a spin ½ nucleus* or *a spin 1 nucleus.* Table 3-1 presents some isotopes of interest to MRI and their respec-

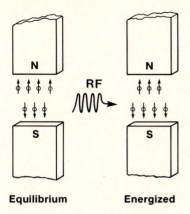

Equilibrium   Energized

Figure 3-2.   At equilibrium more nuclear spins are in the low-energy state with the magnetic field. When energized, more nuclear spins are against the field.

tive spin quantum numbers. Once we accept this quantum mechanical premise, it is easy to use classical mechanics to describe how the NMR signal is generated.

One result of the spin being quantized is that there is a limited number of ways a nucleus can spin. Each of these ways is called a **spin state.** For a spin ½ nucleus, there are only two allowed spin states, $+½$ and $-½$. In general, for a particle with spin **S,** there are $(2 \times S) + 1$ possible states, and each state is one integer value separated from the next. So for a nucleus with spin quantum number of 2, the allowed states are $-2, -1, 0, 1$, and 2.

There is a fundamental law of physics that a spinning mass will induce about itself a magnetic field. The earth is one such example. In general, a spinning mass with charge will induce an even stronger magnetic field. Because the nucleus is a spinning charged particle, a magnetic field is associated with it. This field is given the special name of **nuclear magnetic moment,** and its intensity is related to mass, charge, and the rate of spin of the nucleus. Thus each spin state has a different nuclear magnetic moment. **In the absence of an external magnetic field, each state will have the same energy, but in the presence of an external magnetic field, each state will have a different energy.**

Like most systems, a nucleus in the presence of an external magnetic field will prefer to be in the lower energy state than the higher state. Therefore, the lower state will have more nuclei than the higher state. Such a system of nuclear spins is said to be at **equilibrium** with the external magnetic field. Using electromagnetic radiation with an energy exactly equal to the energy difference between two nuclear energy states, one can disturb this population difference by causing some nuclei of a lower energy state to absorb energy and join the higher energy nuclei as shown in Figure 3-2. The system of energized nuclear spins will slowly return to its original population difference while emitting a signal that can be observed. This is the **NMR signal.**

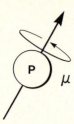

Figure 3-3.   A representation of the nuclear magnetic moment, μ, of a hydrogen nucleus.

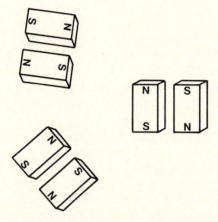

Figure 3-4.   The behavior of small bar magnets is to align parallel with opposing polarity.

CLASSICAL MECHANICAL DESCRIPTION

From the classical mechanical point of view, the nucleus is simply a charged particle that is spinning. The spinning motion will generate a magnetic field parallel to the axis of spin. This magnetic field is shown in Figure 3-3 and is given the same special name of **nuclear magnetic moment** that was described quantum mechanically. It is referred to with the Greek letter mu, μ. For any individual nucleus, the orientation of the axis of rotation, and so the direction of the nuclear magnetic moment, will be random and can be pointing in any direction.

For magnetic resonance imaging, the question is how this nuclear magnetic moment will interact with an externally applied magnetic field. Classically, when two magnets are near each other, a force will be generated that tends to make the two magnetic fields become parallel and pointed in the opposite direction. For bar magnets, this force is manifested by the magnets rotating to align opposite to each other, as shown in Figure 3-4. However, the nucleus is a spinning particle, and so its actual movement in response to an

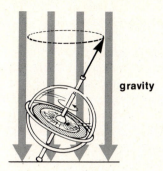

Figure 3-5. The motion of a spinning gyroscope in the presence of gravity.

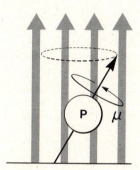

Figure 3-6. The precession of a nuclear magnetic moment in the presence of an external magnetic field.

applied force such as the external magnetic field, **B**, is the same as that produced by a gyroscope; it moves perpendicular to the applied force. This phenomenon is illustrated in Figure 3-5. In the case of the gyroscope, the interaction is mass-mass, the mass of the earth and the mass of the gyroscope.

Similarly, when a nuclear magnetic moment is placed in the presence of a large external magnetic field, which will be referred to as B_0, its axis of rotation will **precess** about the applied magnetic field, as seen Figure 3-6.

We can calculate exactly how fast such a nucleus will precess by the Larmor equation:

$$\omega = \gamma B \qquad \qquad \text{(3-1)}$$

where ω is the frequency of precession (MHz),
γ is the gyromagnetic ratio (MHz/T), and
B is the strength of the external magnetic field (T).

This equation demonstrates that there is a strictly linear relationship between the frequency of precession, ω, and the strength of an applied magnetic field, B_0. The gyromagnetic ratio is different for each type of nucleus and must be measured for each. Thus it is an empirically determined fudge factor used to convert field strength to precessional frequency. The values vary widely and can be found in Table 3-1 for several nuclei of interest to MRI.

This important relationship is used to explain many phenomena for both MRI and NMR spectroscopy. It is important to remember that the key factor is not the strength of the external magnetic field but what magnetic field is experienced by the nucleus, as modified by many other environmental influences. For spectroscopy, this includes the contribution from the magnetic fields generated by the motion of the bonding electrons, which results in **chemical shifts.** It also includes time-varying magnetic fields that contribute to T2 and field gradients that result in **T2*.** Each of these parameters will be dealt with later.

For high-resolution spectroscopy, magnetic field strengths are often described in terms of the Larmor frequency at which hydrogen atoms resonate. Thus a 2.35-T magnet is often referred to as a 100-MHz magnet, and a 11.7-T magnet is a 500-MHz magnet. Such odd-numbered field strengths are often employed to get the resonant frequency of hydrogen atoms to multiples of 30 or 100 MHz. For the imaging world, this convenience has not yet been achieved, and field strength values such as 0.5 T, 1.0 T, and 1.5 T are common, even though this leads to hydrogen resonant frequencies such as 21, 42, and 63 MHz, respectively.

NET MAGNETIZATION

We have been describing the behavior of individual nuclei in the presence of an external magnetic field. Because it is impossible to measure the action of individual nuclei, in the NMR experiment any signals received or data collected are the result of a bulk phenomenon from many nuclei, maybe as many as 10^{26} nuclei, the approximate number in a patient. We never observe a single, isolated nucleus, just collections of similar or identical nuclei as an aggregate. Fortunately, the bulk signals accurately reflect the behavior of each of the individual nuclei, and so one can deal with the **net magnetization, M,** which is just the sum of the individual nuclear magnetic moments, μ:

$$M = \Sigma \mu \qquad\qquad \textbf{(3-2)}$$

One can now consider the properties of this net magnetization during various circumstances. Because M is just the sum of many μ's, the general behavior of M will be identical to the behavior of the individual μ's. First, consider the long-neck bottle of beer shown in Figure 3-7 on a desk in Houston, Texas, where the earth's magnetic field is negligible. Because the orientation of the spin axis of each nucleus is random, the orientation of an individual nuclear magnetic moment pointing in any given direction will be canceled by another nucleus, with its magnetic moment pointing exactly opposite to the first. Therefore, the sum of a large number of nuclear magnetic moments will average out to zero, or M = 0. This agrees with our everyday observation that a long-neck beer bottle is totally nonmagnetic.

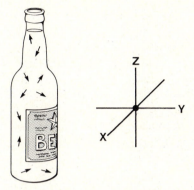

Figure 3-7.   The net magnetization of beer in a long-neck bottle in the absence of an external magnetic field is zero.

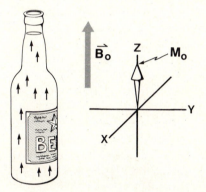

Figure 3-8.   The net magnetization of a long-neck beer bottle in the presence of an external magnetic field has magnitude and direction.

Vector Diagrams

Shown also in Figure 3-7 are three axes—X, Y, and Z—drawn perpendicular to one another to describe a coordinate system. The illustration shows the cartesian coordinate system used by mathematicians to diagram phenomena in space. For NMR such a coordinate system is used to construct **vector diagrams.** A vector is a quantity that has direction. If one speaks of traveling 50 mph, that is a **scalar** quantity. If one speaks of traveling 50 mph in a northerly direction, that is a **vector** quantity. The net magnetization M in Figure 3-7 is a vector quantity whose magnitude is zero. Vector diagrams are very helpful in describing NMR phenomena.

When the long-neck bottle of beer is placed in an intense external magnetic field, as in Figure 3-8, something different happens. Classically, all of the nuclei should precess about the applied field, and the net magnet moment should remain zero. But we know from quantum mechanics that more nuclei will be in one state than another. This nuclear alignment will not occur instantly, but rather over a period of time determined by the molecular nature of beer. Some tissues align quickly and others more slowly. One result of this alignment is that the net magnetization will not be zero. The explanation is that when normal interactions between nuclei occur that reorient the axis of the nuclear spin, the applied field will provide a small preference for the spins to align with the field. This is a small force compared with normal thermal interactions, and only a small number of spins align with the external magnetic field. The result can be illustrated as the vector in Figure 3-8, which shows that net magnetization exists along the Z axis, which is parallel to the external field.

If the long-neck bottle of beer is left in the magnet for a long time, the number of spins oriented with the field will have stabilized to an **equilibrium** value. This value is referred to as M_o, or the **equilibrium value of the net magnetization vector,** and it is the largest value that is possible. Because by convention the applied external magnetic field is parallel to the Z axis of the conventional cartesian coordinate system, this magnetization can also be referred to as M_z, or the Z component of the net magnetization. At equilibrium the x and y components of net magnetization are zero, so $M_x = M_y = O$, because all of the equilibrium magnetization is along the Z axis.

The intensity of the NMR signal is directly dependent on the value of M. The larger M_o, the stronger will be the NMR signal. The number of nuclei that contribute to M_o is small, only about one out of every million nuclei are part of the M_o, and so MRI is a technique that is very signal limited and therefore has a poor signal to noise ratio. In addition to the number of contributing nuclei, there are other factors that affect the amount of signal available for MRI. These factors can be summarized by the following:

$$M_o \propto (N\gamma^2 \, B_o/T) \hspace{3cm} \text{(3-3)}$$

where $\propto$ is a symbol for proportionality,
   N is the number of nuclei in the volume of interest,
   T is the absolute temperature of the material under investigation, and
   γ and B_o are as before.

Thus as the concentration of the nuclear species increases, or the volume being sampled increases, the NMR signal increases because N will be greater.

Hydrogen has the highest γ of any nucleus, other than tritium, and so has the second largest signal per number of nuclei. Tritium, therefore, would make an excellent MRI agent, but patients would frown on its use because of its radiotoxicity! For ^{13}C, γ is about one-fourth the value for ^1H, and so for an equal number of nuclei, the signal available is very much less.

At higher magnetic field strength, B_o, the increase in net magnetization will result in a stronger NMR signal and therefore improvement in any MR image. This is the major reason for going to higher magnetic fields for human imaging systems and spectroscopy. It is only one factor, however, albeit a very large one.

As the temperature of any sample decreases, the net magnetization increases. However, because this is temperature in degrees Kelvin, it is necessary to use drastic cooling to obtain any significant increase in the NMR signal. Any gain is usually offset by problems in keeping the sample or patient intact. This relationship is only an approximation but holds for temperatures near room temperature.

Control of Net Magnetization

Unfortunately, the net magnetization along the Z axis, M_z, is invisible to all observers. From the quantum mechanical point of view, it is impossible to measure this magnetization directly, and from the classical point of view, this magnetization is so small relative to the B_o field that induced it that it cannot be measured. This fact will become more apparent later. Essentially, **it is not possible to measure M_z; only M_x and M_y can be measured.**

To observe this net magnetization, M_z it is necessary to **tip** the net magnetization off of the Z axis or to make it point in another direction, preferably in the XY plane. Remember that M, the net magnetization, is the sum of lots of nuclear moments and so will behave in the same way that the individual nuclear magnetic moments behave. Therefore, if the net magnetization is pointing anywhere except exactly along the Z axis, it will precess about the Z axis with the same frequency that the individual nuclear magnetic moments precess, the Larmor frequency. Precession is a form of change of the magnetic field, and this changing magnetic field will induce an electric current in a loop of wire or antenna placed nearby. The signal can be detected, measured, and recorded. But how does one tip the net magnetization off of the Z axis, and what precisely does this mean? *Tipping the net magnetization* is a concise way of saying that the direction in which the net magnetization of the patient is pointing will be altered. So instead of pointing straight up, it will now point somewhere else, actually, anywhere else. It is just as big as it was before but has a new direction.

REFERENCE FRAMES

At this point it is necessary to introduce a **frame of reference** in order to follow the motions of the individual nuclear magnetic moments and the net magnetization vector. The frame of reference that is used is the standard three-dimensional cartesian coordinate system shown in Figure 3-9.

One condition within this system is that the applied magnetic field is always parallel to the Z axis. Thus, although the Z axis is always drawn as up, its actual orientation is determined by which direction the magnetic field is pointing in the particular magnet system employed, as illustrated in Figure 3-10. The B_o field for a permanent magnet is vertical and therefore passes through the patient in the anteroposterior direction. For resistive and super-

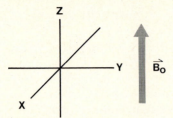

Figure 3-9. The conventional three-dimensional coordinate system used to describe the motion of the net magnetization vector.

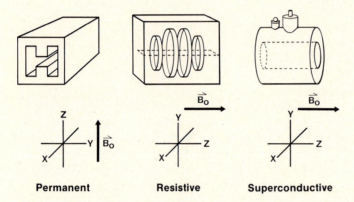

Permanent   Resistive   Superconductive

Figure 3-10. The orientation of B_o and the stationary frame of reference in three types of MR imagers.

conducting electromagnets, however, the B_o is parallel with the axis of the body and therefore passes through the patient from top to bottom.

Laboratory Frame

We will examine how to do this from the point of view of someone standing next to the magnet. This viewpoint is referred to as the **stationary** or **laboratory frame** of reference because all motions are compared to someone standing still in the laboratory.

To tip the net magnetization off the Z axis, a second magnetic field with special properties must be used. The key property is that the extra magnetic field must precess about the applied magnetic field with the same frequency as the nuclei, which is the Larmor frequency. If it does not, there will be effectively no interaction between the applied rotating magnetic field and the nuclear spins. This phenomenon is called **resonance** because of the requirement that the extra magnetic field precesses at exactly the correct frequency or else nothing will happen to the net magnetization vector.

From the Larmor equation, we know that it must precess with a frequency in the megahertz range. Locating a magnetic field with this property

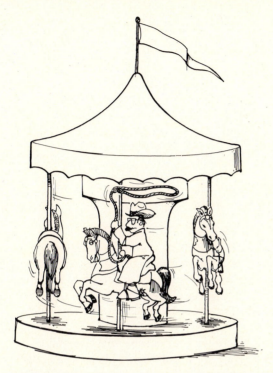

Figure 3-11.   The carousel serves to explain the rotating frame. The only way to carry on a conversation with a friend is to jump on the carousel and rotate with him.

may seem difficult, but it is in fact easily obtained. Recall that an electromagnetic emission, such as a radio emission, is composed of an oscillating electric field positioned 90 degrees to an oscillating magnetic field, as was shown in Figure 2-25.

The magnetic field component of a radio emission at the Larmor frequency is effectively a magnetic field rotating at the Larmor frequency. The precessing nuclear magnetic moments will be affected by the magnetic field component of the radio emission. Thus a rotating magnetic field is produced to tip the net magnetization vector into the X-Y plane by irradiating the sample with radio waves.

Rotating Frame

The next problem is that the net magnetization is precessing so fast now that it is difficult to visualize its motion. To solve this problem, a trick is used to make it easy to follow the motion of the net magnetization. An example of this can be found in an amusement park. If your are in line to go on a carousel and a friend is already on the carousel, as seen in Figure 3-11, you have the same problem that is presented by the precession of the net magnetization in the laboratory frame of reference. The rotation of your friend on the carousel

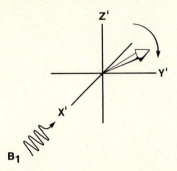

Figure 3-12.   In the rotating frame, a secondary magnetic field, B_1, from an RF emission, will cause net magnetization to rotate in the YZ plane.

relative to you on the ground makes it difficult to carry on a conversation. But if you step onto the carousel, now your friend is stationary relative to you and you can easily decide where to eat lunch. The rest of the world is rotating "backwards" relative to you now, but you have achieved your goal of standing still next to your friend. To easily watch the net magnetization, we must now "step onto the carousel."

The solution is to use a frame of reference that exactly matches the motion of the net magnetization. This is a reference frame that is precessing about the Z axis of the original frame of reference and has its Z axis coaxial with the original Z axis. This new frame of reference is called the **rotating frame.**

The laboratory frame of reference has axes labeled X, Y, and Z, and to avoid confusion, the rotating frame uses axes X', Y', and Z'. Unfortunately, because nearly all vector diagrams use the rotating frame of reference, and everyone knows this, most leave the primes off the axes for the rotating frame. This is done in the remainder of this book.

Within the rotating frame of reference, the net magnetization does not precess and so is easier to follow. Let us now follow the motion of the net magnetization when the second magnetic field is turned on. In the rotating frame of reference, the extra magnetic field, called **B_1,** is stationary and is usually aligned along the X' axis, as in Figure 3-12. It can, however, be aligned along the Y axis just as easily. This new magnetic field will cause the net magnetization to precess around in the YZ plane with a frequency of γB_1. If one is fast enough, B_1 can be turned off when the net magnetization has reached any given location in the YZ plane. One such point is the +Y axis. At this point, all of the net magnetization has been moved into the horizontal plane and so will generate the maximum NMR signal possible.

The conditions of strength of B_1 used to accomplish this are called a 90-degree RF pulse because the net magnetization was moved throughout an arc of 90 degrees. These conditions are the time and intensity of the RF pulse. Because each imaging system has its own combination of these parameters to do this, the universal nomenclature is to say that a 90-degree RF pulse was applied rather than to describe the RF power and pulse duration used. Another interesting stopping point is the $-Z$ axis or rotation of the net magnetization through an arc of 180 degrees. The combination of RF power and duration of the pulse that does this is called a 180-degree RF pulse. We will return to RF pulses in Chapter 5.

SUMMARY

Nuclear magnetic resonance phenomena are governed by quantum mechanical principles. However, they can be adequately described by classical mechanics. Individual nuclear magnetic moments, μ, are collectively described by the net magnetization vector, M. In the presence of an external magnetic field, μ will precess at the Larmor frequency. By exciting the spinning population of nuclei with a proper RF pulse at the Larmor frequency, M will precess in the XY plane.

The preceding phenomena occur in the laboratory frame of reference. To describe what happens to M in an understandable fashion, one employs the rotating frame of reference. To employ a rotating frame of reference, one must visualize the X-Y plane spinning about the Z axis at the Larmor frequency. This simplifies the vector descriptions of M.

Chapter
FOUR

NMR Signals

Chapter 3 concluded with an explanation of net magnetization, vector diagrams, and reference frames. It is necessary to restate some of this discussion
in order to properly develop the origin of the radio signal that results in the
magnetic resonance image. Furthermore, most of the future discussion will involve the rotating frame of reference, not the stationary frame.

First consider more closely how the NMR signal arises. The two basic
properties of a nucleus that are important to this signal are the **nuclear magnetic moment** and **spin.** When a sample is placed in an external magnetic
field, as indicated by B_0 in Figure 4-1, the nuclei in the material attempt to
align with this field because of the magnetic moments of the nuclei. The nuclei
act like tiny bar magnets, each seeking to orient itself with the strong external
magnetic field.

The spin of the nucleus adds a complicating factor. Instead of each nucleus acting like a simple bar magnet, it behaves like a spinning bar magnet.
The result is that, rather than just aligning with the external field, the nucleus
wobbles around the direction of the external field. This wobble is called
precession. In NMR the rate of precession—that is, how fast the nucleus wobbles—depends on the type of nucleus and the strength of the external field.
The relationship between these factors is given by the Larmor equation, which
was introduced earlier.

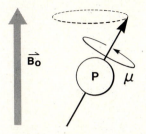

Figure 4-1. In the presence of an external magnetic field, nuclei align with the field and precess at the Larmor frequency.

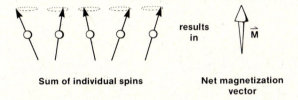

Sum of individual spins   Net magnetization vector

Figure 4-2. The nuclei aligned with the external magnetic field precess randomly at the same frequency. This results in the net magnetization represented by the vector M.

NET MAGNETIZATION

Of course, any patient who is placed in an MR imager consists of a multitude of nuclei. Many of these nuclei will attempt to align with the external field and will be precessing at the Larmor frequency, as diagrammed in Figure 4-2. Notice that although all the nuclei shown are oriented in an upward direction, the exact direction in which they point at any instant is slightly different, since they are at random positions in their wobble. The net result is that when we look at the material as a whole, the individual magnetizations sum to a **net magnetization (M)** parallel to the direction of the external magnetic field.

Equilibrium

In the preceding situation, **the net magnetization does not precess** but is a vector of constant magnitude pointed in the direction of the external magnetic field, which by convention is the Z direction. The horizontal or X and Y components of all the individual nuclear wobbles have canceled because they were randomly oriented and therefore there is no net magnetization in the XY plane. This state of the net magnetization is called **equilibrium.** The nuclear spins are said to be at equilibrium with the external magnetic field.

The magnitude of the net magnetization at equilibrium along the Z axis, symbolized as M_0, is determined by several physical factors. The more nuclei available for alignment, the larger will be M_0. The more of those nuclei available that in fact do align will be determined by the strength of the external magnetic field. Finally, a large gyromagnetic ratio results in a large M_0. There-

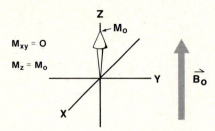

Figure 4-3. At equilibrium there is no XY component to net magnetization, and the Z component is at its maximum value, M_o.

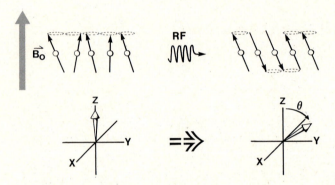

Figure 4-4. An RF pulse at the Larmor frequency will cause the net magnetization vector to tip through an angle, θ.

fore, N, the number of nuclei available, B_o, and γ contribute to M_o. **The larger M_o, the stronger will be the NMR signal.**

Unfortunately, the component of M along the Z axis cannot be measured directly. Only components of the net magnetization vector in the XY plane—that is, M_{xy}—can be detected by the NMR receiver. Therefore, at equilibrium no signal is received from the patient since the net magnetization vector points only in the Z direction and has no component in the XY plane, as seen in Figure 4-3.

To receive a signal from a patient, the magnetization vector is tipped away from the Z axis so that it has some nonzero component in the XY plane. This tipping is done by sending a burst of electromagnetic energy tuned to the nuclei's Larmor frequency. If the energy is not at this frequency, the nuclei will not absorb it and will not be tipped.

It turns out that for typical magnetic fields and for the nuclei of interest, such as hydrogen, the Larmor frequency corresponds to electromagnetic radiation lying in the radio range. Thus, if we send into our patient a burst of radio waves tuned to the precessional frequency of, say, the hydrogen nuclei, some of those nuclei will absorb energy from the radio waves and the magnetization vector will be tipped away from the Z direction, as diagrammed in Figure 4-4.

Tip Angle

Here the net magnetization vector has been tipped an angle θ from the Z axis because individual nuclei have absorbed RF energy and shifted to the high-energy state. Recall that the high-energy or excited state is against the external magnetic field. As long as the radio energy is beamed at the sample, the net magnetization vector will continue tipping. When the RF stops, the tipping of the magnetization vector stops. Consequently, the net magnetization vector can be tipped to any angle by application of a suitable RF pulse.

RF PULSES

Hard and Soft Pulses

The angle through which the net magnetization vector is tipped is controlled by two factors. First, how fast the net magnetization vector tips is controlled by the strength of radio pulse. A strong RF pulse will tip it rapidly, whereas a weak RF pulse will tip it more slowly. Second, the final tip angle is controlled by the duration of the RF pulse. It is the product of these two factors—the RF pulse intensity and duration—that determines the final tip angle.

Thus, for example, a 90-degree pulse can be achieved by either a strong, short duration RF pulse or a weaker RF pulse lasting a longer time. In any case the duration of even the longest RF pulse used in practice is still very short, rarely exceeding 100 μs. This is the reason for calling the burst of RF radiation a **pulse.** Strong, very short RF pulses are called **hard pulses,** and weaker but longer RF pulses are called **soft pulses.**

XY Magnetization

Regardless of whether the RF pulse is hard or soft, what is important is how far the net magnetization vector has been tipped. For this reason, both hard and soft pulses are most commonly labeled not by their strength and duration but by the angle through which they **tip** the net magnetization vector. Net magnetization can be tipped through any angle. A 90-degree RF pulse and 180-degree RF pulse are most often used in MRI, and these are shown in Figure 4-5. A 90-degree RF pulse rotates the net magnetization vector from equilibrium onto the XY plane. Similarly, a 180-degree RF pulse rotates the net magnetization vector from equilibrium to the $-Z$ axis.

The importance of RF pulses in NMR is that this is a mechanism by which one can introduce an XY component to the net magnetization. When the net magnetization vector is tipped, M_z shrinks, whereas M_x and M_y grow. Remember that the net magnetization in the XY plane, M_{xy}, is the only magnetization that can be detected as a signal from the patient.

Consider the net magnetization vector shown in Figure 4-6. This net magnetization vector has absorbed energy from an RF pulse and is no longer at equilibrium. Notice that the components of the net magnetization vector are different from those at equilibrium. M_z is smaller than M_o, and M_{xy} is no longer zero. The nuclear spins are said to be **partially saturated.** If the net magnetiza-

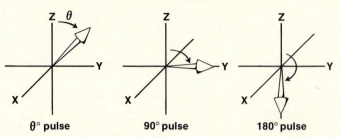

Figure 4-5.   90- and 180-degree RF pulses are always used in MRI. Smaller tip angles are used for fast imaging.

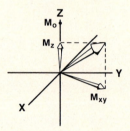

Figure 4-6.   Tipping net magnetization from the Z axis reduces M_z and increases M_{xy}.

tion were totally in the XY plane, the spins would be **saturated.** This terminology is used to identify one of the MRI RF pulse sequences as partial saturation.

M_{xy} Precession

After being excited by an RF pulse, the net magnetization vector does not remain stationary but undergoes a complex motion made up of two parts. First, the magnetization vector begins to precess, just as if it were an individual nucleus. This occurs because the individual nuclear magnetic moments that were precessing randomly are caused to precess together, as was demonstrated in Figure 4-4. This precession is also at the Larmor frequency. Thus, if one were to look at the XY component, M_{xy}, by looking down onto the XY plane, M_{xy} would be seen rotating at the Larmor frequency, as shown in Figure 4-7.

Return to Equilibrium

In addition to this precession, the net magnetization vector seeks to realign itself with the external magnetic field. That is, the magnetization vector slowly returns to its equilibrium position as the saturated nuclear spins individually flip back to their normal state of alignment with the external magnetic field. This is shown in Figure 4-8 as the regrowth of M_z along the Z axis. The net

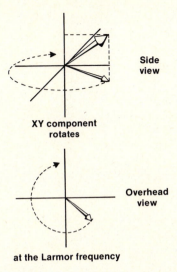

Side view

XY component rotates

Overhead view

at the Larmor frequency

Figure 4-7. Following an RF pulse that tips net magnetization from the Z axis, the XY component, M_{xy}, rotates at the Larmor frequency.

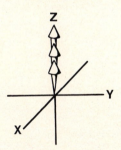

Figure 4-8. Following an RF pulse, the Z component of net magnetization, M_z, returns to equilibrium along the Z axis.

result of these two motions—precession and return to equilibrium—is a corkscrew or spiral pattern in three-dimensional space, as represented in Figure 4-9. The XY component precesses at the Larmor frequency and shrinks gradually until it disappears. The Z component gradually grows until finally it reaches its maximum value at equilibrium, M_o.

Both these changes in component magnitude—the shrinking of the XY component and growth of the Z component—are **independent** of each other. This is because the net magnetization vector is not like a rigid pencil that is rotated over by the RF pulse and then pivots back to equilibrium. Rather, it changes size as it rotates, resulting in a complex motion. **In general the XY component shrinks at a much faster rate than the Z component returns to equilibrium.**

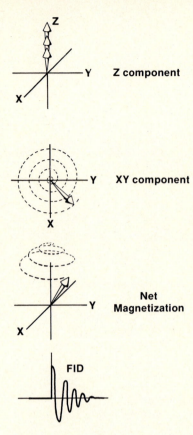

Figure 4-9. Regrowth of M_z and precession with shrinkage of M_{xy} result in a complicated corkscrew-like motion that results in return to equilibrium and the NMR signal—an FID.

Only M_{xy}, however, is responsible for the NMR signal. A receiving antenna outside of the patient views this corkscrew-like motion as an oscillating magnetic field alternately approaching and receding. The antenna is unaware of the return of net magnetization along the Z axis to M_o. The electric current induced in the antenna by the oscillating magnetic field has a waveform like that shown in Figure 4-9, and it is the basic NMR signal.

FREE INDUCTION DECAY

With all this complex motion of the net magnetization vector going on, what then can be observed? As mentioned earlier, the only part of the net magnetization vector that can be observed is the XY component. As long as M_{xy} is not zero, an oscillating signal will be received. The strength of the signal received is proportional to the size of the XY component. As M_{xy} decays to zero, the NMR signal decays to zero. This decaying NMR signal, which is received following an RF pulse, is called a **free induction decay (FID).**

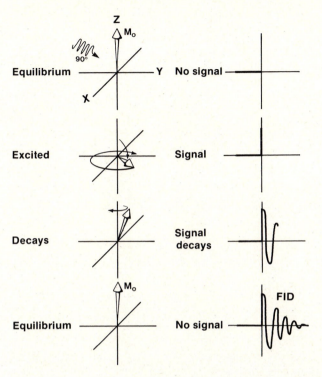

Figure 4-10.   Equilibrium followed by excitation followed by return to equilibrium with emission of an RF signal is the simplest NMR experiment.

Figure 4-10 diagrams in detail the production of the NMR signal following a 90-degree RF pulse. When the net magnetization vector is at equilibrium, there is no signal. The effect of the 90-degree RF pulse is to rotate the net magnetization vector onto the XY plane. At this point a strong signal is received, since there is now a large XY component to the net magnetization vector. As M_{xy} rotates in corkscrew fashion, an oscillating NMR signal is received. The oscillation of the signal is at the same frequency as the rotation of M_{xy}, namely, the Larmor frequency. As the net magnetization vector returns to equilibrium, the XY component shrinks, which is reflected in a gradual decrease in signal. Finally, at equilibrium the NMR signal is again zero. This sequence of events is shown in Figure 4-10 and constitutes the simplest NMR experiment.

RF PULSE DIAGRAMS

In terms of the macroscopic world, two events occur during an NMR experiment. First, an RF pulse, say a 90-degree RF pulse, is transmitted into the patient. Second, an RF signal is received from the patient. This signal is the FID. It is common in NMR literature to diagram these two events as shown in Figure 4-11. There are two lines of information to the diagram. The horizontal

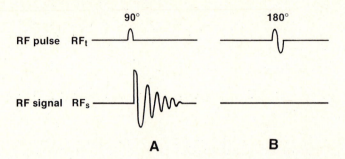

Figure 4-11.   Simple RF pulse diagrams for **A**, a 90-degree, and **B**, a 180-degree RF pulse. The top line represents the transmitted RF pulse (RFt), and the bottom line represents the RF signal received (RFs).

axis in both cases is time. One line, labeled **RF pulse,** or **RFt,** is the RF signal transmitted into the patient. The other, labeled **RF signal,** or **RFs,** is the FID received from the patient.

RF pulses transmitted into the patient are usually indicated on the RFt line by a round bump, which is one-half cycle of a sine wave. The label above the pulse, 90 degrees, indicates that the pulse is a 90-degree RF pulse. A 180-degree RF pulse is indicated by a full sine wave cycle with 180 above it. Note that following a 180-degree RF pulse there is no FID because there is no XY component to the net magnetization.

The signal from the patient is indicated by a plot of the intensity of the signal versus time. For the simple case given here, the diagram is correspondingly simple. In more complicated situations involving dozens of pulses and many signals, such diagrams are complicated but can be extremely descriptive. In MRI additional lines are added to indicate excitation of the gradient magnets necessary for producing images. For now it is sufficient to become familiar with this simple two-line form of an **RF pulse diagram.** This is the forerunner of the musical score to be discussed in Chapter 10.

What about the size and shape of the FID? The size, or amplitude, of the FID is equal to the amplitude of M_z at the start of the experiment. This amplitude is usually equal to and always dependent on M_o, the equilibrium value. Therefore, the amplitude of the FID is determined by the same parameters that influence M_o, namely, the number of spins involved, B_o and γ.

RF PULSE SEQUENCES

Although the FID is the basic NMR signal, it is difficult to use in practice. To get the FID, one must transmit a strong RF pulse at the Larmor frequency into the patient. The FID, which is a very weak RF signal also at the Larmor frequency, immediately follows this. Thus one must listen for a very weak signal after a very strong excitation pulse. Obviously, the RF receiver cannot be left on continuously, otherwise it would be damaged by the blast of energy of the RF pulse. Furthermore, in most systems, much of the electronics and frequently even the antenna are shared by both the RF transmitter and the RF receiver. Thus switching from transmit mode (for the RF pulse) to receive mode (for the FID) is required.

This switching is electronic and is very fast, but still some finite delay is involved. The result is that some of the initial part of the FID is lost. The situation is much like the dead time present in an ultrasound system. Thus, to get additional signals from the patient, more than one RF pulse is used. This grouping of two or more RF pulses is called an **RF pulse sequence.** The term **pulse sequence** is universally used and includes not only the RF pulses but also the gradient magnetic field pulses to be described later.

Many complicated pulse sequences are used in NMR. However, in imaging there are three that are very basic—the **spin echo** sequence, the **inversion recovery** sequence, and the **partial saturation** sequence. Only the first two are discussed here. The purpose of this introduction is to familiarize the reader with the nomenclature that accompanies these pulse sequences. What they do and their effect on the MR image will be detailed in subsequent chapters.

Spin Echo or CPMG Sequence

As indicated, the FID can generally not be used in practice because the first part of the signal may be missed and because of a low signal-to-noise ratio. However, a ghost echo of the FID can be generated if the 90-degree RF pulse is followed at some later point by a 180-degree RF pulse. The mechanism whereby this ghost echo signal arises is discussed in Chapter 6. However, the important point to make here is that this echo signal, called a **spin echo,** does not follow immediately on the heels of the 180-degree RF pulse but trails it. Thus, switching from transmit mode to receive mode can be done without missing any of the signal. The time between the 180-degree pulse and the spin echo is equal to the time between the 90- and the 180-degree pulses. The time between the initial 90-degree pulse and the spin echo is called the **TE** time (time-to-echo). By controlling the time for the 180-degree RF pulse, the time of the spin echo—that is, TE—is controlled and can thereby be prescribed.

If the spin echo is followed by another 180-degree pulse, another spin echo can be generated whose TE is once again measured from the initial 90-degree pulse. This pulse sequence—a 90-degree RF pulse followed by one or more 180-degree RF pulses—is called a **spin echo (SE)** or Carr-Purcell-Mei-boom-Gill (CPMG) sequence, after the original developers of the sequence. The sequence is illustrated in Figure 4-12.

Inversion Recovery

Another very common sequence is called the **inversion recovery (IR)** pulse sequence. The IR sequence adds a 180 RF pulse before the 90-degree RF pulse. This 180-degree RF pulse tips the net magnetization vector through 180 degrees onto the $-Z$ axis, that is, inverts it. No signal arises. After a delay, called **TI** (inversion-delay-time), a 90-degree RF pulse is given to tip the net magnetization vector onto the X-Y plane and produce a signal. Once again, spin

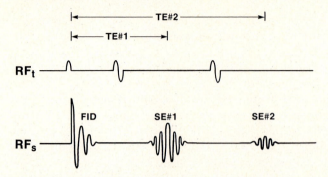

Figure 4-12.   A CPMG RF pulse sequence is used to generate spin echoes and is commonly called a spin echo RF pulse sequence.

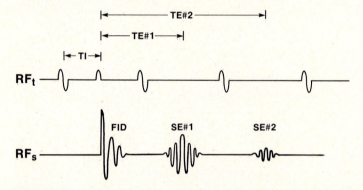

Figure 4-13.   Spin echoes are also produced with the inversion recovery pulse sequence.

echoes are created by adding one or more 180-degree RF pulses. The entire sequence is diagrammed in Figure 4-13.

Repetition Time

In MRI the data from one pulse sequence are not sufficient to generate an image. Rather, one must repeat the sequence many times, for example, 128 or 256 times, to obtain enough data for an image, much as CT must acquire many views to calculate and reconstruct an image. These repetitions usually are spaced out by a sizable delay. The time from the start of one sequence to the start of the next sequence is called the **repetition time (TR).** The importance of TE, TI, and TR to image production will become apparent in subsequent chapters.

SUMMARY

Net magnetization, M, is induced in a patient by a strong external magnetic field, B_o. The magnitude of M at equilibrium, M_o, is determined by the density of nuclear spins, the strength of B_o, and γ. An RF pulse, either hard or soft, is transmitted into the patient to tip M onto the XY plane and saturate the nuclear spins. The component of M in the XY plane, M_{xy}, generates the NMR signal during return to equilibrium.

The principal NMR signal is a free induction decay, but it is very difficult to detect. Therefore, additional RF pulses are transmitted to form spin echoes. The spin echoes are the NMR signals used to make an image. Spin echo and inversion recovery are two popular RF pulse sequences used to make spin echoes. The timing of the RF pulses is identified by TE, TI, and TR. These times control image appearance.

Chapter
FIVE

NMR Spectroscopy

Magnetic resonance imaging evolved out of industrial and scientific application of NMR high-resolution spectroscopy. A knowledge of spectroscopy is not required for an understanding of MRI, but it helps. This chapter deals with NMR spectroscopy in the very simplest of terms. It should provide the imaging physician and technologist with a brief look into the future. One of the potential, significant advantages to MRI is the possibility of performing in vivo NMR spectroscopy to aid in diagnosis.

The first issue to understand is the meaning of the term **spectrum.** A spectrum, sometimes called a **frequency distribution,** is a convenient graphical means of presenting specific frequency- or wavelength-related information. Two spectra that should be familiar are those associated with the emission of light from rare-earth radiographic intensifying screens and the absorption of that light in the emulsion of radiographic film. These spectra are shown in Figure 5-1.

Ultraviolet absorptiometry is an analysis that results in a spectrum of absorption of light as a function of its wavelength. In visual transmission spectroscopy, the X axis is the frequency of light that irradiates the sample and the Y axis is the percentage of light that penetrates the sample. If this is done at many slightly different wavelengths or frequencies, the resulting graph is called a spectrum. For NMR spectroscopy, the X axis of the spectrum relates the radio frequencies used to irradiate the sample or patient and the Y axis is the amount

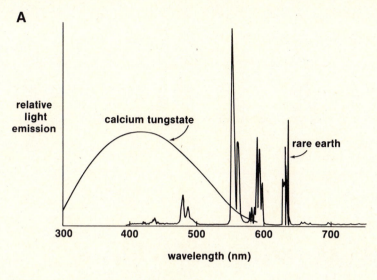

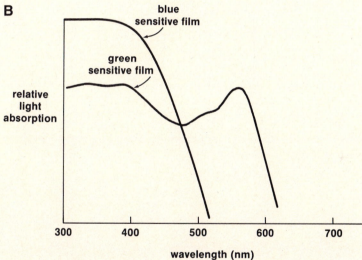

Figure 5-1.   The spectrum of light, **A**, emitted by radiographic intensifying screens and, **B**, that absorbed by a photographic emulsion are familiar examples of spectra.

of the signal produced by the sample at each frequency. Each type of spectrum is shown in Figure 5-2.

The NMR spectrum is obtained from the free induction decay (FID). Recall that the FID is the NMR radio signal emitted at the Larmor frequency from an excited sample. The FID is a plot of signal intensity versus time, as seen in Figure 5-3. If a mathematical process known as **Fourier transformation (FT)** is conducted, the FID is transformed into an NMR spectrum. The graphical

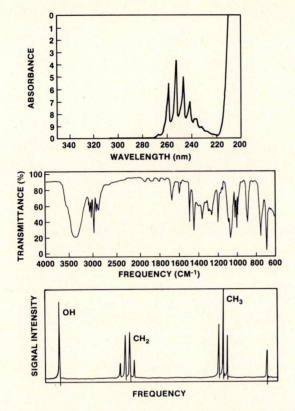

Figure 5-2.   Three examples of a spectrum are ultraviolet absorption, infrared transmission, and nuclear magnetic resonance.

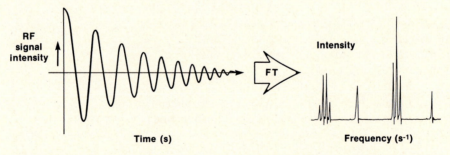

Figure 5-3.   The NMR spectrum is the Fourier transform of the FID.

rendition becomes one of signal intensity as a function of inverse time or frequency.

Fourier transformation is used to analyze sine wave functions mathematically. Knowledge of FT is not necessary for an understanding of MRI. The reader should simply consider it a black box that accepts an FID and generates an NMR spectrum.

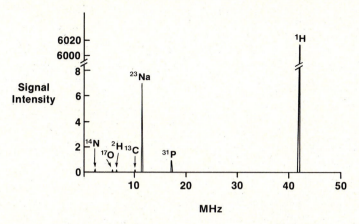

Figure 5-4.   The hypothetical NMR spectrum of the human body at 1 tesla.

NUCLEAR SPECIES

Shortly after the discovery of NMR one principle became well known; each isotope in the periodic table has its own resonant frequency at a given magnetic field strength. If you recall the Larmor equation, the resonant frequency depends only on the gyromagnetic ratio and the magnetic field strength. Each isotope has its own gyromagnetic ratio and the values vary by almost a factor of 100.

The gyromagnetic ratios of several isotopes of MRI interest were given in Table 3-1. If a total NMR spectrum of the body could be produced, it would include many nuclear species and might appear as in Figure 5-4. The gyromagnetic ratio for hydrogen is larger than the ratio of carbon 13 by a factor of four. This large difference in gyromagnetic ratios makes it possible to obtain signals from only one nuclear species at a time. Therefore, hydrogen signals can be obtained without interference from carbon, phosphorus, sodium, or any other NMR-sensitive nucleus that may be present. Fluorine is not normally found in the body; therefore, its signal, which would otherwise appear near the hydrogen signal, is normally zero.

CHEMICAL SHIFT

Even within a single nuclear species, more than one peak may be present in an NMR spectrum. Such a condition is called a **chemical shift.** The reason for the difference in resonant frequency for a single nuclear species is intimately related to the chemical structure of the molecule in which that particular nucleus is bound. Remember that each nucleus is surrounded by a cloud of electrons. Because these electrons are moving charged particles, they will generate their own magnetic fields that will add to or subtract from the applied external field. These additions and subtractions are noticed by the nuclei, and so the exact resonant frequencies are altered slightly.

However, because electrons are very small and each one carries only a small charge, their effect on the nucleus is small compared to the size of the

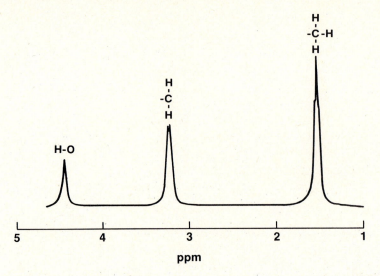

Figure 5-5. The hydrogen NMR spectrum of ethanol consists of three peaks corresponding to the three types of hydrogen atoms according to how each is bound in the molecule. Each peak consists of finer peaks representing the chemical shift of individual nuclei.

external magnetic field. Thus, for each chemically different nucleus in a sample, a unique NMR spectrum will be generated.

As a further example, consider ethanol, whose structure and hydrogen NMR spectrum are shown in Figure 5-5. In this molecule, there are three types of hydrogen atoms, two types of carbon atoms, and one type of oxygen atom. These types of atoms are characterized according to the manner in which they are bound in the molecule. Thus for ethanol there will be three peaks or lines in the hydrogen (or proton) NMR spectrum, two peaks in the carbon NMR spectrum, and one peak in the oxygen NMR spectrum.

Dependence on Magnetic Field

The magnitude of the chemical shift varies with the strength of the external magnetic field used to obtain the NMR spectrum. One might think that the difference in frequency units between these peaks would be independent of the strength of the magnet used, but this is not the case. As the strength of the magnet is increased, the frequency difference, and therefore the separation between peaks, increases in a linear fashion. Figure 5-6 illustrates this property.

The PPM Scale

To simplify interpretation of an NMR spectrum, a system was adopted to report these slight differences in Larmor frequency in a way that was independent of the size of the magnet used. The system used is the parts per million or **PPM scale**, where ppm is the difference in frequency divided by the resonant frequency of one of the peaks all multiplied by one million.

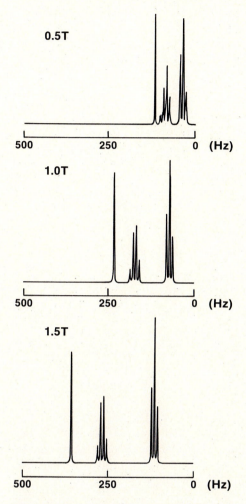

Figure 5-6. The ethanol spectra of hydrogen at three magnetic field strengths show that chemical shifts resulting in peak separation become more obvious at higher field strength. The frequency scale is relative to a standard.

So if one peak resonated at 100,000,000 Hz and another resonated at 100,000,500 Hz, they would differ by 500 parts in 100 million, or 5 ppm. For hydrogen atoms, most peaks differ over a range of about 10 ppm, whereas carbon 13 resonances cover about 200 ppm. Additionally, for many nuclei an arbitrary reference compound has been chosen and given an absolute chemical shift of 0.00, from which all other resonances are measured. For hydrogen and carbon 13, the reference is **tetramethyl-silane (TMS).**

Relative to the reference, chemical shifts can be positive or negative depending on whether the resonance is at a higher or lower frequency than the standard TMS. On old NMR spectrometers, the frequency of the operation was

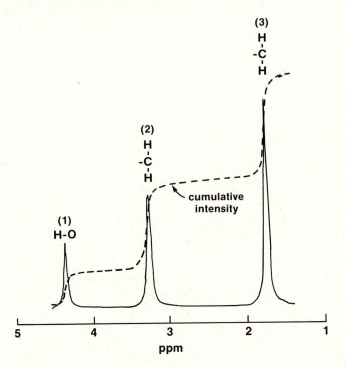

Figure 5-7. The hydrogen NMR spectrum of ethanol contains three peaks, whose sizes are proportional to the number of nuclei with equal Larmor frequency.

constant and the strength of the magnet was changed. Those peaks that resonate at higher frequencies also resonate at lower field strengths, or **downfield.** Peaks with lower resonant frequencies at constant field will resonate at higher fields, or **upfield,** if the frequency is constant. Thus peaks at higher frequencies are downfield, and peaks at lower frequencies are upfield.

Nuclear Abundance

One other property of NMR spectra is that they contain information about the relative amounts of each type of nucleus in a sample. This quantity is described not in the height of the individual peaks but in the area under each peak. Thus for ethanol the methyl (CH_3) signal will have three times the area of the hydroxyl (OH) peak, and the methylene (CH_2) peak will have twice the area of the hydroxyl peak. This property is illustrated in Figure 5-7. Such observations provide information about how much of an isotope is present in a sample.

J-Coupling

J-Coupling is another property of NMR spectra that is very useful. In addition to the chemical shift information being provided, an individual peak may be split into several peaks, making an even finer, more precise spectrum, as seen in Figure 5-8. This splitting is called J-coupling and is caused by other nearby

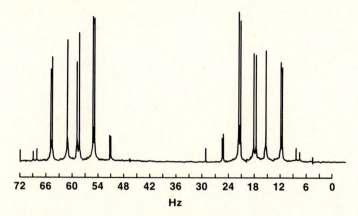

Figure 5-8. This hydrogen NMR spectrum shows fine structure as a result of J-coupling.

nuclei communicating with each other. For each neighboring nucleus that is chemically different, an additional peak will be present in the spectrum. Unlike chemical shifts, which vary with the strength of the magnet, **J-coupling is independent of the external magnetic field strength.** This additional information is very useful to chemists trying to determine the structure of an unknown molecule.

The figures included in this chapter were chosen for simplicity and clarity, not completeness. Organic chemistry and biochemistry have millions of known molecules. In most cases, the NMR spectra are much more complicated than those shown here. However, a trained NMR spectroscopist can understand and explain these spectra in terms of molecular structure and configuration. One word of caution is in order: NMR spectroscopy is a demanding but rewarding complex intellectual proposition, as is magnetic resonance imaging. The expectation that the best features of both can be combined into imaging spectroscopy must be tempered with reality. The combined technique is years from routine clinical application.

MEDICALLY IMPORTANT NUCLEI

This combination of NMR spectral information has been very useful to chemists for the past 35 years, but it is just now attracting the interest of the medical community. By the application of in vivo NMR spectroscopy, it may be possible to obtain various spectra from patients and so gain information about the chemistry of life. So far, little progress has been made toward making any of the spectroscopic tools clinically useful, but that should change in the next few years.

Hydrogen

The hydrogen spectrum is dominated by the NMR signal from water. There is some contribution from fat, depending on the tissue studied. The relatively

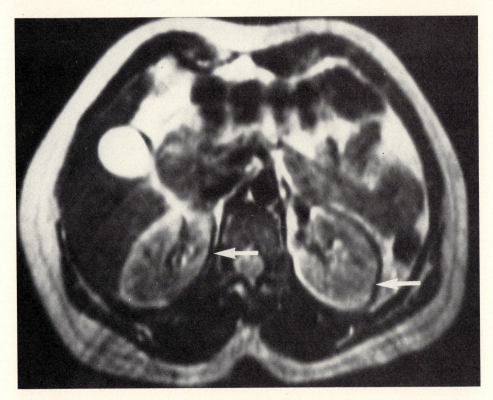

Figure 5-9.   The observed curvilinear rim of decreased signal intensity adjacent to the renal cortex is an artifact due to the chemical shift between hydrogen in water and hydrogen in fat. (Courtesy George Oliver, St. Johns Mercy Medical Center, St. Louis.)

strong signal is what makes hydrogen imaging so attractive and rather easy. There is signal from only one chemical species—water—for many tissues and two—water and fat—for others. However, the presence of these two signals can produce problems at high field strengths. At low fields, the difference between the fat resonance and the water resonance is small enough that it is overwhelmed by the gradients used to make the image. At higher magnetic fields, this difference is not overwhelmed by the imaging gradients, and distinct fat and water images are produced that are slightly offset from each other. The resulting image contains a **chemical shift artifact** such as that shown in Figure 5-9. The water and fat signals are about 10,000 times stronger than the signal from any other metabolite, and therefore it is difficult to use hydrogen spectroscopy to study metabolism.

Phosphorus

Another nucleus that is currently receiving much attention for following metabolism is phosphorus 31. Phosphorus 31 is a well-behaved NMR nucleus and

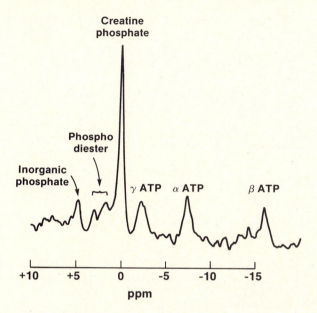

Figure 5-10. A representative phosphorus 31 NMR spectrum.

the natural isotope present in 100% abundance. It is found in several important metabolites, particularly adenosine triphosphate (ATP), the main energy carrier inside cells. It is also present in adenosine diphosphate (ADP), a by-product of ATP; adenosine monophosphate (AMP), a building block of ADP and ATP; creatine phosphate (CrP), the immediate storage form for high-energy phosphates in many tissues; and inorganic phosphate (Pin), the raw material for building the previous high-energy phosphates. These signals dominate the in vivo NMR spectrum for most tissues and provide a window into the energy state of the tissue. A representative phosphorus 31 spectrum is shown in Figure 5-10. Possible applications include diagnosing metabolic disorders, assessing the damage done by a stroke or heart attack, and serving as a research tool for studying the effects of drugs and other treatments.

Carbon

Another nucleus attracting attention is carbon 13, whose NMR spectrum is shown in Figure 5-11. Carbon 12 is the abundant isotope of carbon, constituting about 99% of the naturally occurring carbon. However, carbon 12 has no NMR signal because its spin quantum number is zero. Carbon 13 has a spin quantum number of one half and is another well-behaved NMR nucleus. Unfortunately, it constitutes only 1% of the naturally occurring carbon. Its scarcity makes it attractive for NMR spectroscopy, since synthetic compounds can be enriched in carbon 13. These compounds act as tracers and can be used to follow metabolic pathways both in research and in clinical applications.

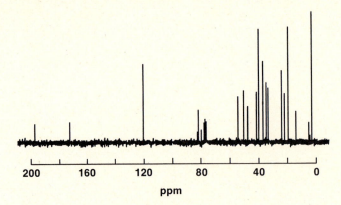

Figure 5-11. A representative carbon 13 NMR spectrum.

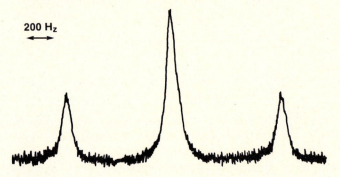

Figure 5-12. A representative sodium 23 NMR spectrum.

Sodium

Sodium is abundant in the body primarily as sodium chloride and other salts. Sodium 23 is the common isotope, with a spin quantum number of 5/2. Its spectrum is shown in Figure 5-12. Spectroscopically, there are plans to try to use it as a marker for intracellular versus extracellular conditions based on differences in relaxation time.

Fluorine

Fluorine represents a unique opportunity for spectroscopy in living systems, including patients. It is a well-behaved NMR nucleus with 100% natural abundance, has almost the same inherent sensitivity as hydrogen, and resonates at almost the same frequency as hydrogen, so existing imagers could be used with only minor modifications. However, it is almost entirely absent from the human body. For this reason, it is the perfect tracer for NMR studies. The only fluorine signal that will be detected comes from the fluorine that is deliberately introduced before the measurement. A representative NMR spectrum is shown

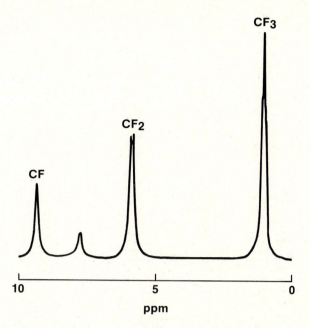

Figure 5-13.   A representative fluorine 19 NMR spectrum.

in Figure 5-13. Forms that are useful include the new perfluoro artificial bloods that would act as a marker for blood vessels and chemically modified compounds such as fluoroglucose to monitor metabolism. Research into these applications is currently under way at various centers.

SUMMARY

The FID obtained during an NMR experiment can undergo Fourier transformation into an NMR spectrum, which is a plot of signal intensity versus frequency. The NMR spectrum is useful for identifying chemical structure. It is known that normal tissue and malignant tissue exhibit differences in their NMR spectra, and it is hoped that in vivo spectroscopy will aid in diagnosis.

   The appearance of the NMR spectrum is dependent on several conditions. At high external magnetic fields the same nucleus will have a slightly different Larmor frequency, depending on its molecule. This is called chemical shift. The NMR scale is simplified from frequency to ppm. The size of individual peaks in the spectrum are in direct proportion to the number of similar nuclei. J-coupling results in the fine structure of each peak. Spectra from several medically important nuclei are presented.

Chapter SIX

MRI Parameters

The previous chapter on NMR spectroscopy was a bit of a diversion. It is helpful to know something about NMR spectroscopy in order to understand MRI, but it is not essential. It is essential, however, to understand the three principal NMR parameters: **spin density, T1 relaxation time,** and **T2 relaxation time.** Each of these is fundamentally different and independent of the others. A closer look at what these basic NMR parameters represent and how they are measured is necessary for an understanding of MR image appearance.

SPIN DENSITY

Back in Chapter 3, equation 3-3 described how the strength of the net magnetization is related to several parameters. It is reasonable to expect that one of the parameters that affects the strength of the NMR signal might be the number of hydrogen nuclei within the volume of the sample. For example, if no hydrogen nuclei are present, we should expect no signal. Conversely, if the sample is rich in hydrogen, we might expect a strong NMR signal. However, this reasoning is true only to a certain extent.

One of the most important aspects of NMR is that the signal is not just dependent on the presence or absence of hydrogen nuclei but is also very sensitive to the environment of the hydrogen nuclei. How hydrogen is bound within a molecule also determines the strength of the NMR signal. For imaging it turns out that hydrogen, which is very tightly bound, creates no usable sig-

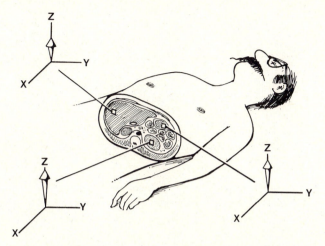

Figure 6-1. M_0 and signal intensity are proportional to mobile hydrogen concentration or spin density. These three voxels each have different spin densities.

nal. Thus the signal received should be thought of as arising from ''mobile hydrogen,'' that is, hydrogen nuclei that are more loosely bound such as those in liquids. A good example of this effect is bone. Bone always appears black on an MR image because it gives no signal. This is not because there is no hydrogen present—indeed there is some—but rather because the hydrogen nuclei are so rigidly bound that they produce no detectable signal and thus appear like air, which of course has little hydrogen.

The measure of the concentration of mobile hydrogen nuclei available to produce an NMR signal is called **spin density (SD)**. The higher the concentration of mobile hydrogen nuclei, the stronger will be the net magnetization vector at equilibrium, M_0, and the more intense will be the NMR signal. A strong NMR signal will result in a better MR image.

Figure 6-1 shows three pixels highlighted in the cross section of a patient. Each represents a voxel containing different tissue with different concentrations of mobile hydrogen nuclei. The tissue with the highest spin density will have the largest value of M_0. Table 6-1 reports relative values of spin density for several tissues. These values are approximate because they are averages from a number of sources.

Having just been told that a large M_0 is necessary for a strong NMR signal, you will be disappointed to be told again that the M_z is not detectable. This has an important consequence. In a magnetic resonance imager, the radio receiver detects only the XY component of the net magnetization vector—that is, M_{xy}. Because M_{xy} at equilibrium is zero, the magnetic resonance imager receives no signal. A patient, whose nuclei are resting at equilibrium in an external magnetic field, creates no NMR signal. To be able to receive some sort of signal from a patient, one must cause the net magnetization vector to have a component in the XY plane.

TABLE 6-1.   Relative values of mobile hydrogen nuclei, spin density, for various tissues

Time	Relative Spin Density
Muscle	100
White matter	100
Fat	98
Cerebrospinal fluid	96
Kidney	95
Gray matter	94
Spleen	92
Liver	91
Blood	90
Pancreas	86
Cortical bone	1–10
Lung	1–5
Air	<1

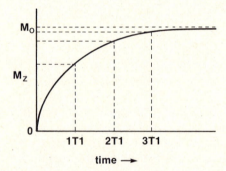

Figure 6-2.   The growth of M_z with time following exposure to a strong magnetic field is dependent on the T1 relaxation time.

T1 RELAXATION TIME

At this point let us return to our patient to examine the transition from the no magnetic field condition to the intense magnetic field condition of a magnetic resonance imager. Discontinuities are rare in nature. Therefore, it is safe to assume that although conditions may change rapidly, such as when we suddenly position the patient in the magnet, the net magnetization will not change rapidly. In fact, the Z component of the net magnetization, M_z, changes rapidly at first and then relatively slowly. This change is shown graphically in Figure 6-2 and is described mathematically in Appendix A for the interested reader.

Once equilibrium is reached and M_z equals M_0, this condition of net magnetization will continue indefinitely unless the situation is disturbed. Suppose

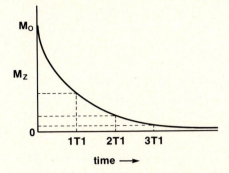

Figure 6-3. M_z shrinks with a time constant T1 when removed from a strong external magnetic field.

TABLE 6-2. Approximate T1 relaxation times at a field strength of 1.0 T for various tissues

Tissue	T1 (ms)
Fat	180
Liver	270
Renal cortex	360
White matter	390
Spleen	480
Gray matter	520
Muscle	600
Renal medulla	680
Blood	800
Cerebrospinal fluid	2000
Water	2500

the magnet was turned off or the patient removed from the magnetic field. The result of such a move is shown graphically in Figure 6-3. As the individual nuclear magnetic moments reposition themselves randomly, the net magnetization along the Z axis disappears so that M_z goes to zero.

The time constant that describes the rate at which the Z component of the net magnetization will return to its equilibrium value, M_0, is the **T1 relaxation time**. For tap water T1 is about 2500 ms. For tissues **in vivo** T1 can be as short as 100 ms for fatty tissues and as long as 2000 ms for bodily fluids such as spinal fluid. Table 6-2 presents representative T1 values for several tissues of interest. In general, **the T1 of diseased and damaged tissue is longer than for corresponding healthy tissue.**

One can write an equation to describe how M_z grows with time toward equilibrium. It turns out that this growth has an exponential form. The farther the Z magnetization (M_z) is from equilibrium (M_0), the faster it will approach equilibrium, and as the system of nuclear spins gets closer to equilibrium, M_z approaches more slowly. As a rule of thumb, the system of nuclear spins will get two thirds of the way to equilibrium in one T1 period. A consequence of this is that it takes about five times T1 for a spin system to return to equilibrium once it has been disturbed away from equilibrium. When repetitive samplings are made, either for imaging or for spectroscopy, this places a limit on the amount of magnetization available for the next sampling, as will be discussed later.

T1 is also called the **longitudinal** or **spin-lattice relaxation time**. The term longitudinal refers to events occurring along the axis of the net magnetization vector. T1 relaxation describes the growth and decay of M_z, and therefore it is longitudinal in nature.

When a patient is in the magnet at equilibrium, the net magnetization vector is constant and of maximum magnitude, M_0. If we disturb the nuclei by directing an RF pulse at the patient, the nuclei absorb energy and the net magnetization vector changes in direction or magnitude. This new magnetization state of the patient is unstable in that the nuclei wish to realign with the external magnetic field and return to equilibrium. The regrowth of the Z component, M_z, is the T1 process and represents a return of the system to the stable equilibrium state.

To return to equilibrium, the nuclei must give up the energy they gained from the transmitted RF pulse. The hydrogen nuclei are not isolated but are bound with other atoms to form a molecule. This binding arrangement is sometimes called a **lattice**. The regrowth of M_z is accomplished by transferring energy mainly to other atoms in the molecule or to the molecule as a whole. That is, the energy is given up by an interaction between the individual hydrogen nuclei (spin) and the surrounding molecule (lattice). Hence, T1 is sometimes called the spin-lattice relaxation time.

Pixel intensity in a magnetic resonance image is a complicated function of the T1 relaxation time. Whether a given pixel appears bright or dark depends on the pulse sequence employed. Generally, **on T1-weighted images tissue with short T1 will appear bright and tissue with long T1 will appear dark.**

T2 RELAXATION TIME

Figure 6-4 plots the magnitude of the Z and XY components of net magnetization versus time following application of a 90-degree pulse. Note that they are very similar in shape. Actually, they are both exponential in form, much like radioactive decay. The T1 relaxation time is usually much longer than the T2 relaxation time. The equations describing these graphs are developed in detail in Appendix A. In the same way that M_z is controlled by T1 relaxation, so is **M_{xy} controlled by T2 relaxation.** The constants, T1 and T2, play a role analogous to radioactive half-life and control the rate of decay of the Z and XY components of the net magnetization vector, respectively. They are each a fundamental property of tissue.

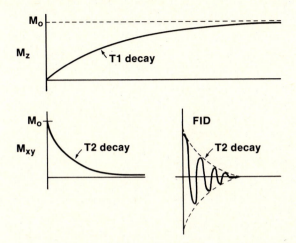

Figure 6-4. As M_z relaxes back to M_0, M_{xy} relaxes back to zero, usually much more quickly because T2 relaxation times are much shorter that T1 relaxation times. It is the M_{xy} relaxation that is detected as an FID or spin echo.

A large value for T1 or T2 indicates a long, gradual decay, and a small value indicates a rapid decay. As an example, the T1 and T2 for tap water are roughly 2000 ms, indicating that the signal would take several seconds to decay. This is much like a struck bell, which rings for several seconds before the sound dies.

As mentioned the decay of M_z and M_{xy} is independent, and thus the decay constants, **T1 and T2, are also independent of one another**. However, T2 is usually much less than T1 and never exceeds T1. Because the NMR signal received is proportional to M_{xy}, it also decays according to T2, and the envelope of the FID is exponential in T2, as shown in Figure 6-4.

It may seem strange that the T1 decay in Figure 6-4 is represented by an increasing value with time, whereas the T2 decay is represented by a decreasing value. That's because the regrowth of M_z to M_0 is actually a decay from the excited state to the equilibrium state, while M_{xy} is being reduced to zero.

Analogous to T1, T2 is sometimes called the **transverse or spin-spin relaxation time**. Because T2 relaxation represents loss of XY magnetization, it represents energy loss in a plane perpendicular to or transverse to equilibrium magnetization, M_0. M_0, of course, is along the Z axis. This is the origin of the terminology *transverse relaxation*.

T2 decay also involves the loss of energy by the nuclei. The main reason the XY component of the net magnetization vector shrinks is because the nuclei are interacting with each other. In any material above absolute zero in temperature, molecules and atoms are in constant motion. At room temperature this motion is rapid so that the nuclei are continually passing near each other and banging into one another as it were. This continual jostling among nuclei allows one nucleus to lose energy to other nuclei. This is the principal mechanism for the loss of the XY component of the net magnetization—the

TABLE 6-3.   Approximate T2 relaxation times at a field strength of 1.0 T for various tissues

Tissue	T2 (ms)
Muscle	40
Liver	50
Renal cortex	70
Spleen	80
Fat	90
White matter	90
Gray matter	100
Renal medulla	140
Blood	180
Cerebrospinal fluid	300
Water	2500

transfer of energy from one spin to another. Hence, T2 is also called the **spin-spin relaxation time.**

Pixel intensity in an MR image is also a complicated function of tissue T2 relaxation time. The pulse sequence employed will determine the T2-related brightness of pixels. **Generally, on T2-weighted images, tissue with long T2 will appear bright and tissue with short T2 will appear dark.** Table 6-3 presents approximate values of T2 relaxation times for various tissues.

Phase Coherence

Now that the three fundamental NMR parameters that affect the NMR signal have been discussed, let us perform a simple experiment to see if some of these effects can be observed. Once again we position the patient in the magnetic resonance imager. Following a 90-degree RF pulse, the net magnetization vector is tipped onto the X-Y plane. Thus there is a large XY component, M_{xy}, which will be detected as a signal. As M_{xy} decays as a result of T2 relaxation, the signal is expected to likewise decay, until finally, when equilibrium is once again reached, the signal has died to zero.

Because the decay of the NMR signal follows the decay of M_{xy} exactly, one should be able to calculate T2 from the FID. However, when this experiment is actually performed, unexpected results are obtained. After excitation with a 90-degree RF pulse, the FID, instead of lasting for several seconds, will decay much more rapidly. The T2 obtained from such a measurement is called **T2 star (T2*)** and is much less than the true T2. This relationship is shown in Figure 6-5.

What has occurred? Why can't the T2 be determined directly in this manner? To answer these questions, we must again turn our attention to the nuclei in the magnetic field of our magnet. The trunk of the patient in the imager is

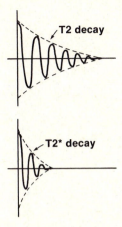

Figure 6-5. Theoretically, M_{xy} should decay as T2. The actual decay is much shorter and is called T2*.

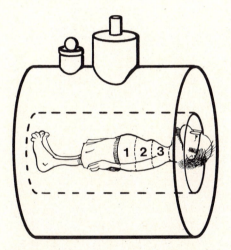

Figure 6-6. To visualize T2 and T2*, consider a patient in an MR magnet whose trunk is divided into three regions.

approximately 50 cm long. For illustration, mentally divide that length into three regions, as in Figure 6-6, and consider the nuclear spins that lie within each of these three adjacent regions in the magnet. Following the 90-degree RF pulse, at time 0, the net magnetization vectors of the three regions are all tipped onto the XY plane along the Y axis. This situation is illustrated in Figure 6-7. Remember that even though the patient is considered divided into three regions the received NMR signal is still from all the tissues of the patient. Therefore, the signal is the vector sum of the net magnetization vectors of the three regions. Because the three magnetization vectors are all pointing in the

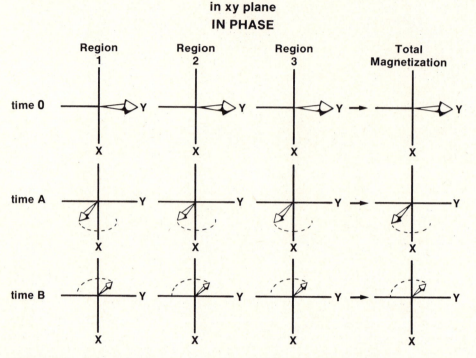

Figure 6-7. In a perfect magnet loss of M_{xy} will be the same throughout a homogeneous patient.

same direction, they add maximally and produce a large signal, as shown in the upper right corner of Figure 6-7.

At some later time, A, the three net magnetization vectors of Figure 6-7 have changed. First, they are shorter in length because of T2 decay. Second, they have rotated around to point in a new direction—they are precessing. The rate of precession is the same for each of the three net magnetization vectors, because this is controlled by the magnetic field strength in the three regions and B_o is the same in each region. The net result is that each M_{xy} has shrunk in length and changed in direction, but they all still point in the same direction. Their sum is smaller than at time 0, and this reduction in length is due only to T2 relaxation.

At some later time, B, the net magnetization vectors have shrunk even further in length because of T2 and point in still another direction as a result of precession. However, they still all point in the same direction. Once again, their sum is smaller still owing to T2 relaxation.

The result is the NMR signal known as an FID. The envelope of the decaying signal is indicated by the dotted line in Figure 6-8, and it decays with a time constant, T2. This condition, in which all the spins turn together so that at any instant they are all pointing in the same direction, is called **in phase**. Another way of saying it is that the spins have maintained **phase coherence**.

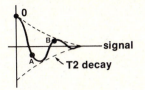

Figure 6-8. The envelope of the FID obtained from a perfect magnet describes T2 relaxation. The times 0, A, and B refer to Figure 6-7.

The key assumption in the preceding description is that the magnetic field in the three regions of the patient is exactly the same. This makes the net magnetization vectors all rotate at precisely the same rate and therefore remain **in phase**. In real life it is not possible to build such a perfect magnet. Although the magnets used in MRI are of very high quality, the magnetic fields are not perfectly homogeneous. The field strength varies slightly from place to place in the imaging aperture. Even this very small inhomogeneity in magnetic field intensity has a profound effect on the NMR signal.

T2* Relaxation

If the preceding NMR experiment is repeated but this time with a realistic, not-quite-perfect magnet, a different FID results. Once again a 90-degree RF pulse is transmitted into the patient, and the net magnetization vectors in the three regions are all tipped together into the XY plane along the Y axis, as shown at time 0 in Figure 6-9. At this point the net magnetization vectors are all parallel and add maximally as before. However, as time progresses, something different occurs from the previous situation. Consider how the net magnetization vectors will be at time A.

Each vector has shrunk by the same amount as a result of T2 decay, so they are all still of equal, albeit shorter, length. Each has also precessed in the magnetic field. However, because the magnetic field is slightly different in the three regions, the distance each vector has rotated is different and they now point in slightly different directions. For example, the magnetization vector in region 1 is in a slightly higher field and precesses at a slightly faster rate. Therefore, at time A it has rotated a little further than its neighbor in region 2. By contrast, the magnetization vector in region 3 is in a slightly lower magnetic field and therefore has precessed more slowly. It points in a different direction.

Thus, when these three net magnetization vectors are added, the total net magnetization vector is smaller because of two effects. One effect is the standard T2 effect, which has shortened all three net magnetization vectors equally. The second effect is the fact that they no longer all point in the same direction owing to inhomogeneities in the magnetic field. Therefore, the total net magnetization vector is shorter than for the perfect magnet system.

At time B the effect of the variations in the magnetic field on the direction of the net magnetization vectors is even more pronounced. The higher-field net magnetization vector on the left is even farther ahead, and the lower-field net magnetization vector on the right has fallen farther behind. The sum is

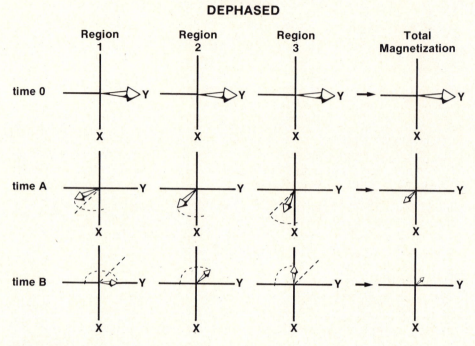

Figure 6-9. In an imaging magnet field, inhomogeneity causes M_{xy} to decay more rapidly than expected. The result is T2* relaxation.

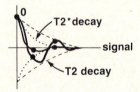

Figure 6-10. The envelope of the FID obtained from an imaging magnet describes T2* relaxation. T2* is much less than T2 because of magnetic field inhomogeneities.

almost zero. The resulting NMR signal, shown in Figure 6-10, therefore, is decaying much more rapidly than T2 alone would cause. The small variations in the magnetic field are causing the net magnetization vectors in different regions to precess at different frequencies. That is, the spins in different regions rapidly lose their **phase coherence**. They **dephase**.

Although this discussion has used a three-compartment model, it should be clear that the actual situation involves a multicompartment model. The inhomogeneity in the magnetic field causes each individual nuclear spin to precess differently so that **T2* is very much shorter than T2**.

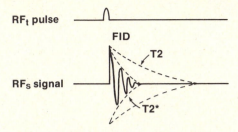

Figure 6-11. Following a 90-degree RF pulse T2* relaxation is observed rather than T2.

Thus the T2* measured in such an NMR experiment is a combination of two factors—the real T2 of the tissue under examination and magnet inhomogeneities. Unfortunately, in practical magnets, the effect of magnet inhomogeneities far outweighs that of decay, owing to the T2. One ends up measuring the imperfections of the magnet rather than the T2 of the sample.

HOW TO MEASURE T2

The RF pulse sequence diagram shown in Figure 6-11 results in the type of signal received from a conventional imaging magnet. The dotted line indicates how the FID would decay in a perfect magnet, and a more realistic, shorter FID is shown.

If in real-world magnets one cannot count on the FID decaying according to the T2 of the sample, how then can the true T2 be measured? Several methods have been developed, all of which employ additional pulses following the initial 90-degree RF pulse. The most common of these is the spin-echo pulse sequence, introduced in Chapter 4. To understand the effect of a spin-echo sequence in this case, consider the following analogy.

Suppose the net magnetization vectors in the three regions of the patient are represented by three runners on an oval track. At time zero they all leave the starting line together, as diagrammed in Figure 6-12. A perfect magnet system is represented by the case in which all the runners run at exactly the same speed, so that at some later time, say time A, the runners are still exactly together and in step, as seen in Figure 6-13. However, in a real magnet the net magnetization vectors dephase because they are precessing at slightly different rates. This situation is diagrammed in Figure 6-14; the runners start out together, but now each runs at a slightly different speed, so that after time A they are no longer together.

Is there some way to cause the runners to come back together even though they each run at a different speed? Suppose a new rule is introduced to the race. Suppose that at time A in Figure 6-14 a whistle is blown and all the runners immediately have to turn around, reversing direction, and run back toward the starting line. If the race is now run making use of this rule, the scene will change. The runners start out together but soon begin to sepa-

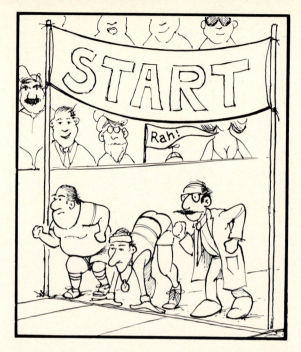

Figure 6-12. Immediately following a 90-degree RF pulse all spins begin at the same starting line just like runners in a race.

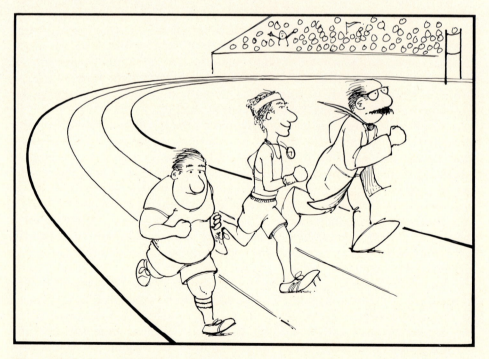

Figure 6-13. A perfect magnet is analogous to a perfect race. In a perfect magnet, M_{xy} remains in phase. In a perfect race, the runners remain in step.

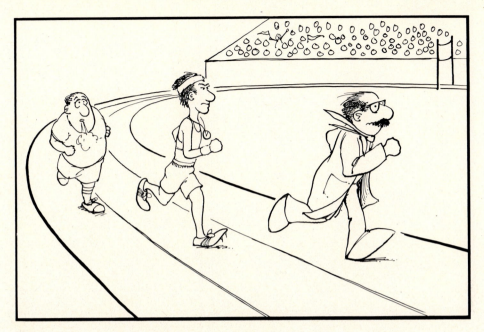

Figure 6-14.   In an imaging magnet, M_{xy} dephases rapidly. In a real race, competitors run at different speeds.

rate, that is, **dephase**. Now at time A the whistle is blown and all the runners reverse and start running back toward the starting line. Suddenly the fastest runner, who was far ahead, is behind, and the slowest runner, who was behind, is in the lead. Remember that even though they have changed directions they have not changed speed. Therefore, even though he is now behind, the fastest runner is still running faster than the others.

A little thought will reveal that running toward the starting line is exactly the reverse of the start, when they ran away from the starting line. This means that as the runners cross the starting line, as seen in Figure 6-15, they will again be precisely together—they are **in phase** again. They will cross the starting line at a time exactly twice that of when the whistle was blown, namely, at time 2A. For example, if the whistle was blown at 20 seconds, then "rephasing" of the runners would occur at 40 seconds.

Of course, if one continues to follow the race, the runners will again **dephase**, as shown in Figure 6-16. However, they can then be forced to rephase by blowing the whistle at time 3A, which will cause them to come together at time 4A. The process can be repeated any number of times. Each time the runners will rephase, and the information lost because of the difference in runners' speeds is recovered. The difference in the runners' speeds is analogous to the dephasing that occurs as a result of magnet inhomogeneities.

In a magnet these reversals of the runners are accomplished by using a 180-degree RF pulse. Such a pulse causes all the net magnetization vectors to flip 180 degrees, in essence reversing their direction. The spins will then begin

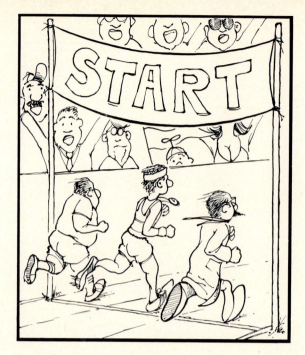

Figure 6-15. If the runners in Figure 6–14 reverse direction at time A, they will cross the starting line at precisely the same time, 2A. They are back in phase.

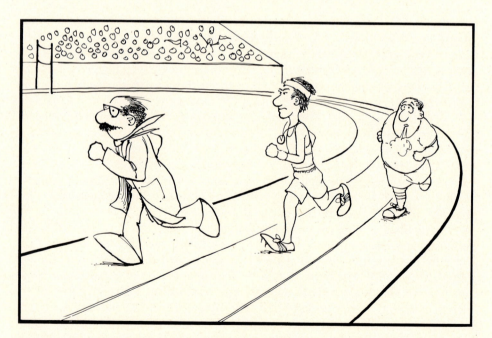

Figure 6-16. After time 3A the runners are again out of phase but not running quite so fast. A whistle blown at 3A will cause the runners to reverse direction again and rephase at time 4A.

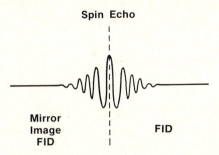

Figure 6-17. The spin echo consists of an FID and its mirror image.

to rephase, and as they do, we will begin to receive a signal. The maximum signal will occur at the point when they are exactly again in phase. If the 180-degree RF pulse were at time A, the maximum rephasing would occur at time 2A.

This NMR signal is a **spin echo,** as shown in Figure 6-17. The spin echo is an RF signal that first increases in intensity to a maximum and then decays back to zero. The decay side of the spin echo is an FID, and the increasing side is the mirror image of an FID.

The key point that allows rephasing of the runners is that even though the runners' speeds are different they are constant. There is a systematic difference between the runners, and we can reverse the effect of this difference. In the same way, we can recover the loss of signal owing to magnet inhomogeneities because the inhomogeneities are constant, fixed by the construction of the magnet. A region of the magnet that is slightly lower in field strength will remain so, unless, of course, the magnet is physically changed.

However, any random changes cannot be recovered in this manner. For example, if one of the runners stumbles momentarily on the track, the distance he lost is not recoverable by reversing directions; he will still end up a little behind or "out of phase" when the runners "rephase." In a similar manner the effects of true T2 relaxation are not recovered by the 180-degree pulses. Thus the induced spin echoes reflect a removal of the magnet inhomogeneity but not the removal of true T2 relaxation. The peaks of the spin echoes will all be smaller because of true T2 alone, and this allows us a method to calculate true T2.

If the peaks of multiple spin echoes are plotted against the time they occur, as in Figure 6-18, the result is a decay curve that reflects true T2 relaxation. Each time a 180-degree RF pulse is employed, a spin echo will result, each echo being smaller than the previous. The time from the 180-degree RF pulse to the echo is always equal to the time from the 90-degree RF pulse to the 180-degree RF pulse. The envelope of the multiple echoes shown in Figure 6-19 describes the true T2 relaxation time. This is similar to finding the half-life of a radioactive sample from sequential measurements.

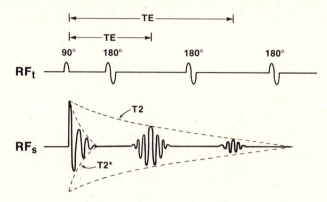

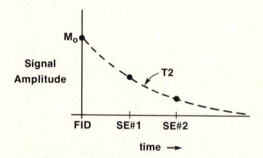

Figure 6-18. T2 relaxation time is measured from the envelope of multiple spin echoes.

Figure 6-19. A plot of the peak heights of multiple spin echoes allows determination of the T2 relaxation time.

HOW TO MEASURE T1

T1 is not so easily measured because it represents magnetization along the Z axis that cannot be sensed directly. Consider the case when a 180-degree RF pulse is transmitted into the patient so that the net magnetization vector is inverted. Once again, this is an unstable state, and the net magnetization vector seeks to regain its alignment with the external magnetic field. It does this by shrinking in the −Z direction until it disappears and then grows in the +Z direction until finally it returns to the equilibrium state. This happens because each individual proton dipole is flipping back to the low-energy state. The situation is diagrammed in Figure 6-20.

A plot of the magnitude of the net magnetization vector versus time results in the curve shown in Figure 6-21. This curve can be fitted by an equation containing the T1 relaxation time. Appendix A describes the mathematics involved.

The problem with this approach is that after the 180-degree RF pulse a signal is never observed. Remember that in order to receive a signal the net

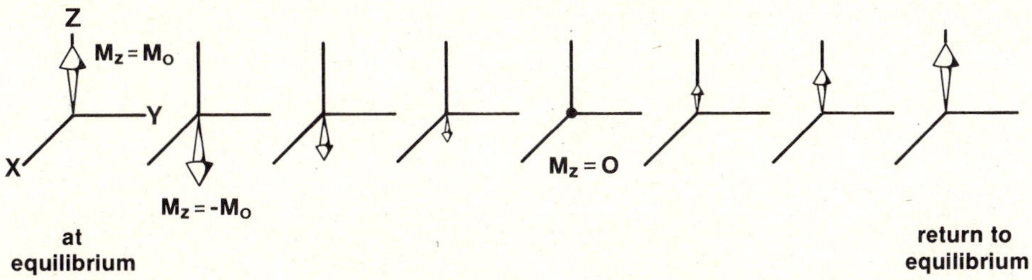

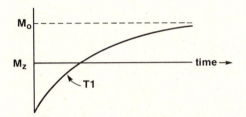

Figure 6-20. A 180-degree RF pulse inverts the net magnetization along the Z axis so that M_z equals $-M_0$. With time M_z returns along the Z axis to its equilibrium state of M_z equals M_0.

Figure 6-21. If the value of M_z at various times during return to equilibrium is plotted, the T1 relaxation time can be obtained.

magnetization vector must have a component in the XY plane. Following a 180-degree RF pulse the decay occurs only along the Z axis with no component in the X-Y plane. Thus no signal is observed.

For a signal to be detected, the 180-degree RF pulse must be followed by a 90-degree RF pulse in order to tip the net magnetization onto the XY plane where it can be observed. Suppose the 180-degree RF pulse is immediately followed by a 90-degree RF pulse, as shown in Figure 6-22. Following the 180-degree RF pulse no signal is detected. But if the net magnetization vector is given an immediate 90-degree RF pulse, it is rotated onto the X-Y plane along the $-Y$ axis and a signal is received.

The situation is now exactly the same as described previously, and the signal is an FID that starts out in the negative direction and decays according to the T2* relaxation time. What is important is that the initial magnitude of the FID is exactly equal to the length of the net magnetization vector following the 180-degree RF pulse.

Now the situation must be changed a little to estimate the T1 relaxation time. Instead of the 90-degree RF pulse being given immediately after the 180-degree RF pulse, a short time is allowed. This results in the situation shown in Figure 6-23. The delay time between the 180-degree and the 90-degree RF pulses was introduced in Chapter 4 as **T1,** for **inversion delay time.** Because there is now a little time before the net magnetization vector is rotated onto

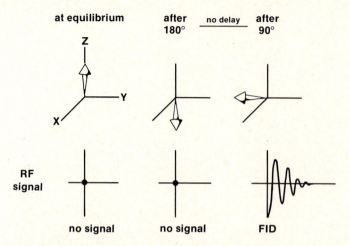

Figure 6-22.   A 180-degree RF pulse followed immediately by a 90-degree RF pulse will produce an FID whose amplitude is equal to M_0. This is equivalent to a single 270-degree RF pulse.

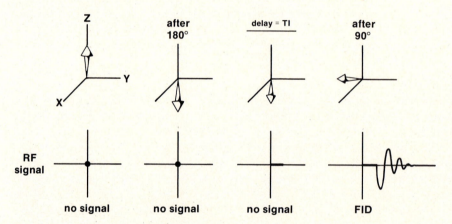

Figure 6-23.   If a short time is allowed between the 180- and 90-degree RF pulses, a reduced-amplitude FID is produced.

the XY plane, the net magnetization vector has a chance to decay somewhat because of T1 relaxation. Thus, although still starting out negative, the FID received, is smaller than that in Figure 6-22. The initial magnitude of the FID is once again equal to the size of the T1-decayed net magnetization vector owing to the interval T1.

If this process is continued, choosing longer and longer delay times for T1, as shown in Figure 6-24, RF signals will be received that can be interpreted for T1. In Figure 6-24, *C*, the inversion time (T1) is just long enough to catch the net magnetization vector at the point when it is zero, switching from $-Z$

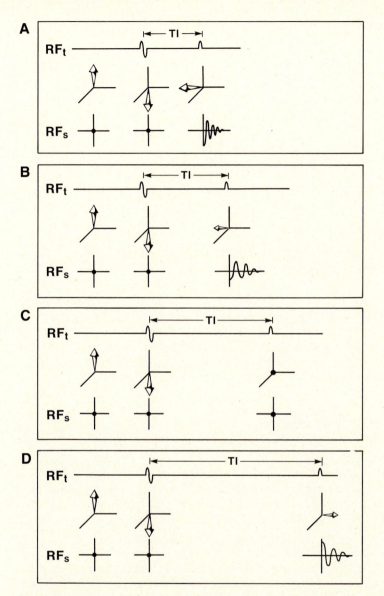

Figure 6-24. As T1 is increased, the magnitude of the FID is reduced by T1 relaxation until it is zero. With still longer T1s, the FID amplitude increases as M_z returns to M_0.

to $+Z$, therefore, when the 90-degree RF pulse is given, there is no signal. In Figure 6-24, *D* T1 is long enough so that the net magnetization vector is back along the $+Z$ axis and the FID has a positive initial magnitude.

The results of this type of sequential experiment are used to determine T1. By the plotting of the initial magnitude of the FID in each case versus the

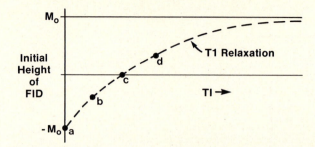

Figure 6-25. A plot of FID amplitude versus inversion time can be used to determine T1 relaxation time. The letters of each data point correspond to Figure 6-22.

inversion time, as shown in Figure 6-25, a curve like that in Figure 6-2 is obtained. This should be no surprise. As was pointed out, the initial height of the FID is exactly the same as the length of the net magnetization vector after a delay of T1. Thus the plot is actually the length of the net magnetization vector at the various times chosen by T1. By fitting these points to the curve given by the equation in Appendix A, one can obtain a value for T1. This pulse sequence, a 180-degree RF pulse followed after a delay of T1 by a 90-degree RF pulse, is called an **inversion recovery** pulse sequence because it inverts the net magnetization vector and then allows it to recover somewhat before measurement. As before, the discussion has been simplified somewhat by assuming that FIDs are the measured NMR signal. In actuality, spin echoes are measured.

T1 VERSUS T2 MEASUREMENTS

There are several differences in the techniques used to measure T2 and T1. The T2 relaxation time can be obtained by the use of a single RF pulse sequence, whereas a minimum of two inversion recovery pulse sequences are required to determine T1. Further, to apply this technique accurately, one must be sure that the net magnetization vector starts out at equilibrium. Because of this, **the T1 measurement often requires a significantly longer time than the T2 measurement.**

For the T2 measurement, one need only wait long enough to obtain a sufficient number of points along the T2 decay curve. Because the T2 relaxation time of most biological tissues is roughly 50 to 350 ms, enough data can easily be obtained to fit the T2 curve in less than 1000 ms. On the other hand, to obtain a value for T1, one must repeat the inversion recovery pulse sequence at least twice, using two different T1 times. Between these two one must wait long enough for the net magnetization vector to return to equilibrium. If enough time is not allowed between the two inversion recovery sequences, the net magnetization vector going into the second sequence will not have recovered its height completely following the first sequence. Thus it will start out shorter than it should for the second sequence, and the received signal will be correspondingly smaller.

This ultimately results in an erroneous value for T1. To allow the net magnetization vector to return to equilibrium between the inversion recovery pulse sequences, the repetition time, TR, between them must be at least four or five times T1. Most biological tissues have T1s of several hundred milliseconds. This means that several seconds are required to obtain two T1 points. Furthermore, to increase accuracy, one must add more points to the T1 curve; each repetition requires another wait of four or five T1s. On the other hand, using the spin echo sequence, one can obtain several points for the T2 curve with little increase in time. Thus from a time standpoint, it is easier to obtain data for an estimate of T2 than for a T1 determination.

SUMMARY

There are three principal MRI parameters: spin density, T1 relaxation time, and T2 relaxation time. Each independently influences pixel brightness in an MR image but not in a simple manner. Spin density refers to the number of mobile hydrogen nuclei in tissue that are available to contribute to the NMR signal.

T1 relaxation is also known as longitudinal or spin-lattice relaxation. The T1 relaxation time is the time constant that controls growth of M_z in the presence of an external magnetic field. T2 relaxation is also known as transverse or spin-spin relaxation. The T2 relaxation time is the time constant associated with loss of M_{xy}.

T2 relaxation is confounded by T2* relaxation, which is much shorter and results from inhomogeneities in the magnetic field. T2 relaxation time can be measured with a spin-echo pulse sequence involving multiple echoes. Determination of T1 relaxation time requires multiple inversion recovery pulse sequences and therefore more time.

SEVEN

MRI Hardware

Now that the basic physics of magnetic resonance imaging has been covered, the equipment used in the process will be discussed in this and the following two chapters. A magnetic resonance imager contains three major components, each of which consists of several subsystems. The major components are the **gantry,** the **operating console,** and the **computer.** In this regard, a magnetic resonance imager is similar to a CT scanner. Here, however, most similarities cease. These principal components are shown in Figure 7-1.

The gantry contains the main magnet and several other electromagnetic devices essential to MRI. Unlike with CT, **there are no moving parts in the gantry.** The operating console resembles a CT console, and although many of the control designations are similar, they also serve very different functions. The operator rarely has any direct contact with the computer. Simply put, the computer is larger and faster than those employed in CT.

THE GANTRY

The Main Magnet

As was introduced in Chapter 2, three methods are used to produce the strong magnetic field required for MRI. There are permanent magnets and two types of electromagnets: resistive and superconducting. We will consider briefly the permanent and resistive types but will focus mainly on superconducting mag-

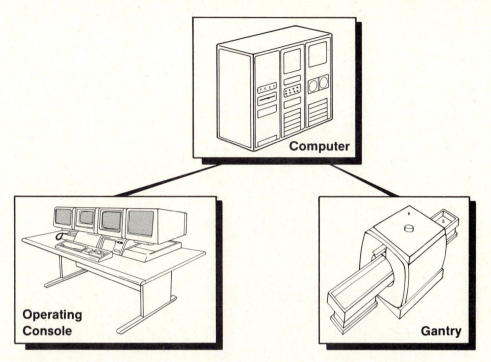

Figure 7-1. The principal components of an MR imager are the gantry, the operating console, and the computer.

netic resonance imagers. Currently more than 95% of all clinical imagers are of the superconducting type.

PERMANENT MAGNETS. Permanent magnets for imaging can be made with field strengths up to about 0.3 T. Such an imager is shown schematically in Figure 7-2. The magnetic field is produced by brick-size ferromagnetic ceramic materials that are rendered magnetic by charging them in the field of an electromagnetic. Once magnetized, these bricks are then carefully oriented into an array, up to one meter on a side, containing two to five layers. The fabrication of such a large magnet made from smaller magnets is not a trivial task. The forces exerted are enormous, and if one brick is positioned incorrectly, contrary magnetic fields can result and cause the whole assembly to fragment violently.

Two such bricklike magnet assemblies are positioned opposite one another at a distance of approximately 50 to 100 cm, depending on whether the imager is to be for head only or for head and body.

A **pole face** is positioned on each exposed magnetic pole. These pole faces are carefully machined pieces of iron designed to help orient and shape the magnetic field in order to increase the homogeneity of the field within the imaging volume. Often there are **adjusting screws** or other shimming devices to further define the homogeneity of the magnetic field.

In physical contact with each magnet is an **iron yoke,** which serves three

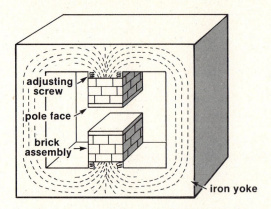

Figure 7-2. A schematic view of a permanent magnet designed for MRI.

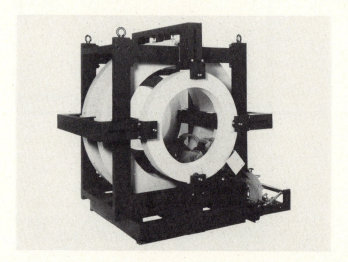

Figure 7-3. A four-coil resistive electromagnet for MRI. (Courtesy Bruker Medical Instruments.)

purposes. First, it provides a mechanical frame for assembly and stability. Second, it confines the fringe magnetic field. The lines of the magnetic field are concentrated in this iron yoke much as they are in the core of the high-voltage transformer of any x-ray generator. Third, by containing the fringe field, the yoke also intensifies the magnetic field in the imaging aperture. Without such a yoke, the magnetic field strength of such an assembly would be very low. The yoke is usually fabricated of soft iron laminated and bolted together like a transformer core.

RESISTIVE ELECTROMAGNETS.   The main magnetic field in a resistive magnet system is produced by a large, classical electromagnet. The most prominent design is a four-coil magnet, as illustrated in Figure 7-3. The two outside coils are wound in a smaller diameter to render the magnetic field more uniform in the imaging volume between the two large internal coils.

Another design is solenoidal, with windings concentrated on the periphery of the solenoid, again to homogenize the magnetic field within the imaging volume. Other designs have also been introduced but have yet to be employed in significant numbers.

Resistive magnetic resonance imagers can produce magnetic field strengths up to about 0.3 T. Beyond that, power consumption and cooling requirements become excessive. Most resistive magnetic resonance imagers are designed for operation at about 0.15 to 0.25 T.

All of the early MRI investigations were conducted on resistive magnet systems. The shift in emphasis to a higher magnetic field strength resulted in a shift from resistive magnet to superconducting magnet technology. However, good clinical images are regularly produced at 0.1 to 0.3 T on resistive electromagnet systems.

Resistive magnet systems have some advantages. They are less expensive than superconducting systems. Because they operate at lower field strengths, they don't require the precision and homogeneity of a superconducting system. Magnetic field homogeneity of 10 to 50 ppm exists for most resistive magnetic resonance imagers. Shimming this type of magnet is somewhat less difficult than shimming a superconducting system.

Because such a resistive magnet is readily brought up to field strength, it is just as easily turned off. This removes the hazard of ferromagnetic projectiles during nonimaging time. It also makes it relatively easy to remove an object that might become lodged against the magnet.

Siting the resistive magnet imager is somewhat more difficult than siting the permanent magnet imager but certainly less difficult than siting the superconducting imager. The resistive magnet system is the lightest of the three, rarely exceeding 4000 kg (8800 pounds).

The principal disadvantage of this type of imager is electrical power consumption. It is the most power hungry of the three. A 0.2-T imager may require 60 to 80 kW, and this is a continuous power drain when the magnet is on. A power rating of 80 kW is common for good radiographic and fluoroscopic equipment. However, with such x-ray equipment, the power is required for only very short exposure times, not continuously. Additionally, requirements for cooling the magnet must be met. Most such magnets are water cooled with a closed primary loop communicating with a secondary single pass system through a heat exchanger.

SUPERCONDUCTING ELECTROMAGNETS.   Actually, there are only two types of magnets: permanent and electromagnetic. Permanent magnets occur naturally or are synthetic. Electromagnets are created by passing electric current through resistive or superconducting wire. Magnetic resonance imagers based on superconducting magnet technology have the principal characteristic of high field strength. Imagers currently available operate in the range of 0.3 to 2.0 T. The 2-T level is an imposed regulatory limit. Superconducting magnets employed in high-energy physics laboratories now exceed 11 T in field strength.

There are several advantages to superconducting imagers. The high field strengths are essential if spectroscopy is planned; however, the tolerances on field homogeneity are more restrictive at such high field strengths. A 2-T imager should have a magnetic field that varies by no more than 1 to 5 ppm. High field strength results in increased signal to noise, and this increase may allow for shorter imaging times and better image quality. This statement is theoretically true but has not been convincingly demonstrated clinically.

As with the other types of magnetic resonance imagers, there are disadvantages to superconducting imagers. The principal disadvantage may be in site selection. The intense magnetic fringe fields of these imagers make location of such an imager in an existing hospital very difficult. The 0.5-mT (5-gauss) isomagnetic line associated with a 1-T imager extends some 10 m in all directions. With a 2-cm ferromagnetic shield, the 0.5-mT line can be brought in to a distance of perhaps 7 m. However, the cost of such ferromagnetic shielding can easily exceed $100,000.

Another disadvantage of the superconducting imager is its need to keep the electromagnetic coils very cold, and this requires the use of cryogenic gases. Maintenance of the niobium-titanium superconducting wire in a superconducting state requires an environment below its critical temperature, which is about 9.5 K. The coils are therefore immersed in liquid helium, which boils at 4.2 K. The vessel containing the coils and liquid helium is separated from an outer vessel containing liquid nitrogen by a vacuum shield. Liquid nitrogen which, boils at 77 K, is used instead of liquid hydrogen (2 O K) or liquid neon (27 K) because it is less expensive. Further, because of its high boiling point, liquid nitrogen also evaporates more slowly. The liquid nitrogen vessel serves essentially as a shield for the liquid helium. The liquid nitrogen is also protected by a vacuum shield from the laboratory environment. This arrangement of multiple thermal blankets is shown in Figure 7-4. The whole assembly is approximately 3.0 m in diameter, but be cause of the multiple thermal layers, the bore of the assembly is approximately only 1.

These several thermal gradient shields are designed to maintain the superconducting condition of the electromagnet efficiently. Despite rather rigorous designs, both liquids tend to vaporize—the nitrogen more readily than the helium. Boil-off rates of 1.5 L per hour for nitrogen and 0.5 to 1.0 L per day for helium are experienced in many imagers. Nitrogen costs about as much as milk whereas helium costs as much as fine wine. At $10 per liter for helium and $0.50 per liter for nitrogen, the annual cost for supplying such cryogens can exceed $50,000.

Some manufacturers are experimenting with recirculating systems involving condenser technology to allow the cryogenic gases to be reused. Undoubtedly, most manufacturers will be implementing such design features in the future if the cost of such cryogenerators can be reduced.

The cryogenic gases are supplied to the MRI facility in large, thermoslike vessels called **dewars**. The dewars require special handling and storage. Only specially trained service personnel should replenish cryogens because of potential hazards. Figure 7-5 shows such a dewar.

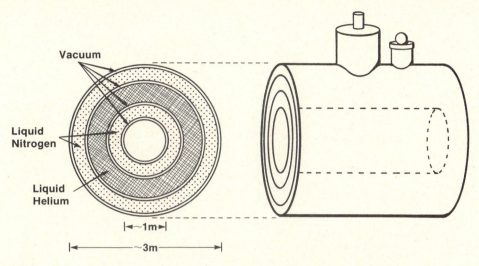

Figure 7-4. Cross-sectional view of a superconducting magnet for MRI.

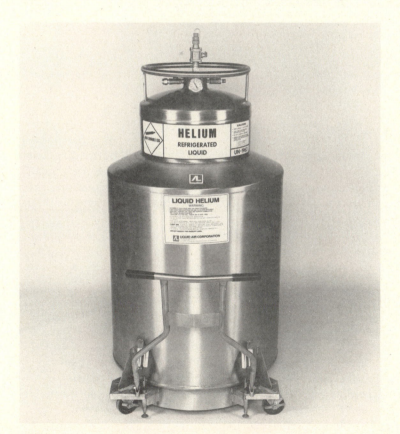

Figure 7-5. Dewar for transporting and storing cryogenic gases. (Courtesy Richard Johnson, Liquid Air Corporation, San Francisco.)

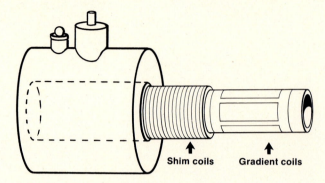

Figure 7-6.   Relative position of the shim coils, gradient coils, and RF probe.

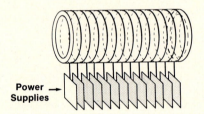

Figure 7-7.   Shim coils are spaced on a drum and energized to make the magnetic field uniform within the imaging volume.

Secondary Magnetic Fields

Magnetic resonance imaging requires on the one hand a uniform magnetic field to produce an FID and spin echo and on the other hand precisely fashioned **gradient magnetic fields to provide spatial location information.** The gradient magnetic fields are produced by secondary electromagnetic coils that are of the resistive type.

In addition to the **gradient coils** that produce the gradient magnetic fields, there are **shim coils** and the **RF probe.** These secondary coils are positioned inside the 1-m bore of the cylinder of the main magnet, as shown in Figure 7-6.

SHIM COILS.   Figure 7-7 shows a drum about 1 m in diameter with 13 separate coils wound around the drum, each attached to its own power supply. These coils are called **shim coils.** The purpose of the shim coils is to make the main magnetic field extremely homogeneous and uniform. The imaging volume in a conventional magnetic resonance imager generally consists of a cylinder with a diameter of approximately 50 cm and a length of 50 to 70 cm along the axis. A conventional six-coil superconducting magnet will normally produce a magnetic field with uniformity of approximately ± 100 ppm. With the use of shim coils, this magnetic field homogeneity can be improved to as good as ± 1 ppm within the 50-cm imaging volume.

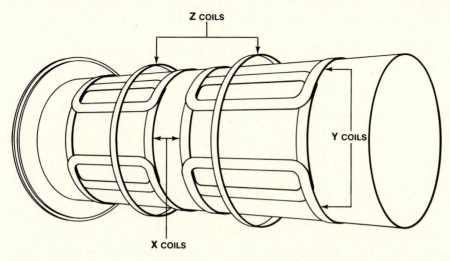

Figure 7-8. This diagram of gradient coils shows that they consist of large band-type conductors.

This improved uniformity is produced by tuning the power to each individual shim coil while at the same time precisely measuring the magnetic field at regions within the imaging volume. The tuning consists of varying the polarity—that is, the direction—and the strength of a direct current through each coil. The electric currents employed vary from approximately 0.1 to 10 A.

This process of tuning each individual coil is called **shimming the magnet.** Depending on the design, as many as 30 shim coils may be available. Much of the shimming is now done automatically under computer control because it can take many hours to do manually. Once a magnet is properly shimmed, it is usually not necessary to repeat the procedure unless there has been a major change in operating technique.

GRADIENT COILS. Inside of the drum on which the shim coils are wound is yet another drum on which are positioned the gradient magnetic coils, or **gradient coils.** The gradient coils consist of three pairs: X gradients, Y gradients, and Z gradients. Figure 7-8 depicts such coils.

Z Gradients: The Z-gradient coils are usually a pair of circular coils, each of which is wound around the drum at each end of the imaging volume, as shown in Figure 7-9. If a DC current with opposite polarity is impressed through the two coils, a very small change in the magnetic field along the Z axis of the imager is produced. The currents employed are usually around 30 A, producing a linear change in main magnetic field strength of about 25 μT/cm. This change in magnetic field strength allows for selection of a slice along the axis of the magnet. **The stronger the Z-gradient currents, the stronger will be the Z-gradient magnetization, and this will result in thinner slices.**

X Gradients: As was shown in Chapter 2, the magnetic field lines of a

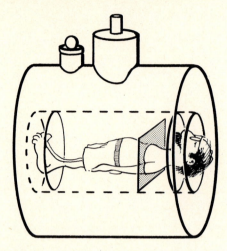

Figure 7-9. Z-gradient coils change the gradient magnetic field along the Z axis, thereby allowing a slice of the patient to be selected for imaging.

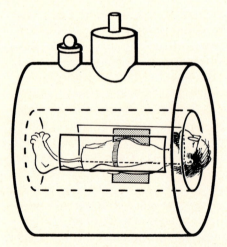

Figure 7-10. X-gradient coils produce a magnetic gradient across the patient. This is usually the frequency-encoding gradient.

coil of wire are along the axis of that coil. As a result, the X- and Y-gradient coils are more difficult to fabricate and position on the drum. Figure 7-10 shows how the X magnetization gradient is induced by a pair of coils positioned on either side of the drum. By convention, these coils are positioned so that the gradient magnetic field is across the patient laterally as shown. The X axis is therefore the horizontal axis across the patient.

    These coils behave in precisely the same way as the Z-gradient coils. DC currents of opposite polarity are applied to produce a magnetic gradient field. The X-gradient currents and the induced magnetic field gradient are similar in

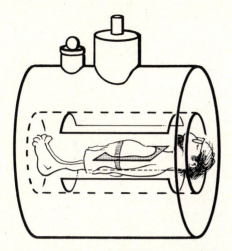

Figure 7-11. Y-gradient coils produce a magnetic gradient through the patient from front to back. They are usually the phase-encoding gradients.

magnitude to the Z gradients. They provide spatial localization along the X axis of the patient, usually by a technique called **frequency encoding**.

   Y Gradients: A magnetic gradient along the Y axis of the patient is produced by a set of coils that look and operate exactly like the X-gradient coils. This is diagrammed in Figure 7-11. By convention, the Y axis is the vertical axis through the patient.

   The Y gradient is normally, though not necessarily, used for **phase encoding** the NMR signal. Together, the Y gradient and the X gradient allow precise determination of where within the imaging plane the contribution to the NMR signal from each voxel originated. The Z gradient is always used for selection of a transaxial plane to be imaged. This is called **slice selection**.

   Combined Gradients: Magnetic fields add vectorially. To select either the transaxial, sagittal, or coronal plane for imaging, only the Z, X, or Y gradients, respectively, will be energized. When energized simultaneously, the currents in the three pairs of gradient coils do not produce three separate magnetic fields, but rather a single composite magnetic field. For one to obtain an obliquely angled plane, as in Figure 7-12, all three gradients would be energized. If the current through each pair of gradient coils is controlled, the plane for imaging can be precisely specified.

THE RF PROBE.   The RF probe is essentially a coil of wire similar to the gradient coils, the shim coils, and the main coils of the magnet. It differs, however, in that it must accommodate a high-frequency AC current, 1.0 to 80 MHz, so that it can produce a radio signal at the Larmor frequency. Furthermore, it must be precisely designed to behave as both a transmitter and a receiver of RF. RF probe design is one of the more critical engineering features of a magnetic resonance imager. It embodies not only considerable science and engineering, but also some art and luck.

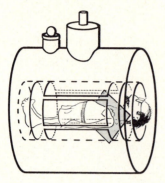

Figure 7-12. When all three gradients are energized at the same time, an oblique plane is identified.

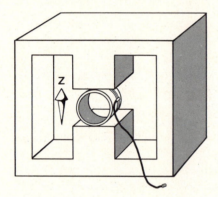

Figure 7-13. A simple circular RF coil can be used with a permanent magnet imager because the probe axis is in the XY plane.

The initial signal for the RF probe comes from a device called a **frequency synthesizer.** It is the master frequency source for the magnetic resonance imager. It provides a tunable frequency band from which the Larmor frequency can be accurately determined for each individual examination.

The simplest RF probe would be a coil of wire wrapped around a patient. The intensity of the emitted RF signal and the sensitivity to the signal received from the patient are approximately equal to the diameter of the coil. Outside of this diameter, signal intensity and sensitivity drop off rapidly. Such a simple type of coil is easily adaptable to a permanent magnet imager, as shown in Figure 7-13. This arrangement adds to the simplicity of a permanent magnet imager and to its theoretically superior signal-to-noise ratio at a given magnetic field strength.

For electromagnetic imagers, however, the main magnetic field is along the axis of the patient rather than transaxial. To be used, the simple coil would have to penetrate through the patient either anteroposteriorly or laterally, as

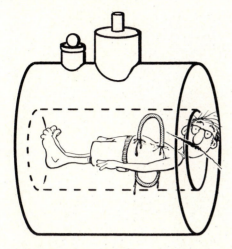

Figure 7-14. RF probes for electromagnetic imagers are complicated because a simple circular coil would have to pass through the patient.

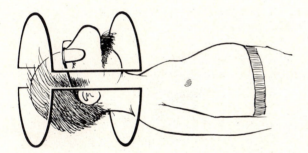

Figure 7-15. The saddle coil is most widely used with electromagnetic magnetic resonance imagers.

shown in Figure 7-14. Because patients object to such treatment, other coil designs and shapes had to be devised.

The most widely used design is a saddle coil, as shown in Figure 7-15. In such a coil, the intensity of emitted RF and the sensitivity of the received signal are nearly uniform within the confines of the coil. The degree of such uniformity results in great measure from the precise spacing of the loops of the saddle.

Quadrature coils, a new development in probe design, are fashioned to improve signal-to-noise ratio. They view the signal as though they were a pair of stereo lenses. The result is better sensitivity to the NMR signal from the patient.

RF probes are designed specifically for head or body imaging, as seen in Figure 7-16. When a smaller probe is used for head imaging, the antenna is more sensitive, resulting in an increased signal-to-noise ratio. However, when

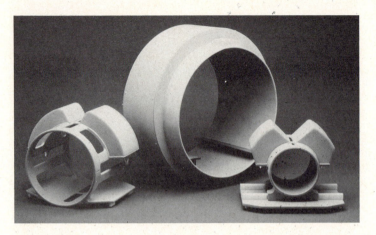

Figure 7-16. A head, body, and extremity RF probe. (Courtesy Diasonics.)

probes are changed between patients, some time is consumed to tune the new probe to the patient.

SURFACE COILS. For most imagers, the RF probe serves as both the transmitter of the RF and the receiver of the NMR signal. One notable exception that is gaining in favor as an imaging device is the **surface coil**.

A surface coil is a specially designed coil that is usually flat and has multiple turns of wire. It may be encased in a rubberized plastic matrix to make it somewhat pliable. The coil is placed on the surface of the patient at that anatomic region under investigation.

Surface coils come in many different sizes and shapes and are usually fabricated for specific anatomic regions. A minimal complement of surface coils, as shown in Figure 7-17, would include individual coils for cervical, lumbar, and thoracic spine; extremity joint; breast; hand and foot; orbit; inner ear; and tempormandibular joint.

When in use, the surface coil lies inside the RF probe, usually in contact with the patient. It is normally used in the receiver mode only, whereas the RF probe behaves as the transmitter. This requires that the two coils be electromagnetically **decoupled** from one another so that they do not interfere with sensing the weak NMR signal.

The advantage of using a surface coil lies in its improved spatial resolution. A surface coil image of the lumbar spine, for instance, such as that shown in Figure 7-18, would have a pixel size of less than 1 mm for a 256 matrix. Because less volume of tissue is being imaged, the pixel size for a given matrix with a surface coil is always less than that for a whole-body RF probe.

The disadvantages of surface coil imaging include limited field of view and positioning. Because the surface coil is smaller than even the head RF probe, it has a smaller sensitive volume, which results in a restricted field of view. Surface coil positioning requires more time. To maximize the signal from

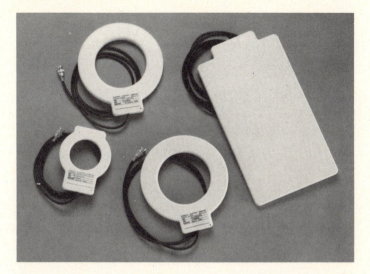

Figure 7-17.   Typical surface coils available for MRI. (Courtesy General Electric.)

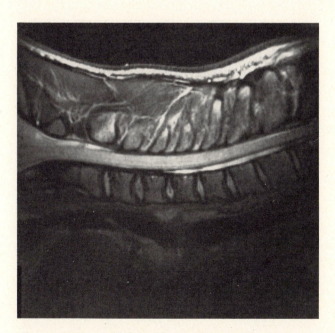

Figure 7-18.   A high-resolution image of the lumbar spine. (Courtesy Larry Rothenberg, Memorial Hospital, New York City.)

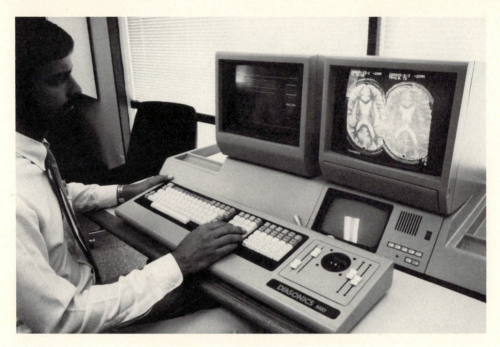

Figure 7-19. An MRI operating console. (Courtesy Diasonics.)

the small volume, the technologist must pay more attention. The surface coil must be as orthogonal or perpendicular to the XY plane as possible for maximum sensitivity. Just a slight tilt in the coil, say 10 degrees off orthogonality, can result in significant loss of signal. With experience, technologists learn to position surface coils easily and quickly.

THE OPERATING CONSOLE

The operating console of a magnetic resonance imager appears similar to that of a CT scanner, but there are substantial differences. Figure 7-19 shows such a console, with a rendering of the operating keyboard. In general, we will find two sets of controls on the operating console; one set is for image acquisition and the other for image processing. Some controls are activated by special function keys, but most are under computer command. The operator responds to a video prompt by keying commands through the alphanumeric keyboard. As with CT, in addition to the operating console, physicians' viewing consoles are also available for MRI.

Many similarities exist between CT and MRI consoles. In general, the operating controls associated with start-up and image processing are very similar. The image acquisition controls are very different. The principal control functions on the console of a magnetic resonance imager are as follows.

Start-up

1. **Power on/off**—Usually a keyswitch or pushswitch to energize the system.
2. **Emergency off**—A scram control that should never be used with a superconducting magnetic resonance imager.
3. **Intercom**—Allows communication with the patient.
4. **CRT controls**—Several knobs to control brightness, contrast, and power to the video monitor.
5. **Annotation**—Alphanumeric and special function keys to input patient and image data for final hard-copy images.

Image Acquisition

1. **Tuning controls**—Several keystrokes under computer command designed to adjust the resonant frequency of the system to accommodate the patient or part being imaged.
2. **Pulse sequence**—The operator usually has a choice of partial saturation, inversion recovery, or spin echo.
3. **Repetition time (TR)**—Increasing TR lengthens the scan time. However, with longer TR, more slices per scan are possible with multislice pulse sequence techniques.
4. **Inversion time (TI)**—Used with an inversion recovery pulse sequence. **The longer the TI, the more T1-weighted will be the image.**
5. **Echo time (TE)**—Used with inversion recovery and spin echo pulse sequences. **The longer the TE, the more T2-weighted will be the image.**
6. **Number of views**—Usually 128 or 256. More views result in better spatial resolution but require a longer scan time.
7. **Number of acquisitions**—Sometimes labeled number of signals to average or signal averaging. The more NMR signal acquisitions, the better the image, because the signal-to-noise ratio increases as the square root of the number of acquisitions. Scan time increases directly as the number of acquisitions.
8. **Field of view**—Reducing the field of view will increase the spatial resolution but may require more signal acquisitions to maintain an adequate signal-to-noise ratio.
9. **Slice thickness**—Reducing slice thickness will increase the spatial resolution by reducing partial volume effects. More acquisitions may be required to maintain an adequate signal-to-noise ratio.

Image Processing

1. **Window width/level**—Used to set the contrast and shades of gray for the displayed image. The ranges are usually much wider for MRI than for CT.

2. **Cursor on/off**—To place a cursor on the image and provide for joystick, trackball, or mouse manipulation of the cursor.
3. **Region of interest (ROI)**—ROI for calculation of area of measure and average and standard deviations of pixel values.
4. **Zoom**—Used to magnify the image. Some systems provide fixed magnification factors, and others have continuously variable factors. This is an electro-optical zoom. Reconstructive zoom is not possible in MRI, as it is in CT.
5. **Profile/histogram**—Plots the pixel values along an identified axis as either a line graph or a histogram.
6. **Highlight**—This control selects pixel values within a given range for special attention. They may appear white or black or blink.
7. **Collage**—Provides for the simultaneous display of multiple images or portions of an image on one video screen. Particularly helpful in MRI because so many images are acquired.

THE MRI COMPUTER

Computers generally come in one of three sizes: microcomputers, minicomputers, and mainframe computers. The explosion in computer technology has erased some of the previous distinguishing factors among these three types of computers. In radiologic imaging, including MRI, minicomputers are generally used. An earlier version of a minicomputer would have required several instrumentation racks. Now, however, some minicomputers are found in single desk-size cabinets.

The basic requirement for a computer in MRI is that it must be large and fast. The capacity to store data for manipulation must be large because of the nature of the NMR signal and the number of signals required for an image. The computer must be fast to handle the high rate of data acquisition and to accommodate the enormous number of calculations required to produce an image. Image processing times in excess of 15 seconds are no longer acceptable to most physicians and technologists.

Storage Capacity

MRI produces quantities of data far in excess of those encountered with other medical imaging modalities. A typical electrocardiogram-gated MR cardiac examination might produce 50 images of 128 by 128 pixels each. If each pixel is 2 bytes deep, this amounts to 1.6 MB (megabytes) of data. A three-dimensional head scan might yield spin echo images at TEs of 24, 72, 120, and 168 ms, with each image 256 by 256 pixels, 1 byte deep. A 31-slice acquisition therefore would produce 124 images occupying 8.1 MB. A typical personal computer has a disk storage capacity of 0.36 MB or a floppy diskette and a usable main memory of 0.5 MB. Consequently, such microcomputers will never find application in MRI. The minicomputers required for MRI have 1 to 10 MB of main memory and secondary memory provided by a 100- to 1000-MB disk.

Computer Speed

Not only must the storage capacity of the computer be large, but the computer must also perform computations quickly. In one common 2DFT image reconstruction method, computation of a single 256-by-256 image requires 512-by-256 **fast Fourier transforms (FFT)**. Each FFT requires 2048 complex multiplications, and these are the most time-consuming part of the FFT algorithm. A complex multiplication may be computed using four real multiplications. The 256-by-256 2DFT image therefore needs about 4.2 million multiplications.

For the maximum precision resolution in the data to be preserved, the FFT should be computed using floating-point numbers. A floating point operation, such as a real multiplication, is referred to as a **flop**. The image will thus require 4.2 million flops. To reconstruct the image in 15 seconds would require approximately 300,000 flops per second. Only with the assistance of an **array processor** can such a computational rate be achieved. Typical array processor speeds range from 0.5 to 20 MFLOPS for all but the most expensive hardware. These advertised speeds are based on idealized situations; practical performance is slowed by limitations on the rate at which data may be moved on and off the disk and by movement of the data in and out of the array processor.

The Operating System

Image reconstruction is not the only chore to be handled by the computer. Data acquisition is often organized by the same computer that performs the image reconstruction. The program that controls such a computer is called the **operating system**.

For the computer to perform several tasks at once, such as data acquisition, image reconstruction, and calculated image preparation, the operating system must be **multitasking**. A multitasking operating system allows the computer hardware to be shared by several programs. Obviously, this sharing slows each program somewhat. A good operating system minimizes the impact of sharing by knowing when each program does not need to use the computer. An example occurs during the latter part of TR, when the acquisition program is just waiting for the nuclear spin system to recover to equilibrium. Another example is the interval between when the reconstruction requests the raw data of an acquisition from the disk and when those data are delivered.

For a physician to review completed studies on one console while an examination is being performed from another, the operating system must be **multiuser**. This means that the operating system allows several users simultaneous access to the computer. A multiuser operating system is inherently a multitasking operation system. Ideally, each computer user thinks that he or she has the full computer at his or her own disposal and does not notice the other users of the system. When the manufacturer does not provide a multiuser operating system, the physician's console often has its own computer, which communicates efficiently with the main console computer.

SUMMARY

A magnetic resonance imager consists of three main components: the gantry, the operating console, and the computer. The operating console and the computer are similar in appearance and function to those used in computed tomography. The operating console will have similar key commands for start-up and image processing but very different key commands for image acquisition. The computer will be bigger and faster than that used in computed tomography.

The gantry contains no moving parts, just kilometers of wire wound on different drums to produce the precisely fashioned magnetic fields that are required. The main magnet provides the strong B_0 field that establishes the basic Larmor frequency. Shim coils are precisely tuned to make a very homogeneous B_0 field. Gradient coils are energized in pulse fashion to provide spatial localization of the NMR signals. The RF probe transmits the energizing RF pulse and receives the NMR signal.

Chapter
EIGHT

The Purchase Decision and Site Selection

Much discussion and publicity have been given to the fact that placing a magnetic resonance imager in a hospital is not at all like fabricating a new radiographic-fluoroscopic room or adding a special procedures suite. Indeed, more rigorous constraints govern where and how the imager can be located. Consequently, the sequence of events surrounding the acquisition of a magnetic resonance imager are more critical than that for radiographic equipment.

The first consideration is not where to place the imager, but rather what kind of imager to purchase. Only after the type of imager has been decided on should the site selection be analyzed. The third phase in this process concerns the actual construction details, which, of course, must wait until the site is selected.

SELECTING THE IMAGER

MRI devices not only are used for imaging but also may be configured for chemical shift spectroscopy as a potential aid to diagnosis. In deciding what

TABLE 8-1. Representative characteristics of MRI systems

	Permanent Magnet	Resistive Magnet	Superconducting Magnet
Field strength (T)	0.1–0.3	0.15–0.3	0.3–2.0
Cost ($ × 10^6)	0.5–1.5	0.8–1.2	1.2–2.5
Approximate size (m)	1.5 × 2.0	2.1 × 2.3	2.3 × 3.0
Weight (kg × 1000)	4.5–30	5.5–9.0	4.5–8.1
Power requirements (kW)	20	80	25
Distance to 0.5-mT fringe field (m)	<1	1–5	5–20

imager to buy, one must first decide if NMR spectroscopy is to be an application of the installation.

Clinical application of NMR spectroscopy is highly speculative at this time. Spectroscopy has been used to great advantage on biologic specimens in the laboratory, but its application in the clinic in vivo has yet to be demonstrated as efficacious. Therefore, spectroscopy is probably inappropriate for any imaging facility other than a research institution. We are probably still many years away from being able to demonstrate the clinical application of NMR spectroscopy.

For those few institutions where NMR spectroscopy is of interest, the decision as to the type of imager is automatic. A superconducting magnetic resonance imager of high magnetic field strength is required. Today, that would suggest that a 1.5-T or 2-T MRI system be obtained. However, for such application, a new facility will probably be required because existing structures are probably unsuitable.

Type of Magnet

If spectroscopy is not intended, an imager based on permanent or resistive magnet technology may be considered in addition to a superconducting system. Table 8-1 summarizes some characteristics, including field strength, associated with these three types of MRI systems. Each type of magnetic resonance imager has certain advantages and disadvantages, summarized in Table 8-2, but it is becoming clearer that when this initial phase of MRI development is over, no single system is going to dominate. Clinically efficacious images can be produced by each of these imaging systems, and it seems certain that none is going to prevail as obviously superior to the others. We will probably see MRI develop similarly to CT imaging. There is no intrinsic basis to suggest that fourth-generation CT technology is superior to third-generation technology or vice versa.

TABLE 8-2.   Comparative advantages and disadvantages of various MR images

Magnet Type	Advantages	Disadvantages
Permanent	Low capital cost Low operating cost Negligible fringe field	Limited field strength Fixed field strength Very heavy
Resistive Iron Core	Low capital cost Easy coil maintenance Negligible fringe field	High power consumption Water cooling required Potential field instability
Resistive Air Core	Low capital cost Light weight Easy coil maintenance	High power consumption Water cooling required Significant fringe field
Superconductive	High field strength High field homogeneity Low power consumption	High capital cost High cryogen cost Intense fringe field

Similarly, the sometimes emotional debate regarding optimum magnet field strength is not easily resolved. It is not clear whether an optimum magnetic field strength exists for MR imaging; exquisite images can be made with each of the three magnets and with B_0 field strengths ranging from 0.1 T to 2 T. The rapidly developing surface coil technology will probably result in more improvements to image quality and obscure the debate over B_0 field strength. Therefore, the purchase decision will be based on other considerations, some of which, such as service support, upgradability, and corporate commitment, cannot be discussed here.

PERMANENT MAGNET.   The principal advantage to a permanent-magnet magnetic resonance imager is the lack of a significant magnetic fringe field. This allows great flexibility in siting such a system. The 0.5-mT fringe field will certainly not exceed one meter in any direction from the magnet, and therefore, protective measures for adjacent areas are unnecessary.

The principal disadvantage of a permanent-magnet magnetic resonance imager is its weight. The mass of such an imaging gantry will range from approximately 5000 kg for a head-only imager to 30,000 kg for a whole-body imager. The heavier systems may be restricted to location on the ground floor because of inadequate load design of upper floors. Certainly the heavier of such systems are not adaptable to mobile units because of problems like the one shown in Figure 8-1.

RESISTIVE MAGNET.   A resistive magnet can be turned on and off rather simply. At all such sites the magnet is energized throughout the day and turned off at night. Permanent magnets are never off, and because superconducting magnets require considerable time, effort, and expense to deenergize, they are almost never off.

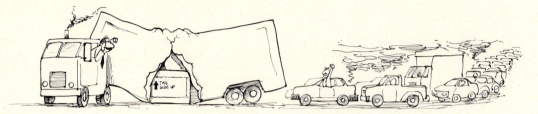

Figure 8-1. Possible fate of a mobile magnetic resonance imager with a permanent magnet.

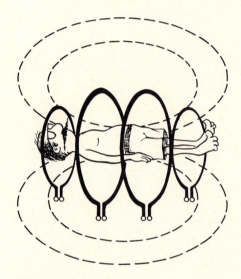

Figure 8-2. A four-coil air core magnet with the B_0 field horizontal. This causes the Z axis and the patient axis to be coincident.

Resistive magnets are relatively inexpensive to purchase. Operating such a magnet can be quite the opposite, however. With electric power costs running to $0.10 per kilowatt-hour in many areas, the operating expense can be considerable.

Two types of resistive magnets are available for imaging: **air core** and **iron core**. The most popular is a four-coil air core magnet such as that shown in Figure 8-2. In this magnet, the B_0 field is along the axis of the patient. Another design, shown schematically in Figure 8-3, has the B_0 field oriented vertically, so that the Z axis is perpendicular to the axis of the patient, as in a permanent magnet imager.

An iron core resistive magnet is diagrammed in Figure 8-4. The yoke of such a magnet confines the fringe magnetic field and permits a stronger B_0 field than that from an air core magnet. If permanent magnets are used as pole pieces and resistive conductor windings are also used, a **hybrid magnet,** which is even stronger, is made.

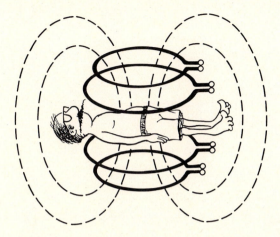

Figure 8-3. A four-coil air core magnet with the B_0 field vertical makes the Z axis perpendicular to the patient axis.

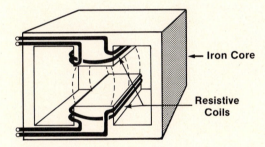

Figure 8-4. An iron core resistive magnet has the advantages of a stronger B_0 field and negligible fringe magnetic field.

SUPERCONDUCTING MAGNET. The superconducting magnet is by far the most widely used because of its field strength. Neither a permanent nor a resistive magnet imager can produce magnetic fields in excess of about 0.3 T. Current superconducting magnets provide imaging fields up to 2 T, and designs for 4-T magnets are appearing.

There are several disadvantages to a superconducting imager. The initial cost is very high, sometimes exceeding $2 million. The magnetic fringe field is intense, which will usually place severe limits on where the imager can be located. Site preparation costs are often excessive for existing buildings. This may require that such an imager be located in a new, relatively isolated location.

The advantages of a superconducting magnetic resonance imager are many. Better image quality is strongly suggested by some. The high B_0 magnetic field is associated with high field homogeneity with most such imagers. The superconductive MRI magnet consumes no electric power, but this advantage is offset by the requirement for cryogenic gases.

Performance Evaluation

The medical radiologic physics community has developed some rather precise testing methods and tools for evaluating image quality in CT. With the large selection of CT systems available, few purchasers would buy a particular system without the assistance of a medical physicist. One should not rely on the specifications published by manufacturers for performance characteristics of such imagers without independent confirmation. Imaging characteristics such as high-contrast resolution, low-contrast detectability, slice thickness, linearity, uniformity, artifact generation, and reconstruction time should be routinely evaluated for CT.

Likewise, these same performance characteristics and more should be evaluated certainly before the purchase of a magnetic resonance imager but also routinely. Unfortunately, the tools and procedures do not yet exist for such precise performance evaluation of magnetic resonance imagers. Some medical physicists have developed test tools for evaluating magnetic resonance imagers, but the process is not yet standardized by published protocols. Nevertheless, the purchaser of an imager should insist that the manufacturer meet published specifications and should make every effort to obtain medical physics assistance to evaluate such performance. Chapter 17 provides more information on performance evaluation and quality assurance.

LOCATING THE IMAGER

Having selected the imager and made arrangements for its acceptance testing, one should next decide where to locate the imager. There are four options. A magnetic resonance imager can be located in new construction, an existing building, a temporary but fixed building, or a mobile van.

If the imager is to be located in a new building such as an imaging center, the siting requirements may not be so rigorous. Most new construction will have been designed around the imager so that only considerations of adjacent imaging apparatus may be necessary. New construction can generally be designed so that shielding of the fringe magnetic field is unnecessary. Exclusion areas are easily identified and controlled.

The decision to locate an imager in an existing building, usually a hospital, will place considerable demands on the precise site location and its preparation. This may preclude the purchase of a superconductive magnet system of high field strength. On the other hand, except for possible weight constraints, permanent magnet systems may be sited nearly anywhere in existing buildings. There are essentially no fringe fields with a permanent or resistive iron core magnet.

Placing the imager in a temporary but fixed location adjacent to a hospital has many attractions. Site preparation costs will be low. The time required to prepare the site will be short, which will allow for placing a system in operation quickly. Patient and visitor access can be closely controlled. This approach is appealing because minimum time and expense are involved and considerable experience can be gained early. This experience can be used to advantage if it is subsequently decided to place a magnetic resonance imager in a permanent location such as a hospital. This sequence of events is already resulting in a used imager market!

Mobile MRI is most attractive to facilities that cannot justify full-time operation because of low patient load. Mobile operation suffers from the time required to shim the magnet and tune up the electronics after each move. This is especially so with superconducting magnetic resonance imagers.

IDENTIFYING THE SITE

Two concerns predominate during site selection for the magnet. First, what will be its influence on equipment and operations in surrounding areas? Second, what characteristics of adjacent areas will adversely affect the operation of the magnetic resonance imager?

Effect of Magnet on Environment

Perhaps the first consideration in selecting a site for a magnetic resonance imager is the influence that the fringe magnetic field might have on equipment and activities in surrounding areas. Any electronic device that operates on the basis of moving electric charges in a vacuum can be influenced by the fringe magnetic field of the imager. Devices such as cathode-ray tubes, image intensifier tubes, electron microscopes, and gamma cameras are all susceptible to MRI fringe magnetic fields.

Recall that a stationary electron has associated with it an electric field. In motion, the electron will have not only an electric field but also a magnetic field. In the presence of an external magnetic field, the magnetic field of the electron will interact with the external magnetic field. This interaction tends to cause the electron to travel from its intended course, moving circularly rather than in a straight line. An electron beam, therefore, as part of sensitive equipment operated in the presence of an external magnetic field will experience a directional deviation, which can severely compromise the operation of the equipment.

Table 8-3 presents some general rules of thumb for determining exclusion limits of sensitive electronic equipment from magnetic resonance imager. This requirement is illustrated in Figure 8-5. It must be recognized that the fringe magnetic field is three dimensional. It extends not only to the space on the same floor but also to the space above and below, as shown in Figure 8-6.

This effect of the magnet on the environment is particularly important for superconductive magnetic resonance imagers. It must also be considered for the resistive air core–type imager, but the fringe field of a resistive iron core or permanent magnet imager will rarely require such consideration.

The intensity of the fringe magnetic field of a superconductive magnetic

**TABLE 8-3.   Exclusion of various types of equipment according to the
strength of the fringe magnetic field**

Strength of the Fringe Magnetic Field (mT)	Devices to Be Excluded
10	Analog watches, credit cards
5	Operator's console, magnetic tapes and diskettes, electric motors, computers
1	Video cameras and monitors, multiformat cameras, dewars
0.5	Cardiac pacemakers, hearing aids image intensifiers, metal detectors
0.1	Gamma cameras, electron microscopes, CT scanners, positron-emission tomography scanners

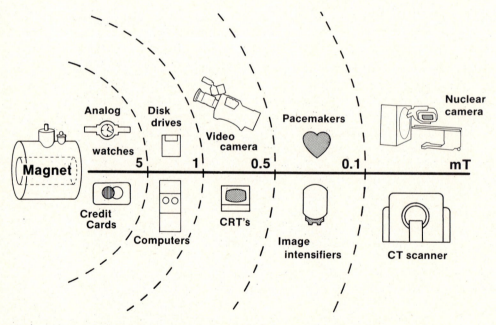

Figure 8-5.   These are the types of objects that should be excluded at several
isomagnetic fringe field strengths.

resonance image is directly proportional to the strength of the B_0 field. For
instance, a 0.5-T imager will have its 0.3-mT fringe magnetic field at a distance
of approximately 11 m. For a 2.0-T magnet, the same fringe magnetic field will
extend to a distance of approximately 18 m. Figure 8-7 shows that the isomagnetic lines in both a plane and side projection are elliptical. The front elevation

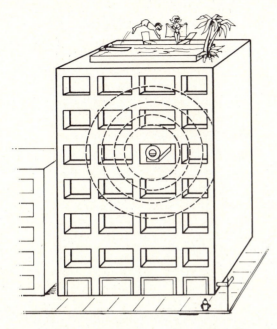

Figure 8-6. The fringe magnetic field is three dimensional. This characteristic will influence the potential locations for such a magnetic resonance imager.

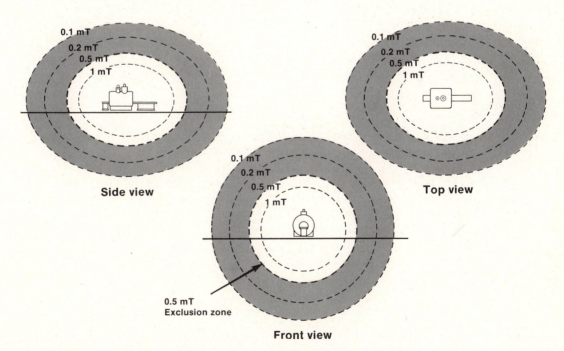

Figure 8-7. The axial fringe magnetic field is elliptical. The transaxial field is circular.

TABLE 8-4.   Axial and transaxial distances to various fringe magnetic fields for several magnet strengths

Fringe Magnetic Field (mT)	Magnet Strength			
	0.5 T axial/ transaxial	1.0 T axial/ transaxial	1.5 T axial/ transaxial	2.0 T axial/ transaxial
1.0	7.0 m/5.0 m	8.5 m/6.7 m	10 m/7.0 m	11 m/9 m
0.5	8.5 m/6.7 m	11 m/8.5 m	13 m/9.7 m	14 m/11 m
0.3	11 m/8.3 m	13 m/10 m	15 m/12 m	18 m/14 m
0.1	15 m/12 m	19 m/15 m	21 m/17 m	23 m/19 m

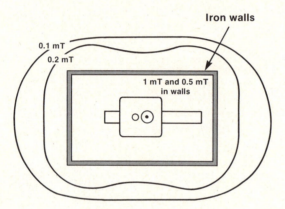

Figure 8-8.   The use of iron shielding will pull the fringe magnetic field closer to the magnet.

shows the circular nature of the fringe magnetic field. Table 8-4 presents the distance from the center of an imager to various isomagnetic levels along the axis and transaxis for imagers of various field strengths.

   If a magnetic shield is employed, as in Figure 8-8, the isomagnetic lines can be pulled closer to the magnet. As a general rule, 10 mm of unsaturated iron will reduce the intensity of the fringe field by about 50%. This rule of thumb is not absolute but varies with the permeability of the iron and the strength of the fringe magnetic field. Figure 8-9 shows some manufacturers' innovative self-shielding approaches to the magnetic shielding problem.

Effect of Environment on the Imager

To produce an image, a very uniform magnetic field must first exist in the imaging volume. Gradient magnetic fields are introduced to shape the magnetic field in a precise, controlled fashion for pixel localization. This shaped field can be disturbed by large stationary ferromagnetic objects that interact with the

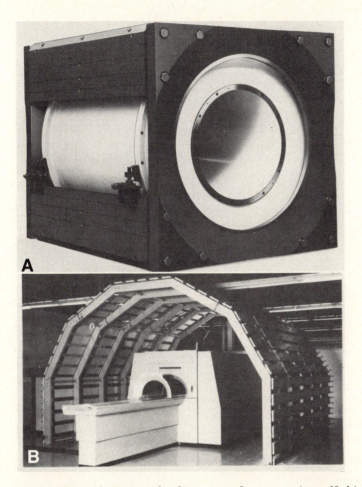

Figure 8-9.   The approach of two manufacturers using self-shielding magnets to shrink the fringe magnetic field. (Courtesy Siemens Medical Systems, Inc., and Phillips Medical Systems, Inc.)

fringe magnetic field of the imager. Smaller ferromagnetic objects that are in motion can be even more bothersome.

It is well understood that when a mass of ferromagnetic material is positioned external to the magnet, such as the iron wall in Figure 8-10, the fringe magnetic field will be deviated into that material. This is the basis for the use of iron as a magnetic shield to protect the environment. What also occurs, however, is a compensating distortion of the magnetic field inside the imaging volume, which results in degradation of the B_0 field.

Such stationary objects can usually be compensated for by shimming the magnet with smaller pieces of iron positioned strategically on the external surface of the magnet. Additional shimming can be done with the **shim coils** described in Chapter 7. Generally, more rigorous site selection in a nonferrous

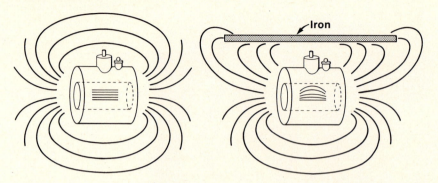

Figure 8-10.   When a large stationary ferromagnetic object is positioned near a magnetic resonance imager, it not only attracts the magnetic fringe field but also degrades B_0 homogeneity.

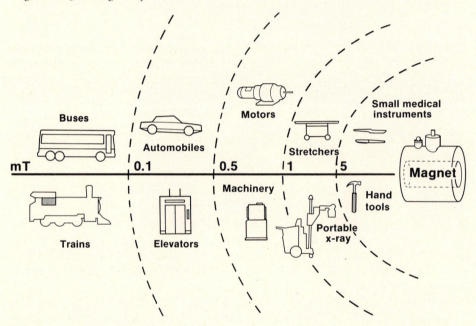

Figure 8-11.   Some ferromagnetic objects should remain outside of fringe magnetic fields because they might become projectiles or degrade the B_0 homogeneity in the imaging volume.

environment is required for magnets of higher field strength because of the requirement for higher field homogeneity. If substantial iron or steel is within the 10-mT isomagnetic line, computer-assisted site modeling will be required.

A more difficult problem results from moving masses of metal. Vehicular traffic, elevators, and motorized dollies in hospitals are examples of such moving masses. It is not possible to protect the B_0 field from such influences, and therefore, this aspect of site selection is critical. Figure 8-11 illustrates what general objects should remain outside of fringe magnetic fields.

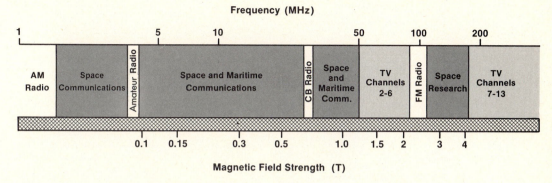

Figure 8-12. Radio frequencies allocated by the Federal Communications Commission in the MRI RF band. (Courtesy Stanley W. Hames, Bechtl Engineers, Inc., San Francisco.)

Equally critical to the operation of a magnetic resonance imager is isolation of the RF signal. The signal detected in the NMR imaging experiment is an RF signal of extremely low intensity, usually less than 100 μV. Broadcast radio signals are an order of magnitude higher and can substantially obscure the NMR signal. These environmental RF signals represent severe noise that limits the detectability of the NMR signal.

The Federal Communications Commission (FCC) identifies the RF band as frequencies ranging from 3 kHz to 300 GHz. Frequencies throughout the range are allocated by the FCC for certain purposes such as navigation, space operation, satellite communications, citizens band broadcast, and commercial broadcast. MRI operates in the RF range of approximately 1 to 100 MHz, where there is considerable other RF activity, as shown by the frequency allocation chart in Figure 8-12. For instance, television channels 2 to 6 broadcast in the 54- to 88-MHz band. Citizen band broadcast is in the 30-MHz region, and much of the rest of the MRI RF band is taken by space and weather communications.

When one designs an x-ray examination room, it is necessary to shield the environment from the potentially harmful electromagnetic radiation, x-rays, that are produced inside the room. With MRI quite the opposite exists. One must shield the imager from the electromagnetic radiation, RF, that exists outside the room. In an x-ray room, lead sheeting up to one sixteenth of an inch thick is installed to absorb the x-radiation. In MRI, the room is lined with copper or aluminum mesh or sheets to absorb external RF.

To improve the NMR signal detection by reduction of environmental noise, MRI rooms are shielded completely by a continuous sheeting or wire mesh of copper or aluminum. Such a design feature is called a **Faraday cage,** for Michael Faraday, the English physicist who first described electromagnetic induction in the 1850s. The shielding must be continuous and include both the ceiling and the floor. It is also important that secure continuous electrical contact is provided. Any breach of electrical continuity will allow environmental

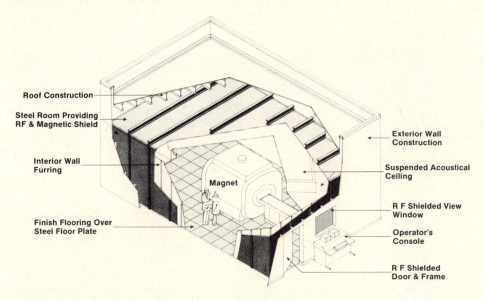

Roof Construction

Steel Room Providing
RF & Magnetic Shield

Interior Wall
Furring

Finish Flooring Over
Steel Floor Plate

Magnet

Exterior Wall
Construction

Suspended Acoustical
Ceiling

R F Shielded View
Window

Operator's
Console

R F Shielded
Door & Frame

Figure 8-13. An MRI room should be shielded to exclude environmental RF by a continuous enclosure of sheet or wire mesh of copper or aluminum. (Courtesy TME, Inc.)

RF to leak into the room and interfere with the NMR signal. MRI facilities should require at least a 90-decibel reduction in signal intensity in the RF range from 1 to 100 MHz.

Figure 8-13 illustrates such a Faraday cage. Note that the entire room, including doors and windows, is shielded from RF. Often the RF enclosure is a room built within a room. All wiring and cables that enter the imaging room must be properly filtered to exclude environmental RF. View windows should be fabricated with sufficiently large mesh so that vision is not compromised and at the same time a continuous RF shield is provided.

Several manufacturers have successfully employed a self-shielded magnet such as that shown in Figure 8-14. The telescoping cage can make total room shielding unnecessary. This approach is not acceptable to all sites, particularly at higher field strengths.

DESIGNING THE FACILITY

Once an imager has been selected and the site identified, the facility can be designed. Many design features are independent of the type of imager selected. Others must take into account certain characteristics of the type of imager. The differences in some characteristics are extensive and will require special consideration in the design of the facility. Because other characteristics are shared by each type of imager, general design criteria may be employed.

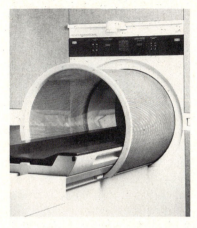

Figure 8-14. The telescoping Faraday cage has been satisfactorily employed by several manufacturers. (Courtesy Picker International.)

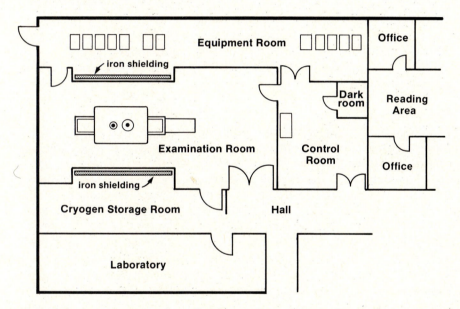

Figure 8-15. A representative plan layout for an MRI facility showing the required support areas.

General Design Criteria

Figure 8-15 is a typical plan layout of an MRI facility as part of an imaging center. A similar layout could be proposed for an existing hospital. Within the immediate imaging area, space must be allocated for the imaging room, computer room, control room, viewing room, and cryogen storage area. A minimum of approximately 150 m^2 is required. In addition, a reception area, office space, and physics/engineering space are necessary.

RECEPTION.   Most MRI facilities are not going to be an integral part of an existing radiology department. Therefore, a reception and waiting area common with radiology may not be available. In such situations a separate reception area will have to be provided for the MRI. Because many MRI examinations are conducted on an outpatient basis, the patient is examined in street clothes, eliminating the need for the many change rooms associated with x-ray examinations. However, some sort of change and security room is required so the patient can remove metal objects and valuables prior to examination.

METAL DETECTOR.   At the threshold of the examination area, space must be reserved for metal detection. Most facilities will choose a threshold-type metal surveillance device similar to those employed in airports for security. An additional wand-type metal detector may be required. Metal detection is important not only for the patient prior to imaging but also for other persons who may enter the facility. Physicians, attendants, and custodial personnel must be instructed about potential hazards from metal projectiles. Magnets and people can be damaged by projectiles from individuals who may not otherwise be adequately advised.

OFFICE SUPPORT.   Office space for physicians, technologists, engineers, and physicists is required, and a darkroom is needed for processing images from a multiformat camera or a laser printer.

PATIENT ACCESS.   The position of the entrance door to the imaging room must be considered. The door should be so positioned so that a patient in distress can be quickly and easily removed from the room without undue manipulation. Such a design feature also permits the easy access of a crash cart, whose implements, of course, will be nonmagnetic.

POWER REQUIREMENTS.   Regardless of the type of imager, approximately 10 kW of power is required for computers, operating consoles, and other electronic devices. An additional 10 to 20 kW is required to power the shim coils, gradient coils, and the RF network. Beyond that, a superconducting imager requires an additional 20 to 30 kW, but only while the imager is being brought up to the design field strength. During operation no power is required for the main magnet coils. A resistive-type imager, however, may require an additional 60 to 80 kW to maintain the main magnetic field.

Construction Materials and Techniques

Because the presence of external ferromagnetic material can degrade the homogeneity of the main magnetic field, construction materials must be selected carefully. Large existing metal objects such as cast-iron waste water lines and electrical machinery may have to be moved. In general, the site should be metal free and vibration stable. This requires special material and construction techniques.

FOUNDATION.   The weight of most imagers requires a substantial concrete pad with reinforcing. Instead of iron reinforcing rods and corrugated iron sheets, some of the available fiberglass-impregnated reinforcing rods and epoxy concrete should be used. A sufficient structural foundation is required not only in the imaging room but also along the route for installation. Post tension or other techniques may be necessary to ensure that the foundation is vibration free. Even subtle vibration can encourage cryogen to boil off and degrade image quality.

Normal construction techniques for walls and ceilings are generally acceptable. Unreinforced concrete or wood stud construction with standard nails is acceptable.

ELECTRICAL SERVICE. Electrical conduits in the imaging room should be made of either polyvinyl chloride or aluminum. Electrical receptacles and fixtures should be aluminum or ceramic. Electrical distribution transformers should not be located within the 3-mT isomagnetic line. Lighting in the scan room must be incandescent; no fluorescent lamps are allowed. The supply should be DC or properly filtered. Dimmer controls should not be mounted within the room. Fixtures should be brass or ceramic.

PLUMBING. Supply lines, floor drains, and soil pipes should be nonferrous. Polyvinyl chloride or copper is acceptable. If building codes require a sprinkler system, only brass or copper components should be used. All sprinkler heads that penetrate the RF shielding must be completely electrically grounded.

PATIENT VIEWING. The ability to view the patient during examination is mandatory. Although closed-circuit television capable of operating in the magnetic field of the room has been developed, it is expensive and not totally satisfactory. Most facilities will find that a direct-view window incorporating the required RF shield will be adequate.

HVAC. Heating, ventilation, and air conditioning (HVAC) are important engineering considerations for an MRI site. The HVAC design must deal with not only the normal space-occupying activities of a conventional office or laboratory but also the special requirements of the imager.

Constant temperature is essential for the stability of the magnet and associated electronic components. The B_0 field of a permanent magnet increases approximately 0.1% per degree. A 10-degree drift could cause an electronic frequency mismatch that would destroy the tuned response at the Larmor frequency. Any computer that accompanies MRI must be provided with a cool, dry environment. Temperature must be maintained between 18 and 20° C at a relative humidity of not more than 40%.

MAGNET COOLING. Permanent magnet imagers have no special cooling requirements beyond those normally needed for electronic and computer components. This feature contributes to the relatively low capital cost and site preparation requirements.

A resistive-type magnetic resonance imager requires a cooling system sufficient to dissipate the enormous heat generated by the electricity used to produce the B_0 magnetic field. A closed primary coolant loop usually containing deionized water flows continuously through the resistive magnet. Heat is extracted from the magnet by the coolant and is then dissipated through a heat exchanger to a secondary cooling system. The secondary coolant is usually a single pass of tap water. For a 0.25-T magnet such a cooling system must be able to remove up to 5000 BTUs per hour. The water consumption is approximately 100 L/m during operation.

A superconducting imager requires cryogens, liquid helium, and liquid nitrogen. Up to 0.5 L/hr of helium and 2 L/hr of liquid nitrogen may be required to maintain the low temperature to support superconductivity. Superconducting magnets require aluminum venting usually through the ceiling for cryogen exhaust. It is desirable to have the liquid nitrogen piped in from a storage tank.

ADDITIONAL FEATURES.   In addition to the preceding design features that are appropriate for any MRI facility, there are special considerations attendant to each type of imager that concern the design of each such facility.

Permanent magnets are small but heavy. A 0.3-T whole-body imager can weigh 40,000 kg. Such a mass will probably preempt its placement anywhere but on ground level. Smaller head and neck imagers weigh not more than 5000 kg and can be located on any level.

Resistive magnet imagers require much electrical power and considerable cooling capacity. Sufficient space for the power supplies and cooling system is necessary.

Superconducting magnet imagers require cryogenic support. Loading, handling, and storage space for cryogens must be provided. The loading dock for cryogen dewars should be outside the 1.0-mT isomagnetic line and easily accessible to the magnet room.

SUMMARY

Establishing an MRI facility involves three giant steps and several mother-may-I's. The imager should be selected first because that in large measure will determine its location. Site selection is the second step. Location in turn will influence the design of the facility, which completes the process.

The principal considerations surrounding site selection and facility design are the intensity of the fringe magnetic field and the nature of the environmental RF. Iron shielding may be required to accommodate the fringe magnetic field in addition to establishing controlled exclusion areas. RF shielding is usually done by incorporating a Faraday cage into the floor, walls, and ceiling of the examination room.

Chapter
NINE

Digital Imaging

When applied to medical imaging, the term **digital imaging** implies that a digital computer is used. MRI could not be performed without the digital computer. This is because the NMR signal does not interact directly with a viewable medium as x-rays do with an intensifying screen phosphor. The NMR signal does not present its information in a form that can be directly viewed electronically as does ultrasound. The NMR signal provides information about the **spatial frequency** content of the image rather than the direct image. Figure 9-1, *A,* is a computer-generated image of two bright balls on a dark background. Figure 9-1, *B,* is a set of projections, called a **sinogram,** from that image of the two balls. This sort of data set is obtained from a parallel-beam x-ray CT scan. Note that the positions and sizes of the objects may be inferred, at least to a limited extent, from the projection data because the data are in the **spatial location** domain, which means the data are related directly to coordinates in space. Figure 9-1, *C,* shows the magnitude data, and Figure 9-1, *D* shows the phase data from the MR representation of the two balls. Because the MRI data are in the spatial frequency domain, it is much more difficult to make sense of the raw data from such a magnetic resonance image.

The digital computer converts this information about the spatial frequency domain into the spatial location of the NMR signal within the patient to produce an image. To explain why MRI is inherently digital, this chapter reviews some characteristics of the digital computer and then examines the details of the formation of magnetic resonance images.

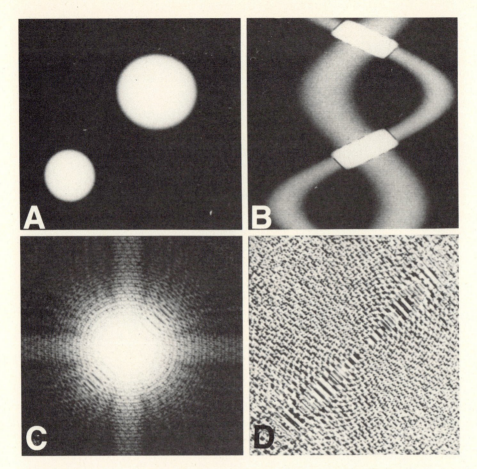

Figure 9-1. **A,** A plane image of two balls. **B,** The sinogram of the two balls. **C,** The magnitude of the spatial frequency representation of the image. **D,** The phase of the spatial frequency representation of the image. **C** and **D** together are the data set that one actually receives in MRI.

THE COMPUTER'S "VIEW" OF THE WORLD

The computer works with numbers. Specifically, it works with binary numbers. The binary number set consists of 0 and 1. Perhaps if humans had only two fingers instead of ten, the binary number system would seem to be more natural than decimal numbers. A single decimal numeral is called a **digit,** the same as fingers are. A single binary numeral is called a **bit**—short for **binary digit.** The computer uses the binary number system because it is so easy to implement with real-world components. One simply defines a 1 to be any voltage above a specified value and a 0 to be any voltage below a specified value. The electronic circuit that does this is called a **flip-flop.**

TABLE 9-1. Organization of binary number system

Decimal Number	Binary Equivalent					Binary Number
0					0	0
1					2^0	1
2				2^1 +	0	10
3				2^1 +	2^0	11
4			2^2 +	0 +	0	100
5			2^2 +	0 +	2^0	101
6			2^2 +	2^1 +	0	110
7			2^2 +	2^1 +	2^0	111
8		2^3 +	0 +	0 +	0	1000
9		2^3 +	0 +	0 +	2^0	1001
10		2^3 +	0 +	2^1 +	0	1010
11		2^3 +	0 +	2^1 +	2^0	1011
12		2^3 +	2^2 +	0 +	0	1100
13		2^3 +	2^2 +	0 +	2^0	1101
14		2^3 +	2^2 +	2^1 +	0	1110
15		2^3 +	2^2 +	2^1 +	2^0	1111
16	2^4 +	0 +	0 +	0 +	0	10000

Binary Number System

When counting in the binary number system, as shown in Table 9-1, one counts 0 to 1 and then counts over again. There are only two digits, 0 and 1, and the computer performs all operations by converting alphabetic characters, decimal values, and logic functions to binary values. That way, although the binary numbers may become exceedingly long, computation can be handled by properly adjusting the thousands of flip-flop circuits in the computer.

In the binary system, 0 is 0 and 1 is 1, but the direct relationship with the decimal system ends there. In fact, it ends at 0 because the 1 in binary notation comes from 2^0. Recall that any number raised to the zero power is 1; therefore, 2^0 equals 1. In binary notation, 2 is equal to 1 plus no 2^0. This is expressed as 10. The decimal 3 is equal to 1 and one 2^0, or 11 in binary form; 4 is one 2^2 plus no 2^1 plus no 2^0, or 100 in binary form. As shown in Table 9-1, each time it is necessary to raise 2 to an additional power to express a number, the number of binary digits increases by one.

Just as we know the meaning of the powers of ten, it is necessary to recognize the powers of two easily. Power-of-two notation is used in radiologic imaging to describe image size, image dynamic range (shades of gray), and image storage capacity. Table 9-2 reviews these power notations. Note the following similarity: in both power notations the number of zeros to the right of 1 equals the value of the exponent.

TABLE 9-2. Power-of-10, power-of-2, and binary notation

Power of 10	Power of 2	Binary Notation
$10^0 = 1$	$2^0 = 1$	1
$10^1 = 10$	$2^1 = 2$	10
$10^2 = 100$	$2^2 = 4$	100
$10^3 = 1000$	$2^3 = 8$	1000
$10^4 = 10,000$	$2^4 = 16$	10000
$10^5 = 100,000$	$2^5 = 32$	100000
$10^6 = 1,000,000$	$2^6 = 64$	1000000
	$2^7 = 128$	10000000
	$2^8 = 256$	100000000
	$2^9 = 512$	1000000000
	$2^{10} = 1024$	10000000000

Example: Express the number 193 in binary form.

Answer: 193 falls between 2^7 and 2^8. Therefore, it will be expressed as 1 followed by seven binary digits. Simply add the decimal equivalents of each binary digit from left to right:

Yes $2^7 = 1 = 128$
Yes $2^6 = 1 = 64$
No $2^5 = 0 =$ No 32
No $2^4 = 0 =$ No 16
No $2^3 = 0 =$ No 8
No $2^2 = 0 =$ No 4
No $2^1 = 0 =$ No 2
Yes $2^0 = 1 = 1$

11000001 = 193

Digital radiologic images are made of discrete numerical values arranged in a matrix. The size of the image is described in the binary system of numbers by power-of-two equivalents. Most MR images are either 128 by 128 (2^7) or 256 by 256 (2^8).

Bits, Bytes, and Words

The computer will use as many bits, zeros and ones, as necessary to express a decimal digit. The 26 characters of the alphabet and other special characters are usually encoded by 8 bits. To **encode** is to translate from ordinary characters to computer-compatible characters—binary digits. Depending on the computer, a string of 8, 16, or 32 bits will be manipulated simultaneously.

Bits are grouped into bunches of eight called **bytes.** Computer capacity is expressed by the number of bytes that computer memory can accommodate. The most popular personal computers employ 8- and 16-bit microprocessors with a minimum of 64 kilobytes (KB) of memory. One kilobyte is 2^{10} or 1024 bits. Note that *kilo* is not metric in computer use. The minicomputers used in radiology have capacities measured in megabytes, where 1 MB = 1 KB × 1 KB = $2^{10} \times 2^{10} = 2^{20}$ = 1,048,576 bytes.

Example: How many bits can be stored on a 64-KB chip whose byte size is 8 bits?
Answer: 1024 bits × 64 KB × 8 bits = $2^{10} \times 2^{6} \times 2^{3} = 2^{19}$ = 524,288 bits

Depending on the computer configuration, 1 or 2 bytes usually constitute a **word**. In the case of a 16-bit microprocessor, a word would be 16 consecutive bits of information that are interpreted and shuffled about the computer as a unit. Each word of data in memory has its own address.

The number of bits determines the resolution or **precision** of the numbers that the computer uses. This means simply that the number of bits determines the total number of elements that the computer can count. This is similar to the U.S. Postal Service zip codes. When the Postal Service wanted to add **resolution** to the zip codes, it added four more numbers at the end of the five-numeral zip code to define the carrier route as well as the postal zone to which a letter is addressed.

An 8-bit computer number can count from 0 to 255 and thus can represent 256 different things (2^8). A 16-bit number can count from 0 to 65,535 and thus can represent 65,536 different things (2^{16}). Regardless of the number of bits that the computer uses, it is limited in the number of elements it can represent. It cannot hold continuous data the way a tape recorder or a phonograph record can. In the digital computer, limited resolution and limited storage affect the manipulation of data. MRI is limited in the same way and hence is truly digital imaging.

Quantization or Resolution

PRECISION. The limited number of elements that the computer can count restricts the **precision** with which the computer can store values. For proper interpretation some quantities must be specified with great precision. However, imprecision is a fact of daily life, and people live comfortably with acceptable degrees of imprecision. When one asks, ''How far is it to Dallas?,'' a satisfactory answer would be to the nearest mile or so. We don't need to know the distance to the nearest foot or inch. One does not ask your height to the nearest micron but rather to the nearest inch. Age is not given precisely to the minute but usually only to the year. Such limits of precision are totally satisfactory in everyday life. Considerably more precision is required for MRI.

In the design of a computer system, the required resolution in the data is determined first. Suppose that differences of 0.01 volt must be distinguished in an NMR signal, either an FID or a spin echo. An 8-bit computer word allows for 256 discrete steps or a voltage range from 0 to 2.55 volts. A 16-bit computer word gives a voltage range from 0 to 655.35 volts.

A voltage range from 0 to 24 volts is typically needed in MRI. Thus, 12 bits (2^{12}) = 4096 would be required because 12 bits allow a range from 0 to 41.96 volts. Eleven bits (2^{11}) = 2048 would provide only a range from 0 to 20.48 volts, which would not be sufficient. Sixteen or 24 bits are commonly used to allow extra bits for the results of computations. For example, if one adds 22 volts to 23 volts, 12 bits is not enough to hold 45 volts and an additional bit is required. Although more than ample, the 32-bit word is becoming more popular as the price of 32-bit computing hardware drops.

DYNAMIC RANGE.   One area in which the resolution of the data affects medical images is the number of gray levels used to display an image. This is referred to as the **dynamic range** of an imaging system. An imaging system that could display only black or white would have a dynamic range of 2^1, or 2. Such an image would be of very high contrast but would display very little information. Although the value of each pixel is unimportant, the range of values is extremely important in determining the final image. Dynamic range in magnetic resonance imager corresponds to the numerical range of each pixel. Visually, dynamic range refers to the shades of gray that can be represented.

The dynamic range of the human eye is between 2^4 and 2^5, or 16 to 32 shades of gray, stretching from white to black. The dynamic range of the NMR signal emitted by the patient exceeds 2^{10}. Although humans cannot visualize such a dynamic range, a computer with sufficient capacity can. The higher the dynamic range, the more gradual will be the gray scale representing the range from maximum to minimum signal intensity. The greater the dynamic range, therefore, the better the image.

Early image displays were capable of only 4 bits (2^4), or 16 gray levels, whereas newer displays provide 8 bits (2^8), or 256 gray levels. However, the data may have more than 256 values. In CT the Hounsfield numbers have a range of 2000; in radioisotope scintigraphic imaging, one might have thousands of counts in a pixel in a first-pass study; and in MRI T1 and T2 values have ranges of several thousand. Despite this, the human visual system can resolve no more than 32 gray levels, and so in a display system somewhere between 16 and 256 gray levels are sufficient to ensure no visual loss of information.

To see the significance of the concept of an acceptable degree of imprecision, consider an MR image displayed with different numbers of gray levels. In Figure 9-2, the same image is displayed with 8, 7, 6, 5, 4, 3, 2, and 1 bits of gray-scale resolution. These bit values correspond respectively to 256, 128, 64, 32, 16, 8, 4, and 2 shades of gray. With an insufficient number of gray levels available, there is a visual loss of gray-scale resolution. That loss is perceived as **false contouring,** in which boundaries appear in the image where there should be none. However, resolution is not the only limitation implicit in working with digital computers.

Sampling

When the computer stores data, it must be able to **address** the data. In the same way that there is a limited number of postal zones in the United States that can have a unique five-digit zip code, there is a limited number of memory

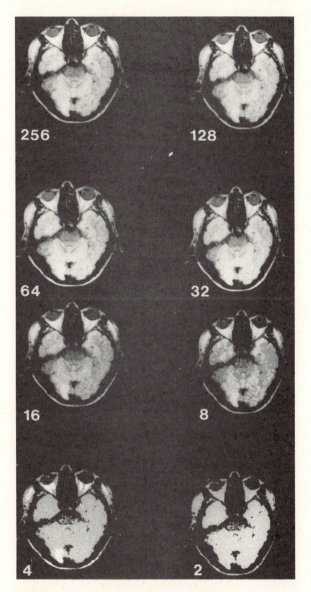

Figure 9-2. Different gray-scale resolutions in an image display. For many people, the loss of gray scale resolution does not become visible until one has only about 16 shades of gray. Then, one sees apparent edges or contours in the image where there should be none.

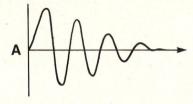

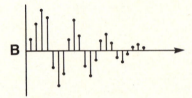

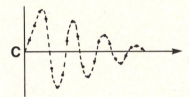

Figure 9-3.   **A,** A continuous FID. **B,** A sampled version of the FID. The computer would store only the values taken at the regularly spaced indicated points along the horizontal axis. **C,** The connect-the-dots reconstruction of the original signal from the sampled values.

locations that can be used for image storage. This limitation is imposed by the limited number of bits in the memory address. Consequently, for the image to be stored in the computer, the image information must be sampled.

The process of sampling involves taking occasional values, or samples, of information from the NMR signal. This is illustrated in Figure 9-3, in which a continuous FID is represented by a set of values taken at a regular interval. In this instance the sampled data set is similar to a **connect-the-dots** picture.

Sampling is a familiar process. The business pages of the newspapers give the closing prices for stocks each day. Even though the price of a stock may change during the day, only its price at the end of the day and the range of its price during the day are given. A television picture is not a continuously changing image but rather a rapid succession of static images, displayed at the rate of 30 images per second. Obviously, there is no loss of important information about the action on the television screen even though one sees only 30 samples per second rather than continuous motion.

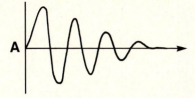

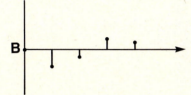

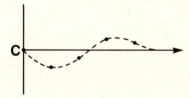

Figure 9-4. **A,** A continuous FID. **B,** A sampled version of the FID in which the samples are taken too far apart in time. **C,** The connect-the-dots representation of the "undersampled" shows that the higher frequency has been "aliased" into a lower frequency.

There is a direct relationship between the speed with which changes are occurring and the rate at which sampling is performed, so as not to lose any useful information. The faster things are changing, the faster one must sample to be able to describe all of the details of that change accurately with the data stored in the computer. Things that change rapidly are said to contain **high frequencies,** and things that change slowly are described as containing predominately **low frequencies**.

Sampling must be rapid enough so that the signal being sampled does not change directions more than once between samples. If the sampling is not quick enough, as shown in Figure 9-4, a quickly changing process may appear to change slowly. When a rapidly changing signal is **undersampled** and appears to change slowly, the process is said to be **aliased** because of the misleading nature of the sampled data. Aliasing results in a permanent loss of information. An example of an aliasing artifact, not uncommon in CT, is shown in Figure 9-5.

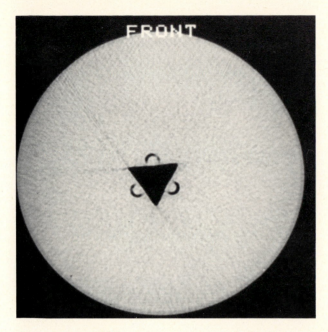

Figure 9-5.   This is a CT scan of a plastic cylinder containing an air-filled triangular section. The dark streaks appearing off the edges of the triangles are the result of aliasing. (Courtesy Edward L. Nickoloff, Columbia University, New York City.)

Using a digital computer imposes two opposing constraints. The limited amount of data storage capacity argues for taking as few samples as possible. However, so that information is not **aliased** and lost, the lower limit on the sampling rate is determined by the nature of the signal itself.

MRI also must sample the information about the patient. The number of samples in MRI is limited by the time available to collect the data from a very short signal. The changes of the signal are not only changes in time but also changes in space because the signal originates from various regions of the body. Thus the frequencies to be observed are those of **spatial frequency**.

THE SPATIAL FREQUENCY DOMAIN

Spatial frequency is measured in line pairs per centimeter (lp/cm) or line pairs per millimeter (lp/mm). This numeration is used to identify the spatial resolution of an imaging system. The ability to image a high spatial frequency means the ability to image very small objects. Five line pair patterns are shown in Figure 9-6. The larger patterns are represented by smaller numbers. As spatial frequency increases, object size decreases and becomes more difficult to image. The spatial resolution of the best magnetic resonance imager is about 10 lp/cm or 1 lp/mm. Table 9-3 shows limiting spatial resolution for other medical imaging modalities.

A high spatial frequency reflects many changes in the strength of the

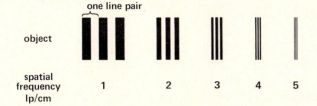

Figure 9-6. These five bar patterns demonstrate the meaning of spatial frequency. The higher the spatial frequency, the smaller the object.

TABLE 9-3.   Representative spatial resolution capability of several medical imaging modalities

Imaging Modality	Object Size (mm)	Spatial Frequency (lp/mm)
Radioisotope scan	10.0	0.05
Ultrasound	2.0	0.25
Intensified fluoroscopy	1.0	0.5
Computed tomography	0.5	1.0
Magnetic resonance imaging	0.5	1.0
Screen-film	0.2	2.5
Human eye	0.05	10.0
Direct exposure film	0.02	25.0

NMR signal within a given region of the patient. A low spatial frequency arises from little or no change in the strength of the NMR signal within that region.

As an example of different spatial frequencies, consider the three businessmen shown in Figure 9-7: a used-car salesman, an undertaker, and a banker. The used-car salesman is wearing a loud, plaid jacket. The undertaker is wearing a plain black suit, and the banker is wearing a pinstripe suit. The pattern of the fabric of the used-car saleman's plaid jacket has many abrupt changes in any square centimeter. Thus there are many high spatial frequencies in that jacket because there are many changes per centimeter, whether the jacket is scanned horizontally across the cloth or vertically. Now, consider the undertaker's solid black suit. Whether one scans vertically or horizontally, there are no changes in the pattern of the cloth, and hence the undertaker's jacket has very low spatial frequencies. In between these extremes is the banker's pinstripe suit. A vertical scan on the back of the jacket reveals no change; therefore, the jacket has very low spatial frequencies vertically. On the other hand, when scanning horizontally across the fabric, one crosses the pinstripes and thus observes some relatively high spatial frequencies. The more closely together the pinstripes are placed, the more changes per centimeter and the higher the horizontal spatial frequency will be.

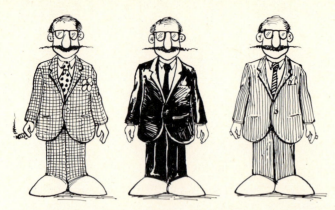

Figure 9-7. Three entrepreneurs and their working attire demonstrate the concept of spatial frequency. The used-car salesman's plaid jacket contains high spatial frequencies both horizontally and vertically. The undertaker's plain black jacket has zero spatial frequency. The banker's pinstripe suit has zero vertical spatial frequency but higher horizontal spatial frequency.

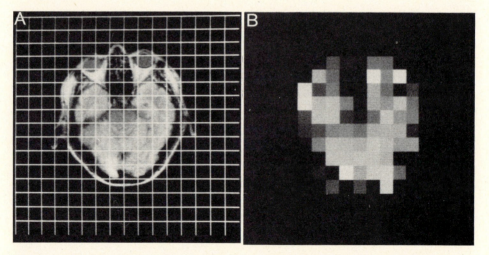

Figure 9-8. **A,** The original image with a sampling grid superimposed. **B,** The sampled values of the original image. Because of sampling in space, the resulting computer image may look blocky.

Image Matrix

Because the computer has a limited amount of memory in which an image can be stored, the image must be sampled in space as well as time. To sample an image in space, one selects the values at the intersections of an imaginary grid, which is superimposed on the image as shown in Figure 9-8, and lets that value represent a small region of the image.

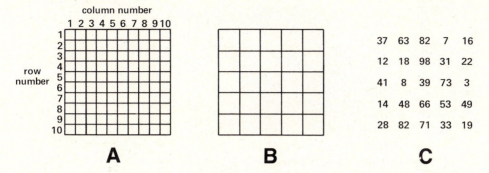

Figure 9-9. Imaginary cells of a matrix are assigned numbers that represent image brightness.

The term **image matrix** refers to a layout of rows and columns, usually containing numbers representing intensity in boxes or cells. Figure 9-9 shows a 10-by-10 matrix of cells, a 5-by-5 matrix of cells, and a 5-by-5 matrix of numbers in imaginary cells. Each magnetic resonance image consists of a matrix of imaginary cells having various brightness levels on the television monitor. The brightness of a cell is determined by the computer-generated number in that cell.

The size of the image matrix is determined by characteristics of the imaging equipment and by the capacity of the computer. Most magnetic resonance imagers provide image matrix sizes of 7 bits (128 by 128) or 8 bits (256 by 256). Spatial resolution of the image will be better with a larger image matrix.

Figure 9-10 illustrates the influence of matrix size on image quality. A 6-bit image matrix (64 by 64) appears definitely "blocky," whereas a 9-bit image (512 by 512) is a good representation of the original analog image. A 10-bit image (1024 by 1024) is indistinguishable from the original. Because the images in Figure 9-10 are rectangular, only half of each image is shown.

To present a sampled image, it is insufficient to display just the sampled points, so **pixels** are used. Pixel is short for **picture element** and is a two-dimensional representation of **voxel**, or **volume element**. A sampled image is just like a mosaic. Each pixel is a rectangular tile having an intensity equal to that of the sample value at that point in the image. This accounts for the blocky appearance of some computer-displayed images.

The spacing of the samples must be sufficiently close so that there are no surprises between samples. For example, if there is a sharp edge or small structure in the object and the samples are far apart, it will be difficult to say where the transition is located in the image and, more important, what the precise shape of a small structure is, as shown in Figure 9-10. **Sharp edges and small structures contain many high spatial frequencies.**

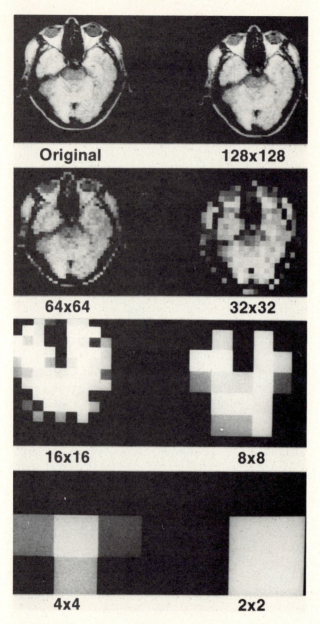

Figure 9-10. The small features and sharp edges in the image that contain much of the high spatial frequency information are progressively obscured as the sampling rate and image matrix are reduced. Note that the fine structures become blurred as their high spatial frequencies are aliased into lower spatial frequencies.

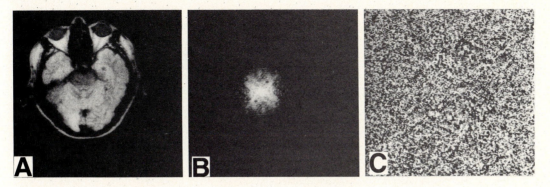

Figure 9-11. The spatial frequency representation of an image. **A,** The original image. **B,** The magnitude map of the spatial frequencies. **C,** The phase map of the spatial frequencies. Note that because the image is predominately positive in intensity, the center of **B** is very bright because the average value in the image is quite large.

Frequency Domain Map

The spatial frequency content of an image is plotted in two dimensions just the way the image itself is displayed. Low frequencies are toward the center of the spatial frequency display, and higher spatial frequencies are toward the edges. This is shown in Figure 9-11.

Horizontal spatial frequencies appear along horizontal lines, and vertical spatial frequencies appear along vertical lines. The intensity of an arbitrary point represents the strength of a particular combination of horizontal and vertical spatial frequencies. Recall that the banker's pinstripe suit was a combination of low vertical spatial frequency and high horizontal spatial frequency.

The information in the spatial frequency representation of the image is exactly the same as the information in the image; it is just being presented in a different way. There are examples of this concept in everyday life. Today's patients will be scheduled in chronological order and will appear that way on the magnetic resonance imager worksheets. However, when they are billed for the procedure, the list is likely to be in alphabetical order or arranged by hospital number. The same information is present; a group of patients received MR examinations. The manner in which the data are presented is different for different purposes. **Whether the information in an image is organized by horizontal and vertical position or by horizontal and vertical spatial frequency does not affect the information itself but only how it is presented.**

SPATIAL LOCALIZATION AND MRI

Although the topic of this book is MRI, computers and spatial frequency and sampling are being emphasized because MRI samples the strengths of the spatial frequencies of the NMR signal in the subject to get the image information. The computer then converts that information from its spatial frequency representation to a representation in spatial location or position. This latter is the

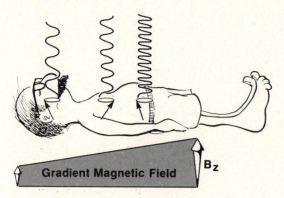

Figure 9-12.   The effect of a magnetic field gradient on the resonant frequencies of spins within the patient. Note that the nuclear spins to the superior side of the patient spin more slowly than those to the inferior side.

usual definition of an image, but the former is the way in which the raw data are presented to the computer.

Several MRI techniques have been developed. The two major approaches differ far more than x-ray CT, which has fan beam and parallel beam acquisition and nuclear medicine **SPECT** (single photon emission computed tomography), which has continuous and step-and-shoot motion. The easier method to understand is **projection reconstruction**. The most popular technique of MRI is **two-dimensional Fourier transform** imaging **(2DFT)**. A variant of 2DFT is called **spin warp,** and an older name is the **KWE method,** recognizing its inventors, Kumar, Welti, and Ernst.

Both projection reconstruction and 2DFT MRI are digital imaging techniques. They differ in the manner in which they sample the spatial frequencies of the patient. The principles of spatial localization demonstrate why MRI is inherently digital, regardless of the particular technique employed.

In a homogeneous magnetic field all of the spins precess at exactly the same rate. This rate is equal to the Larmor frequency. The Larmor equation holds that the frequency of precession is directly proportional to the strength of the magnetic field. Because the frequency, phase, and amplitude of the signal are all that can be measured, it becomes necessary to modify the magnetic field so that the MR signal can reflect its spatial origin.

A magnetic field gradient is used to achieve spatial localization; that is the difference between an NMR spectrometer and magnetic resonance imager. When the strength of the magnetic field varies linearly across the patient, so will frequency of the signal across the patient. Spins on one side of the patient precess faster than spins on the other side. If one could "listen" to the MR signal the way one can listen to a rock band, the distribution of the NMR signal in the patient would be audible just the way the different instruments of the rock band may be clearly distinguished, as illustrated in Figure 9-12.

The magnetic field gradient provides the means to distinguish left from right within the plane of the image, but it does not yield any information about

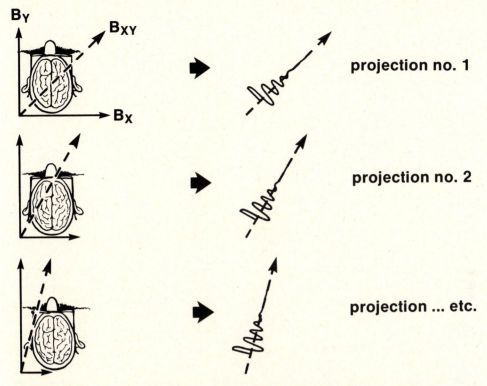

Figure 9-13. The vector sum of two simultaneously applied gradient magnetic fields can be rotated by varying the strength of the individual gradients. Note that the strengths of the X and Y gradients are chosen so that even though the angle of the resultant B_{xy} changes, its strength is always the same.

the distribution of intensity along the direction at right angles to the gradient. To obtain information throughout the plane of the object, two gradient magnetic fields must be used. The gradients are applied simultaneously in projection reconstruction imaging and sequentially in 2DFT imaging. These two major approaches to MRI reflect different ways of coordinating the effect of the two orthogonal magnetic field gradients. The combination of the two gradients allows the whole plane to be sampled. Sampling the spatial frequency representation of the image plane makes MRI inherently digital imaging.

Projection Reconstruction MRI

The projection reconstruction MRI technique is easier to understand because it resembles the way in which data are collected in parallel-beam x-ray CT. As the two orthogonal gradients are applied simultaneously, the direction of the resulting gradient is the vector sum of these two orthogonal gradients. The direction of the resultant gradient may be rotated in the imaging plane by varying the relative strengths of the two orthogonal gradients, as shown in Figure 9-13.

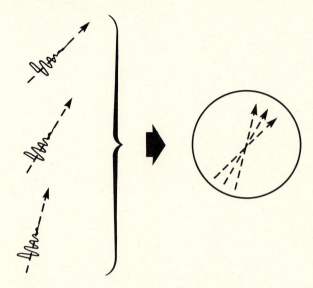

Figure 9-14.   Polar sampling of the spatial frequency representation of the image. Note that the angle of the resultant B_{xy} gradient determines the angle of the sample line in the spatial frequency representation.

A separate NMR signal is acquired for each orientation of the resultant gradient. This NMR signal is a sample of the two-dimensional spatial frequency representation of the image. As the resultant gradient is rotated from acquisition to acquisition, the orientation of the samples in the spatial frequency domain rotates. Thus the spatial frequencies in the image are sampled on a polar grid. This is shown in Figure 9-14.

In MRI nothing moves from acquisition to acquisition. The gradient magnetic field rotates electrically. In CT the x-ray tube and sometimes the detector array also move between acquisitions.

Most image display systems have square pixels, so it is desirable to sample the reconstructed image in rectangular coordinates. The density of samples in the polar sampling is not uniform on a rectangular grid, and thus the NMR signals must be **filtered** to correct for the fact that they contain more information about the low spatial frequencies than they do about the high spatial frequencies. After filtering, the NMR signal is transformed to get a projection. Finally, the filtered projection is back-projected into the rectangular image matrix.

Back-projection is a time-consuming computational chore. Furthermore, the filtering operation tends to emphasize the noise in the projections. For these reasons, the 2DFT technique has become the method of choice for planar MRI.

2DFT Magnetic Resonance Imaging

The 2DFT approach also samples the spatial frequency representation of the image, but it does so on a rectangular grid instead of a polar grid. The 2DFT

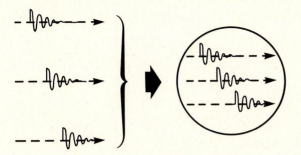

Figure 9-15. Rectangular sampling of the spatial frequency representation of the image. The phase-encoding gradient is changed during each cycle of data acquisition, which determines the horizontal line of the spatial frequency representation.

technique consists of a basic cycle, which is repeated many times, typically 128 or 256. This cycle consists of an RF **excitation pulse,** a gradient pulse called the **phase-encoding gradient,** followed by a steady application of an orthogonal gradient called the **frequency-encoding gradient,** during which time the data are collected. After a suitable delay, the cycle is repeated. The cycle differs in only one respect from one acquisition to the next. **The strength of the phase-encoding gradient is different in each cycle.** This is illustrated in Figure 9-15.

What the phase-encoding gradient does is select a single line in the frequency domain representation of the image. Then, the frequency-encoding gradient forms the NMR signal along this line. Instead of rotating the sampling line around the center of the spatial frequency map, the phase-encoding gradient shifts the NMR signal so that it samples a different line parallel to the others. When the strength of the phase-encoding gradient is changed in other cycles, other lines in the frequency representation are selected. When the whole set of cycles has been performed, a set of lines through the frequency domain has been selected and the frequency information along those lines has been measured. Thus the phase-encoding gradient is used to sample the frequency representation of the image in a rectangular coordinate system. This rectangular sampling is Fourier transformed to yield the image. Because the spatial frequency domain data are already sampled on a rectangular grid, 2DFT replaces the filtering and back-projection steps of projection reconstruction with a simple Fourier transform.

The two most common artifacts peculiar to 2DFT images are the consequences of **undersampling** and **motion.** Undersampling means that not enough cycles are used in the data collection, with the result that the samples are not sufficiently close in the frequency representation of the data. When this happens, the result is for the bottom of the image to appear wrapped around to the top and vice versa. An example of such an artifact is shown in Figure 9-16. The cure for this is to increase the number of cycles in the data collection stage or to reduce the hardware zoom factor.

The effects of motion of the subject on the 2DFT image are complicated.

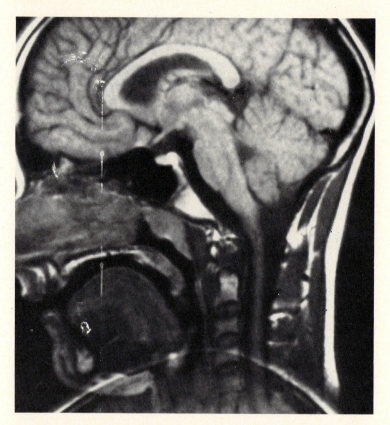

Figure 9-16. Aliasing in 2DFT images can result in wraparound of the structures in the object. (Courtesy R. Mark Henkelman, Ontario Cancer Institute, Toronto.)

However, almost all of the visible effects are in the phase-encoded direction of the image. This is because the frequency-encoding gradient is the same for every cycle, whereas the phase-encoding gradient is different for each cycle. Because the motion effect is related to the strength of the gradients and only the phase-encoding gradient changes in strength, the motion effects are visible only in the phase-encoded direction. This is sometimes useful in identifying the phase-encoding direction. It is necessary to know this because even when the image is cardiac- and respiratory-gated, motion can still produce artifacts. This is shown in Figure 9-17. By selecting the phase-encoding direction correctly, one can minimize the overlap of the artifacts and organs of interest.

SUMMARY

MRI does not produce a signal that can be directly translated into an image. It is necessary to convert from a frequency representation to a location representation. The digital computer performs the mathematics of this conversion or transformation, but it has limited resolution in the numbers with which it

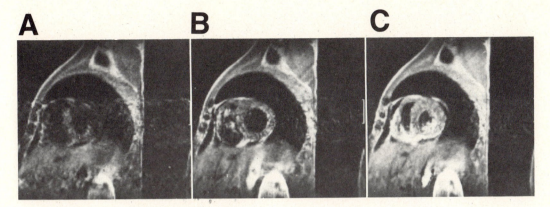

Figure 9-17. The effects of motion on 2DFT images. **A,** An ungated cardiac image. End-diastolic **(B)** and end-systolic **(C)** images of the same heart. The ungated image has very poor definition of the myocardium and prominent streaking artifacts in the phase-encoded direction. The gated images show improvement in the motion artifacts, but these artifacts are not eliminated because the motion, even when gated, causes phase errors, which mislead the 2DFT reconstruction algorithm.

works. One consequence of this limited resolution is that the data must be sampled in order to be stored in the computer.

Fortunately, if the samples are sufficiently close together, there is no loss of information. In the presence of a magnetic field gradient the NMR signal yields a one-dimensional distribution of information. The various techniques of MRI are different schemes for using this one-dimensional measurement to sample the two-dimensional image plane.

Projection reconstruction imaging rotates the sampling line about the center of the spatial frequency representation of the image. The image is reconstructed by filtering the NMR signals, Fourier transforming them, and back-projecting the filtered projections. Two-dimensional Fourier transform imaging samples a line at a time in only one direction of the frequency representation. The direction of the sampling is determined by the direction of the phase-encoding gradient. The information along this line is determined by using the frequency-encoding gradient. When the entire frequency representation of the image has been sampled by repeated cycles of the 2DFT process using different phase-encoding gradient strengths, the sampled frequency representation is converted to an image in the computer by using a two-dimensional Fourier transform.

Chapter
TEN

The Musical Score

PURPOSE OF PULSE SEQUENCES

Having dealt with the physics of NMR and the equipment needed for MRI, let us now turn our attention to precisely how an image is made from NMR signals and what the characteristics of that image are. This and the following five chapters deal with MR image production and characterization.

A pulse sequence in MRI is basically a set of instructions to the magnet telling it how to make an image. In radiography one would give a set of instructions to the x-ray machine by setting the kVp and the mAs. How those dials, especially the kVp control, are positioned influences the contrast of the resulting image. However, regardless of the kVp, the relative order of shades of gray remains unchanged; for example, bone is always whiter than soft tissue. With MRI, one can alter even the relative order of different tissues by changing the timing and magnitude of RF pulses, as seen in Figure 10-1.

In computed tomography one would specify the length of time for the scan, the slice thickness, and the reconstruction algorithm, knowing that these choices influence the spatial resolution of the image. MRI pulse sequences are analogous to the radiography and CT selections made by the operator. They specify the timing and magnitude of RF pulses and magnetic field gradients. **The RF pulses have a great deal to do with image contrast, and the pulsed gradient magnetic fields influence the spatial resolution of that image.**

In MRI as in CT, the image is digital in form, not analog as in radiogra-

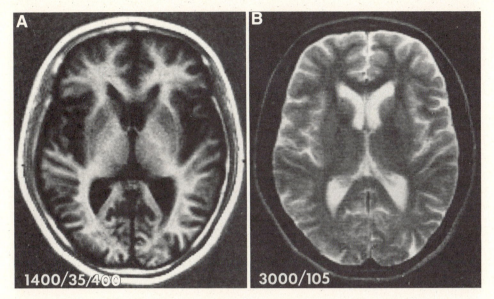

Figure 10-1. These images of the same slice in the same patient illustrate that the timing of RF pulses not only controls contrast but also can even reverse contrast. **A,** A T1-weighted inversion recovery image. **B,** A T2-weighted spin echo image.

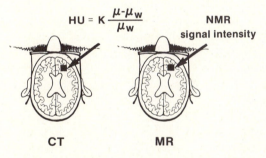

Figure 10-2. Pixel brightness in CT is determined by the x-ray attenuation coefficient, and in MRI it is determined by signal intensity.

phy. The image is essentially a mosaic of pixels, each of which has two properties, namely **character** and **position**. Character refers to the pixel's intensity or color. In a CT image, shades of gray are assigned on the basis of Hounsfield numbers, which relate to x-ray attenuation values as illustrated in Figure 10-2. By convention white is assigned to pixels with high attenuation values, such as bone, and black is assigned to pixels with low attenuation values, such as air. In MRI, the gray scale is assigned on the basis of the intensity of the NMR signal emitted by the protons in a given voxel, also shown in Figure 10-2. White is assigned to pixels with high signal intensity and black to those

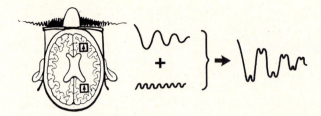

Figure 10-3. During proton relaxation a complicated NMR signal is received and computer processed to form an image.

with low signal intensity. Pixel character and therefore image contrast will be covered fully in Chapter 11. This chapter deals with position.

The pixel's position, or **spatial localization,** is determined by a complex process. When an RF pulse is transmitted into the patient, all the protons in a slice are stimulated at once. Following this RF pulse, the protons in all the individual voxels relax, emitting their radio signals simultaneously as shown in Figure 10-3. Hence the composite NMR signal is very complicated, and determining the source of all the single pixel contributions is no simple matter. Yet the computer is able to do this, provided that the gradient magnetic fields have been used in a systematic way.

RELEVANT FEATURES OF THE MAGNET

In most imagers the main magnetic field, B_0, is horizontal, aligned with the bore of the magnet. This is true for superconducting and resistive magnets but not for permanent magnets. In keeping with earlier discussions, a horizontal orientation will be assumed. Therefore, the Z axis, which by convention is parallel to B_0, runs through the center of the magnet in the direction of the long axis of the patient. Also, by convention X and Y are perpendicular to Z, with X usually horizontal and Y vertical.

The main magnetic field is very strong and is on continuously. Manufacturers go to great lengths to ensure that this B_0 field strength is not only intense but also uniform throughout the imaging volume. Paradoxically, the manufacturers also provide a means of disturbing this field homogeneity but in a very systematic and ordered way. This disturbance is achieved through the use of the paired gradient coils previously described and illustrated in Chapter 7. **These gradient coils are the key feature that distinguishes an MR imager from an NMR spectrometer.**

The gradient coils produce magnetic fields superimposed on the B_0 field that are very much weaker and that are turned on intermittently for only a small fraction of a second in pulse fashion. Each pair of coils produces a small gradient magnetic field along one of the axes. These small gradient magnetic fields add to the main magnetic field, making the latter stronger at one end of an axis than at the other. If two or more pairs of gradient coils are energized at the same time, a gradient magnetic field can be created in any direction, not restricted to the direction of an axis.

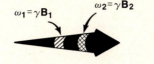

$\omega_1 = \gamma B_1$ $\omega_2 = \gamma B_2$

gradient + RF (excitation) ⟶ **Slice selection**

gradient + emitted signal (relaxation) ⟶ **Pixel localization within slice**

Figure 10-4. Gradients cause slight differences in proton-resonant frequencies, which can be used for selective excitation of a slice and for localization of protons in that slice.

FUNCTION OF THE GRADIENT COILS

The purpose of these magnetic field inhomogeneities—the gradient magnetic fields—is twofold: **slice selection and pixel localization within the slice.** The gradient coils therefore identify pixel position. The Larmor equation, $\omega = \gamma B$, says that hydrogen nuclei in a magnetic field precess at a frequency (ω), which depends on the strength of the magnetic field (B). The γ is a constant that is characteristic of a given nuclear species. For hydrogen it is equal to 42.6 MHz/T. Therefore, if the magnetic field is not homogeneous, protons in a slightly stronger field precess faster than those in a weaker field, as shown in Figure 10-4.

This fact is important for two reasons having to do with proton excitation and relaxation. First, to excite protons in an area of a stronger field, a higher-frequency RF transmission is required to match the resonance frequency of those protons. In this case, **the combination of field gradient inhomogeneity and excitation by a specific RF frequency permits slice selection.** During relaxation the frequencies of the signals emitted by the protons also depend on field strength. When the RF transmitter is turned off and the protons relax back to equilibrium, the FID of the protons at the strong end of a gradient magnetic field has a frequency that is higher than the FID of the protons at the weak end of the field. Consequently, **the presence of a gradient magnetic field during relaxation helps localize the protons within the slice that was selected during excitation.** The following is a more detailed discussion of how these gradient magnetic fields are used.

Slice Selection

If the Z gradient is on, as shown in Figure 10-5, the field strength at one end of the magnet bore is stronger than at the other. The proton Larmor frequency for a 1.0-T magnet is 42.6 MHz. A proton at the strong end may precess at 42.7 MHz, and at the weak end the precessional frequency may be 42.5 MHz. An RF pulse that is exactly 42.7 MHz excites all the protons in the plane perpendicular to the Z axis at the 42.7-MHz position on the gradient line. Everywhere else inside the magnet protons ignore the 42.7-MHz frequency, since it is not their resonant frequency. In this way a single transaxial slice is selec-

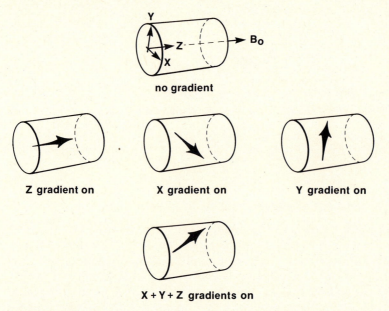

Figure 10-5. Selective excitation along the Z axis results in a transaxial plane. Excitation along the X and Y axes results in parasagittal and paracoronal planes, respectively. When all three gradients are energized at the same time, any oblique plane can be selected.

tively excited. If a gradient along the X axis were used instead of the Z gradient, the slice selected would be in a parasagittal plane. Similarly, a Y gradient would select a paracoronal plane. In fact, one could choose any plane in the body just by turning on the X, Y, and Z gradients together, as in Figure 10-5. For the sake of simplicity, all further discussions will assume transaxial slice selection, but the principles apply to slices in any orientation.

The thickness of the slice selected is determined by the steepness or slope of the gradient magnetic field and the frequency width of the RF pulse. **The steeper the gradient magnetic field, the thinner will be the slice. The narrower the RF pulse, the thinner will be the slice.** Manufacturers take advantage of both these properties for selection of slice thickness.

Pixel Localization Within a Slice

FREQUENCY ENCODING. At this point the protons in a single slice have been selectively excited by energizing the Z gradient at the same time as the RF pulse. When the RF pulse is turned off and all the protons relax back to their equilibrium state, they all give off FIDs with the same frequency, assuming the Z gradient is still on. The individual voxel contributions are all at the same frequency, so they add constructively, as seen in Figure 10-6, *A*, to make a larger-amplitude NMR signal. There is no way of determining the magnitude and location of the individual voxel contributions to the received signal.

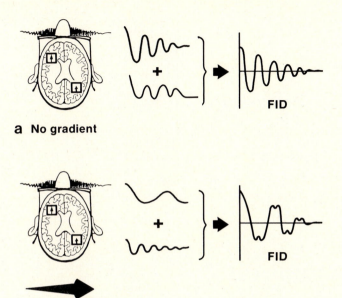

a No gradient

b X gradient on

Figure 10-6. **A,** When there is no gradient, spatial localization of the signal is not possible. **B,** With the X gradient energized during relaxation while receiving an FID, pixel localization by column is possible.

Therefore, one turns off the original Z gradient while receiving the FID and energizes the X gradient, creating a gradient magnetic field that is oriented across the slice in a lateral direction, as shown in Figure 10-6, *B*. The result is the division of the slice into imaginary columns, the width of which establishes the width of one pixel. Now the excited protons experience a different field strength at the time they give off their FIDs. Hence, because of the Larmor relationship $\omega = \gamma B$, the FIDs associated with each column of pixels have different frequencies. These add to make a very complex signal, but at least it contains some information about the source of signal contributions.

The computer uses a Fourier transformation to determine the amplitude of the contribution associated with each frequency and hence with each column in the transaxial slice. This is illustrated in Figure 10-7. The amplitude of each contribution is a reflection in part of the number of protons in a particular column. The X gradient has thereby **encoded** some positional information into the protons in the form of differences in precessional **frequency**. In this case the X gradient is said to be the **frequency-encoding gradient**. The manufacturer may choose to make the Y gradient instead of the X gradient the frequency-encoding gradient, dividing the slice into rows instead of columns.

The job of pixel localization is not finished. Because signals have been assigned only to columns, not to individual pixels, it is necessary to figure out from which rows they were emitted and thereby identify individual pixels. In-

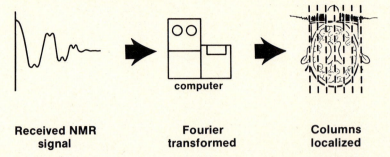

Received NMR
signal

Fourier
transformed

Columns
localized

Figure 10-7.   The FID received while the X gradient is energized is Fourier transformed to provide information about the column of origin of the signal contribution.

tuitively, one expects that turning on a gradient in the Y direction might help sort them into rows. Unfortunately, the procedure is not that simple. If the Y gradient were energized simultaneously with the X gradient, oblique columns would result with still no pixel localization, because simultaneously energized magnetic fields add vectorially to form a single field.

To determine pixel localization in this fashion, one could repeatedly excite the protons and collect the FIDs, typically 128 or 256 times, each time changing the strength of the X and Y gradients and therefore the orientation of the oblique columns. The process bears a resemblance to the translate-rotate procedure used by first-generation CT scanners. With these machines the x-ray tube would translate across the object gathering one projection of data, rotate 1 degree, and then continue translating and rotating through 180 degrees for 180 projections of a slice.

MRI is similar in that many "projections" are required, but instead of translating and rotating, one can change gradient strengths to rotate around the patient collecting projections. With CT, of course, the process is all mechanical; the tube physically rotates around the patient. With MRI the process is electronic and simply involves changing the strength of the simultaneously energized X and Y gradients during signal acquisition with each successive excitation of the protons. Early MR images were obtained by this method followed by **filtered back-projection reconstruction** as discussed in Chapter 9. MR images are no longer obtained like this but rather use the technique of **two-dimensional Fourier transformation (2DFT)**.

A similar procedure is used in the **2DFT** method of image reconstruction, except **the X and Y gradients are energized sequentially**, not simultaneously, and only the Y-gradient strength is varied with each signal acquisition. When the 2DFT methodology is used, the data acquired do not truly form a projection and, therefore, that term is replaced by **signal acquisition**. To understand 2DFT a little better, one must be familiar with the concepts of **phase encoding** and **spatial frequency**.

PHASE ENCODING.   At the end of a 90-degree RF pulse, the net magnetization

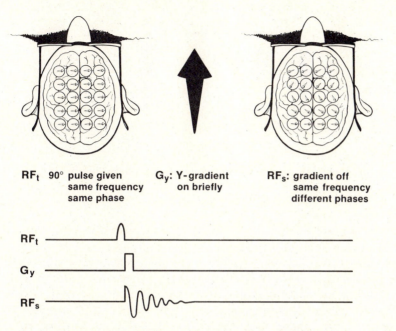

RF$_t$ 90° pulse given
same frequency
same phase

G$_y$: Y-gradient
on briefly

RF$_s$: gradient off
same frequency
different phases

RF$_t$

G$_y$

RF$_s$

Figure 10-8. After a 90-degree RF pulse, the net magnetization vectors are tipped into the X-Y plane and are in phase. During relaxation, in the presence of a Y gradient, the net magnetization vectors precess at different frequencies.

vectors of all the protons in every voxel within a slice have been tipped into the XY plane. Furthermore, the magnetization vectors are in phase; that is they are all pointing in the same direction and rotating in the XY plane at the same frequency as shown in Figure 10-8. These individual net magnetization vectors are rotating in the transaxial XY plane, which was selected by energizing the Z gradients during the transmitted 90-degree RF pulse (RT$_t$).

If a gradient is now applied in the Y direction such that the protons in the upper portion of the magnet experience a stronger magnetic field than those in the lower portion, the upper protons will precess faster than the lower ones. Therefore, the protons in a given column will no longer be in phase with each other. However, any row of protons will experience the same magnetic field strength; therefore, all the protons in a given row will be in phase with each other. The protons that are precessing faster are said to have positive phase with respect to the more slowly precessing protons.

The pulse sequence illustrated at the bottom of Figure 10-8 is the beginning of the **musical score presentation**. Prior to RF excitation, the net magnetization vectors precess with the same frequency but are out of phase. Immediately following a 90-degree pulse, all the net magnetization vectors not only precess at the same frequency but also are oriented in the same direction, which means they have the same phase. If the Y gradient is turned on for a very brief interval, the different rows of protons experience different magnetic

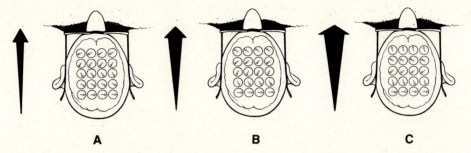

Figure 10-9. As the Y gradient is increased in intensity, the phase shift between adjacent rows increases.

field strengths during that interval. Consequently, they precess at different frequencies. Therefore, at the end of the brief interval, protons in one row are oriented in a different direction from protons in an adjacent row because they now have different phases. If the Y gradient is then turned off, all the protons will again experience the same magnetic field strength and will rotate at the same frequency. However, the different rows will still be oriented in different directions. They are now **phase encoded**. It is as if they retain a memory of that brief interval when the Y gradient sorted them into rows. If the process is repeated using Y gradients of different strength, the amount of phase shift between adjacent rows will be different, as shown in Figure 10-9.

SPATIAL FREQUENCY. The concept of spatial frequency was discussed in Chapter 9. Recall that spatial frequency is usually expressed as line pairs per millimeter (lp/mm) or line pairs per centimeter (lp/cm) and that the NMR signals are obtained in the spatial frequency domain.

The idea of representing an image in terms of spatial frequencies may be difficult to grasp. Perhaps an analogy with music will be helpful. If one listens to an orchestra playing a chord of music, one could say that it contains frequency A (perhaps piccolos) with an intensity A', no frequency B component (perhaps violas), a frequency C component (the basses) with intensity C', and so on. During recording, the orchestra sound is converted to a complex electronic signal that contains all of the frequencies represented. This electronic signal is of no use to the listener until it has been deconverted by the listener's stereo set into sound again. Nevertheless, it is a representation of the original orchestra chord.

Similarly, an image such as that shown in Figure 10-10, *D*, can be represented in terms of spatial frequencies. The image could be said to contain spatial frequency A, 1 lp/cm, with a certain intensity A', which might be very weak as in Figure 10-10, *A*. The image may also contain spatial frequency B, 2 lp/cm, with intensity B', which is stronger as in Figure 10-10, *B*, and spatial frequency C, 3 lp/cm, as in Figure 10-10, *C*, which is even more intense. This frequency representation can be converted, just as the stereo system converted

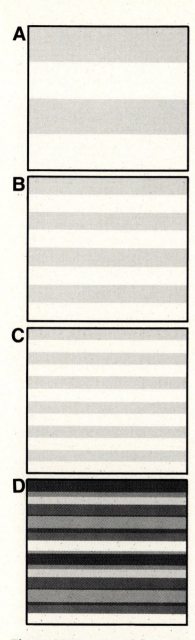

Figure 10-10.   Spatial frequencies **A**, **B**, and **C** can be combined into the composite spatial frequency image (**D**) much like musical instruments in an orchestra.

electronic signals, to reconstruct the image pattern, which is represented by Figure 10-10, *D*.

In 2DFT imaging, the purpose of the phase-encoding gradient is to isolate spatial frequencies. It is as if one could block out all of the instruments in the orchestra with the exception of the piccolos and measure the intensity of only that instrument. Then one could selectively filter out all of the instruments except for the basses and measure their intensity. One could in this way systematically evaluate the intensity contribution from each kind of instrument in the orchestra by selectively filtering all the others.

In MRI the phase-encoding gradient acts as a similar filter, selecting out individual spatial frequencies so that their intensities can be measured. When the Y gradient is set to a particular strength, it causes a certain phase relationship between the rows of protons, which effectively selects out the corresponding spatial frequency within the image as suggested by the shading in Figures 10-10, *A*, *B*, and *C*. The intensity A′ of the signal corresponding to this spatial frequency is determined. This would represent one acquisition in the imaging process. For the second acquisition, a gradient of different strength would be used to select a different phase relationship between the rows corresponding to a different spatial frequency. The intensity B′ of this spatial frequency could also be determined. This process would be repeated typically 128 or 256 times. Here it has been repeated three times, and the composite image contains multiple brightness bands or rows, as seen in Figure 10-10, *D*. In this illustration the pattern is the entire image, which can be conceived as only one pixel wide.

COMBINING FREQUENCY AND PHASE ENCODING. After the phase-encoding Y gradient has been on briefly, it has selected out a single spatial frequency, which can be conceptualized as horizontal line pairs through the image. However, this spatial frequency may be more intense in some areas of the image than in others. So far, though, the phase-encoding gradient has only been able to select out spatial frequency A. Its measured intensity represents the sum of all the contributors to spatial frequency A in the image, as shown in Figure 10-10, *A*. The frequency-encoding X gradient is then turned on to determine how the intensity contributions to that spatial frequency should be distributed into columns. Figure 10-11, *A* shows the resulting distribution for two columns, each one pixel wide. Figure 10-11, *B*, shows the resulting pattern when a phase-encoding gradient pulse of different strength is followed by the frequency-encoding gradient. If this process is repeated 256 times, 256 spatial frequencies will have been isolated and their respective intensity contributions parceled out into columns in the image. Again, this simplistic example results in an image pattern two pixels wide, as shown in Figure 10-11, *D*.

To summarize the steps so far, the Z gradient is turned on at the same time as the RF excitation pulse in order to select a transaxial slice. The Z gradient and RF are turned off, and an FID appears. During the FID, first the phase-encoding gradient and then the frequency-encoding gradient are turned on to enable the computer to assign signal intensities to individual pixels.

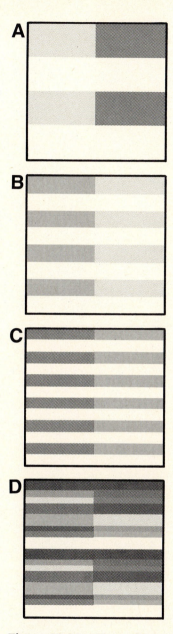

Figure 10-11. By combining frequency encoding for columns and phase encoding for rows, one can produce an image pattern such as **D**, which consists of spatial frequencies **A**, **B**, and **C**, and is two pixels wide. Typically, images with 128 or 256 rows and columns are obtained.

Partial Saturation

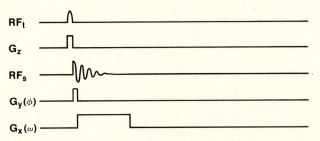

Figure 10-12.   The first signal acquisition of a partial-saturation pulse sequence.

Partial Saturation

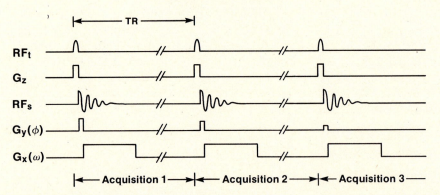

Figure 10-13.   Multiple partial-saturation projections are obtained by varying the strength of the phase-encoding gradient.

To simplify these concepts, it has been assumed in the preceding discussions that FIDs are acquired to make an image. **Actually, spin echoes must be used** instead of FIDs, as will be discussed later.

PULSE SEQUENCE DIAGRAMS

Partial Saturation

To diagram this pulse sequence, one must first indicate when to turn on the RF transmitter, specifying a 90-degree pulse. For single transaxial slice excitation, the Z gradient must be on at the same time as the RF and the frequency of the RF must be specified. A signal, the FID, is emitted immediately after the RF is turned off. If Y is chosen to be the phase-encoding gradient, it is energized briefly at the beginning of the FID. Then the Y gradient is turned off and the frequency-encoding X gradient is energized during signal acquisition before the signal disappears. Such a pulse sequence is diagrammed in Figure 10-12.

Partial Saturation

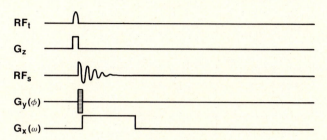

Figure 10-14. The change in intensity of the phase-encoding gradient is represented symbolically in a single pulse sequence.

Is this enough information to make an image? No, this is only one **signal acquisition.** One has to do typically 128 or 256 such acquisitions, depending on the desired matrix size. Each time a new signal is acquired, the only change is in the strength of the phase-encoding gradient, as shown in Figure 10-13.

Figure 10-14 shows a further simplification of the musical score. Because the only change from one projection to the next is the intensity of the phase-encoding gradient, this change is shown symbolically in a single rendition of the pulse sequence.

Finally, one must specify the time interval between each 90-degree pulse, called the **TR interval,** for time of repetition. It can be any length of time, but 50 to 10,000 ms would be a very generous range for clinical use. This time interval, TR, has a great deal of influence on the character of the pixels and hence on the image contrast. It also determines to a great extent the time required for image acquisition.

Question: How long does it take to make an image, assuming a TR of 1000 ms and a 256 by 256 matrix?

Answer: Scan time per slice = (TR) × (number of signal acquisitions)
= (1000 ms) × (256)
= 256 s, or about 4 $\frac{1}{4}$ min.

If the resulting image appears too noisy, one can repeat the whole sequence and combine both sets of data to make one image. This procedure is called **signal averaging.** To improve image quality, one can take any integer number of signal averages at the expense of time.

MULTISLICE.   For a 10-slice head scan, 4 $\frac{1}{4}$ minutes per slice would require 43 minutes of scan time. What could one do to reduce the time? One could decrease the TR, but because the TR is a very important determinant of image contrast, the radiologist may not want a shorter TR. Alternatively, one could cut the number of projections down to 128, but that would result in a larger pixel size, which may reduce spatial resolution unacceptably.

Partial Saturation
Multislice

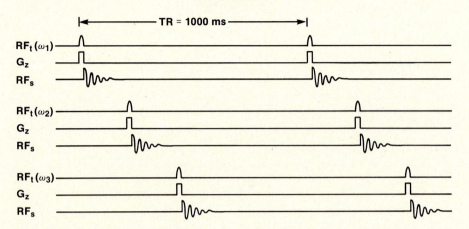

Figure 10-15. Multislice techniques are employed to reduce imaging time.

Fortunately, there is a trick for getting around this problem. One can implement **multislice imaging**. Basically this technique, illustrated in Figure 10-15, takes advantage of the long waiting time required for the specified TR interval.

If the TR interval is 1000 ms and the FID for the first projection is gone after just a few milliseconds, there is a very long waiting period while protons undergo some relaxation before the next excitation. So one takes advantage of that time by energizing the RF transmitter, using a different frequency to excite a different transaxial slice. This pulse does not disturb the first slice because the frequency is not appropriate for it. Because each slice excitation and relaxation require just a few milliseconds, the procedure can be repeated many times before the RF transmitter must go back to excite the first slice again for the next signal acquisition. In this way, a 10-slice examination can be performed in the same time it takes to complete a single slice.

Unfortunately, it has not been possible to confine the excitation process to protons in a single slice having flat surfaces without some spillover excitation of protons in adjacent slices. The significance of this problem is that when it is time to excite the adjacent slice, some of its protons have already been excited and are undergoing relaxation. Hence there is degradation of the image. To avoid the problem of slice overlap, one usually specifies a **gap** between slices. For example, one might allow a 3-mm nonimaged gap between 10-mm-thick slices.

Inversion Recovery

The inversion recovery pulse sequence, illustrated in Figure 10-16, is seldom used in clinical practice in most facilities mainly because it is very time con-

Inversion Recovery

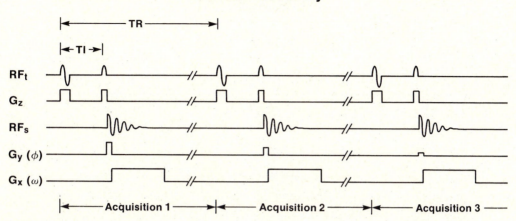

Figure 10-16. The inversion recovery pulse sequence requires a 180-degree RF pulse followed by a 90-degree RF pulse.

suming. This pulse sequence, as the name suggests, is designed to invert the net magnetization vector along the Z axis by giving the spins an inverting 180-degree RF pulse. One then follows the recovery of this vector along the Z axis to equilibrium. Because events that occur along the Z axis cannot be observed directly, it is necessary at some time to tip the net magnetization vector from the Z axis onto the X-Y plane by using a 90-degree RF pulse. This is necessary to detect the NMR signal. The time interval between the 180-degree RF pulse and the 90-degree RF pulse is called the **TI** interval, for time of inversion. As with the other time intervals, the duration of the TI interval has considerable influence on image contrast. As before, the Z gradient must be on during the 180-degree and 90-degree RF pulses for slice selection purposes. The X and Y gradients are on while receiving the FID in order to provide spatial localization within the slice. Although any time interval shorter than the TR can be used for the TI, typical durations for the TI are in the range of 100 to 700 ms.

Multislice techniques, shown in Figure 10-17, can also be used with the inversion recovery pulse sequence. However, the long TI interval severely restricts the number of slices that can be obtained during any given TR interval. For example, if the TR is 1000 ms and the TI is 400 ms, only two slices can be obtained. Therefore, a 10-slice set of images would take five times the 4 ¼-minute scanning time, which would be impractical in a clinical setting.

For instructional simplification, the pulse sequences were introduced with the assumption that FIDs are collected to make MR images. Actually, however, it is not possible from engineering requirements to perform all the necessary gradient switching before the FID is gone. Therefore, for every imaging pulse sequence a spin echo must be acquired. A partial-saturation pulse sequence is actually a partial-saturation spin echo sequence and differs from the true spin

**Inversion Recovery
Multislice**

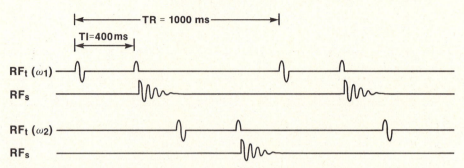

Figure 10-17. Multislice techniques can be employed with the inversion recovery pulse sequence. The number of slices is very limited, however.

Spin Echo

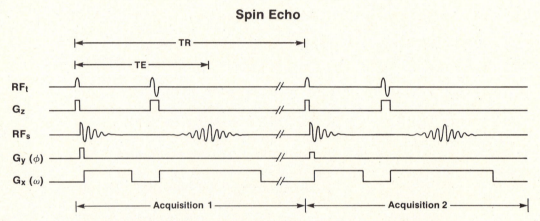

Figure 10-18. The spin echo pulse sequence requires a 90-degree RF pulse followed by a 180-degree refocusing RF pulse.

echo sequence only in that the TE is as short as possible. Similarly, inversion recovery pulse sequences are really inversion recovery spin echo sequences with very short TE.

Spin Echo

The spin echo pulse sequence, illustrated in Figure 10-18, is probably the most commonly used pulse sequence in clinical situations. To get a spin echo, one starts with a 90-degree RF pulse to tip the magnetization vectors into the XY plane. This is followed by a 180-degree RF pulse, which flips the vectors about an axis in the XY plane. After some time, an echo is formed. For the spin echo pulse sequence, as well as the other pulse sequences, echoes are the NMR

Spin Echo
Multislice

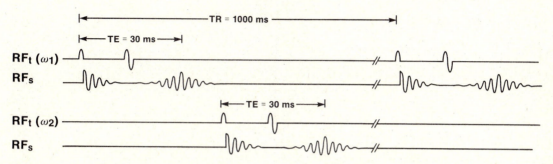

Figure 10-19.   The RF pulse sequences necessary for multislice spin echo imaging.

signals acquired to make an image. As before, the Z gradient is on during the 90-degree RF pulse for slice selection. An FID is emitted when the 90-degree pulse is turned off, but it is ignored. After a time, TE/2 ms, a 180-degree RF pulse is given. The Z gradient is on again during the 180-degree RF pulse so that only those protons that are in the slice of interest will be affected. At a time TE/2 ms after the 180-degree RF pulse the echo occurs. Measured from the original 90-degree RF pulse, the echo appears at time **TE**, for time of echo. Because the spin echoes are the NMR signals acquired to make the image, the X gradient must be on during the spin echo to encode spatial localization information.

Again, the interval from one 90-degree RF pulse to the next, the TR interval, must be specified and is important for pixel character. The other time interval to specify is the time between the 90-degree and 180-degree RF pulses. Actually, the time between the 90-degree RF pulse and the spin echo, TE, is specified, and the computer tells the RF transmitter when to give the 180-degree RF pulse. The TE interval is also an important determinant of image contrast. Typical times for TEs range from about 15 to 180 ms or, for special applications, as long as several hundred milliseconds.

Question: What is the scanning time for a spin echo imaging sequence?
Answer: Scan time = (TR) × (number of signal acquisitions) ×
                  (number of signal averages)
              = 1000 ms (256) (1)
              = 4 ¼ m

For multislice imaging, one must wait until the echo has been obtained, TE, before beginning excitation of the next slice, as shown in Figure 10-19. For TR = 1000 ms and TE = 60 ms, excitation of the next slice can be implemented after about 100 ms. Therefore, a maximum of 10 slices can be excited before time to return to the first slice.

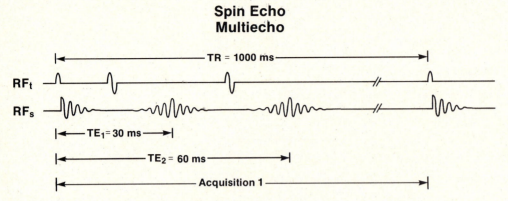

Figure 10-20.   Multiecho imaging allows the acquisition of distinctively different images formed at different echo times.

MULTIECHO.   It is often useful clinically to have images made with different spin echo times. A pulse sequence with TR = 1000 ms, TE = 30 ms, 256 projections, and one signal average takes about 4¼ minutes. It may be desirable to have another image made using the same parameters except for TE = 60 ms, which also would take about 4¼ minutes. However, by using another trick, **multiecho,** one can obtain both images in the same 4¼-minute scanning time, as shown in Figure 10-20. At 15 ms after the 90-degree RF pulse, a 180-degree RF pulse is given, producing a spin echo at 30 ms. Then 15 ms later another 180-degree RF pulse is given, resulting in another spin echo at 60 ms. The 256 30-ms echoes are collected to make one image, and the 256 60-ms echoes are collected separately to make another image. This results in two separate images with very different image contrast because of the different echo times.

Because both echoes are collected within 60 ms, excitation of another slice can begin at about 100 ms. Therefore, 10 slices can be excited within the 1000-ms TR interval. In this way it is possible to generate 20 images in the time previously required to make one. This is a very common imaging technique and has the name **multislice, multiecho spin echo imaging.** A complete representative musical score for such a sequence is shown in Figure 10-21. This is obviously too complicated for most of us to read, but then, so are real musical scores.

SUMMARY

A pulse sequence is a set of instructions that accomplishes two tasks. First, it tells the imager how to collect data in an orderly fashion so that the origin of the signals can be determined—**pixel position**. This is the function of the gradient magnetic fields. Second, it influences image contrast—**pixel character**—by specifying the timing and power of the RF pulses. Many of the parameters that must be specified in a pulse sequence, such as the timing and magnitude

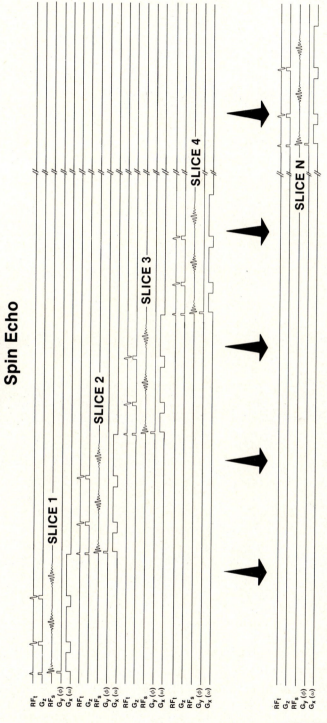

Figure 10-21. Multislice, multiecho spin echo imaging involves an awesome arrangement of RF and gradient magnetic field pulses.

of gradient magnetic fields, are included in the computer software and are not normally under operator control. However, the operator must routinely specify parameters that influence image contrast and quality, including:

1. Type of pulse sequence
2. Time intervals TR, TI, and TE
3. Matrix size (the number of signal acquisitions)
4. Number of signal averages
5. Plane of imaging
6. Slice thickness
7. Spatial separation of the slices

Three of these operator-selected parameters—time intervals, matrix size, and number of signal averages—determine the length of scan time.

There are three basic pulse sequences in use: partial saturation, inversion recovery, and spin echo. Multislice and multiecho techniques help to decrease total scan time.

Chapter
ELEVEN

Magnetic Resonance Images

WHAT IS AN IMAGE?

In the most general sense **an image is a mental picture.** It may be a **visual** image based on direct observation, such as the viewing of the Grand Canyon, or an **imaginary** image, such as the duck elicited by the sound of the oboe in Prokofiev's "Peter and the Wolf." An image can also be **abstract,** such as the famous painting by Tanner, shown in Figure 11-1. Medical images generally fall into the category of visual images; they attempt to represent real objects accurately. A brief discussion of some basic concepts of visual images will be helpful in explaining magnetic resonance images.

Visual Images

All visual images are initially detected by the eye and are due to stimulation of receptor cells in the retina by electromagnetic radiation in the visible region of the spectrum. The two basic types of receptor cells are **rods** and **cones.** These receptor cells can be considered digital detectors that are stimulated by the input of light photons. They respond to such stimulation with an output of discrete electrical impulses called **action potentials.**

    Each retinal receptor is arranged by the optical structure of the eye to be

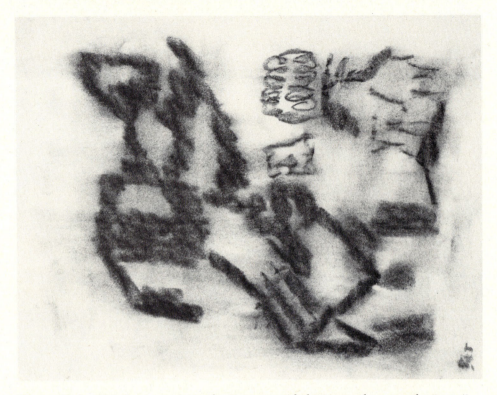

Figure 11-1. This famous painting by Tanner entitled "Stampede across the Pecos" is an example of an abstract image. (Courtesy Raymond Tanner, University of Tennessee.)

sensitive to light coming from a specific region of the visual field and to characterize the nature of that light as to intensity and color. This initial information about the source and character of light is then relayed through complex visual pathways to the occipital lobe, where the most complex processing and analysis of these data are performed, as illustrated in Figure 11-2. In the occipital lobe the myriad of discrete data concerning light impinging upon the retina is reconstructed into the perceived image. Although the final image is often considered to be a continuum of information about light, **it is initially detected, processed, and conceived as a high-resolution digital image.**

Optical Receptors

When light arrives at the retina, it is detected by the rods and the cones. Rods and cones are small structures; there are more than 100,000 of them per square millimeter of retina. The cones are concentrated on the center of the retina in an area called the **fovea centralis.** Rods, on the other hand, are most numerous on the periphery of the retina. There are no rods at the fovea centralis.

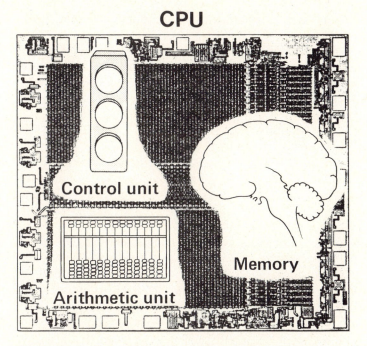

CPU

Control unit

Memory

Arithmetic unit

Figure 11-2. Processing and analysis of signals from the visual receptors occur in the occipital lobe, much like with a computer.

The rods are very sensitive to light and are used in dim lighting. The threshold for rod vision is approximately 10^{-6} mL. Cones, on the other hand, are less sensitive to light; their threshold is only 5×10^{-3} mL, but they can respond to intense light levels, whereas rods cannot. Consequently, cones are used primarily for daylight vision, called **photopic vision,** and rods are used for night vision, called **scotopic vision.** This aspect of visual physiology explains why dim objects are more readily viewed if they are not looked at directly. Astronomers and radiologists are familiar with the fact that a dim object can be seen better if viewed peripherally, where rod vision dominates.

The ability of the rods to visualize small objects is much worse than that of the cones. This ability to perceive fine detail is called **visual acuity.** Cones are also much more able than rods to detect differences in brightness levels. This property of vision is termed **contrast perception.** Furthermore, cones are sensitive to a wide range of wavelengths of light. **Cones perceive color, but rods are essentially color blind.**

The cones of the eye are color receptors of three types, each stimulated by relatively narrow bandwidths of light generally referred to as red, blue, and green. They are sensitive to **brightness** (number of light photons), **hue** (wavelength), and **saturation** (ratio of monochromatic to white light). The human eye can detect approximately 2000 different color combinations or hues compared with perhaps only 20 shades of gray.

Therefore, color images contain significantly more information than black and white images. Imaging techniques such as MRI that intrinsically contain more information are more naturally adaptable to color imaging. In a standard clinical setting when viewing a 14- by 17-inch chest radiograph at 50 cm, the eye can spatially resolve 0.5 to 1 mm, 20 shades of gray, and 1000 different colors. Optimum medical imaging should take maximum advantage of this basic physiologic capability.

Pattern Recognition

The spatial map of light that is a visual image does not have any intrinsic intellectual significance. The intellectual value of such an image is primarily dependent on the mental comparison of an image to the large library of images stored within the brain and the subsequent evaluation of the image as to its meaning.

Most medical imaging is a process of **pattern recognition,** which basically involves comparing one image pattern with another. Evaluation for similarities and differences with known patterns resulting in a "best fit" conclusion or "most likely" diagnosis is illustrated in Figure 11-3. This leads to the inescapable fact that a major factor in diagnostic efficiency is the observer's development of a large **image memory bank**, which at least partially comes from viewing many, many images.

Regardless of the intellectual significance of an image, visual images can be evaluated on the basis of **spatial resolution** and **contrast resolution.** That is, the perception and interpretation of an image are dependent on the **location** of light photons and the differences in **character** of those photons.

LOCATION AND CHARACTER

An image therefore consists of discrete spatial points, each having different light characteristics. This concept was appreciated and emphasized by a group of postimpressionist painters called **pointilists,** who painted pictures made up of dots of different colors. When viewed at close range, the dots are obvious, but at a distance they appear to merge into a continuum of space and color. Figure 11-4 is patterned after the work of a famous pointilist, Georges Seurat, and illustrates this concept. When viewed at a distance, the picture is of a picnic in the Texas hill country and elicits the psychological impression of such a real scene. When viewed at close range, the picture loses its totality, and it becomes simply a matrix of dots. Such artists called these dots points, but these dots are perfectly analogous to what we call pixels. Each pixel has a unique **location** and **character.** The location is the position of each pixel in relationship to others. The character is represented by either brightness or color or both.

Most medical images differ from paintings in what the character of the pixel means. When an object is directly viewed, the pixel character is the actual brightness and wavelength of light reflected to the eye. When a **representational image** is viewed, the pixel character still primarily reflects the light reflected to the eye, but this initial character of light **represents** or stands for

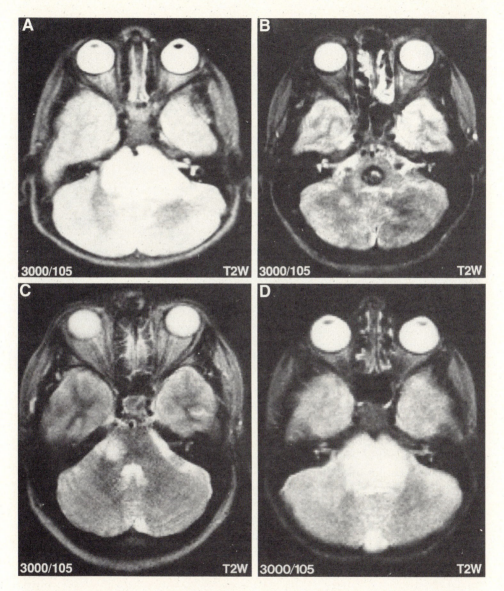

Figure 11-3.   Pattern recognition involves the mental comparison of images in order to fit the ''best-fit'' pattern for diagnosis.   **A,** Clinically unknown case with high-signal mass in brainstem.   **B,** Comparison pattern no. 1—low-signal brainstem lesion without mass. Hematoma.   **C,** Comparison pattern no. 2—eccentric high-signal brainstem lesion without mass. Multiple sclerosis.   **D,** Comparison pattern no. 3—high-signal brainstem mass. Brainstem glioma. Correct diagnosis by comparison.

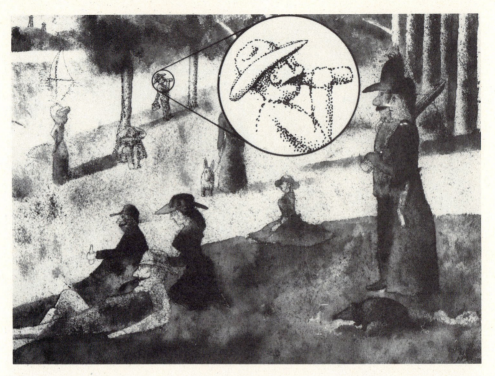

Figure 11-4. This scene of a picnic in the Texas hill country is patterned after the pointillist Seurat's "Sunday Afternoon on the Island of La Grande Jatte." It is essentially a digital image. (Courtesy Frank Scalfano.)

something else. In a realistic painting the pixel character represents the visual light characteristics of actual objects, as in Figure 11-4.

Medical images are **representational.** They represent something else; they are not realistic. They do not attempt to copy a real, directly visualized image. For instance, in the infrared images shown in Figure 11-5 the pixel character represents the radiant heat of an object, a feature we cannot see directly. Equally representational is the temperature map shown in Figure 11-6 in which the various pixels stand for the temperature of a region rather than any geographic feature. Such a representational image can be made whenever any parameter can be measured as a function of location.

Figure 11-5. These infrared images represent emitted radiant heat, which is something our optical receptors cannot detect. In **A** the image is a thermogram of a patient, and in **B** the image is an infrared photograph of the Texas gulf coast. Houston is at the top of the photo and Galveston Bay at the upper right. (Courtesy Alphonso Zermeno, M. D. Anderson Hospital and Tumor Institute, and Mike Gentry, National Aeronautics and Space Administration.)

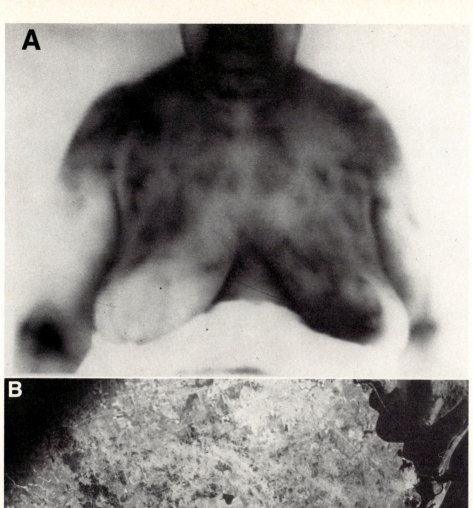

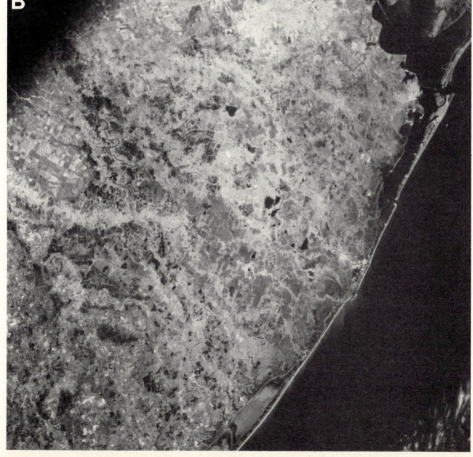

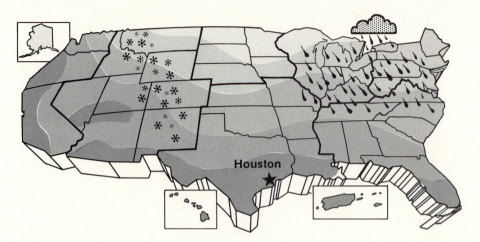

Figure 11-6. This weather map normally published in multicolors is symbolic of regional temperatures. (Courtesy *USA Today*.)

Representational Images

Medical images are **representational** because the character of the pixel does not attempt to reflect the actual visual light feature of the tissue but rather some other physical parameter that has been measured and transformed into the image. The character of a pixel can be made to stand for essentially any measurable quantity that can be spatially defined. Examples include electron density maps (radiographs), radioactive decay maps (radionuclide scans), and hydrogen concentration maps (MR images).

Another obvious difference between most directly observed images and medical images is that medical images are of the interior of a body rather than the surface. The primary clinician does the medical imaging of the surface of the body by direct observation, whereas the radiologist images the inside of the body.

Radiographic Images

Imaging the inside of the body was a major problem in early medicine. Before Roentgen's discovery of x-rays in 1895, the only way medical images of the interior of the body were made was by direct visualization. This obviously required cutting into the subject and viewing the organ or tissue of interest as illustrated in Figure 11-7. Although this type of medical imaging in the form of traditional medical illustration is still important, we usually consider modern medical imaging to mean relatively painless, noninvasive imaging of the inside of the body.

With the discovery of x-rays, it became possible to make images of the interior of the body in a relatively noninvasive fashion. X-ray images have features comparable to the representational images we have discussed. An

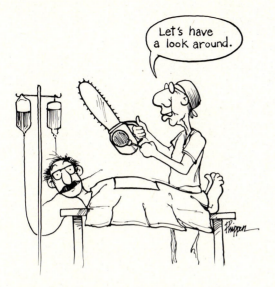

Figure 11-7.   Prior to roentgenography, the interior of the body could be viewed directly only during surgery.

x-ray image has pixels (groups of silver grains) with unique location and concentration differences, which account for pixel character or brightness.

The basic difference between the x-ray image and a direct visual image of the body is in the devices that measure pixel character, or the detectors. In the case of direct visualization, the detectors are the rods and cones of the retina. In the case of a radiograph, the detectors are the silver halide grains of the film emulsion that are sensitive to short wavelength electromagnetic radiation. The number of x-ray photons detected determines pixel character. The amount of x-rays absorbed by the body is physically determined by the x-ray attenuation coefficient, which is principally related to the density of electrons in different tissues. Therefore, a radiograph is essentially an **electron density map** of the body.

However, a radiograph doesn't relay any numerical information about the electron density such as that of the hand seen in Figure 11-8. The informed observer knows only that the blackness or whiteness on the image is related to electron density. The whiter the image is, the higher the electron density. This is very useful information, even if one has completely forgotten about the physics of x-ray interaction and electron density. This concept is used empirically to evaluate the internal structure of the anatomy. Contrast resolution among tissues is determined principally by differences in electron density. For example, bone has a much higher electron density than soft tissue and is therefore highly contrasted to those tissues on a radiograph. The evaluation of bone remains one of the main uses of conventional radiography.

Radiographs differentiate tissues from each other and therefore depict

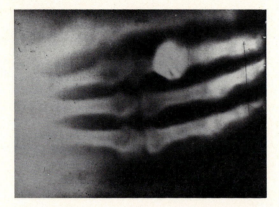

Figure 11-8.   Radiographs are electron density maps of tissue, but they do not provide numerical data. This famous radiograph was taken by Roentgen of his wife's hand. (Courtesy Deutsches Roentgen-Museum.)

gross anatomy. For this reason, the foundation of medical imaging is gross anatomy. However, radiographs can also relate pathologic anatomy by showing abnormal gross anatomy, as reflected by deformities, distortions, absence, enlargement, and reduction of organs and tissues. In addition to providing information about normal and abnormal gross anatomy, radiographs can provide some information about physiology, such as the healing of fractures reflected by calcium deposition in callus formation or the abnormal deposition of calcium in the basal ganglia in patients with hypercalcemia.

MR Images

Unfortunately, most anatomic or physiologic implications of radiographic images are indirect as **there is no intrinsic biologic significance to electron density.** The clinical significance of an x-ray image is based on the recognition of patterns from accumulated experience of empirically evaluated radiographs.

Essentially all forms of medical imaging used the substitution of some primary physical detector system other than the human visual system. The visual system becomes a secondary receptor that interprets the representational images created by the primary receptor system. All medical detector systems create a spatially defined map of the human body as a function of some particular physical parameter. Such medical images, then, are really three-dimensional images. Two dimensions define pixel location, and the third dimension, represented by brightness or color, contains information about the physical character of the tissue.

The physical character of the pixels in an MR image is itself multidimensional. The numerical value of an MRI pixel will be principally determined by the MRI parameters—spin density, T1, and T2. Secondary determinants of MRI pixel values are chemical shift and motion. The weighting given to each of these parameters can be varied greatly from one image to another depending on the timing of the RF pulses and gradient magnetic fields.

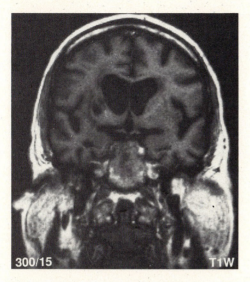

Figure 11-9. The lateral ventricles in this MR image have such high contrast from surrounding brain tissue that further pixel characterization is largely irrelevant.

IMAGE EVALUATION CRITERIA

Spatial Criteria

The primary value of pixel location is to display geometry or gross anatomy. The display of gross anatomy requires not only appropriate pixel positioning but also adequate differences in pixel character to produce sufficient contrast between tissues to allow their separation and recognition. However, most evaluation of gross anatomy is geographic and therefore relatively independent of the imaging technique. For instance, once the lateral ventricles have been displayed on an image such as that in Figure 11-9, the character of the pixels becomes largely irrelevant. The relevant factors for the evaluation of the gross anatomy of the lateral ventricles, or any other structure, are basically the geometric factors—**size, shape,** and **position.** In viewing the image, one would reference the size, shape, and position of the lateral ventricles to normal, based on one's experience.

Evaluation of the spatial aspects of an image is relatively straightforward. As shown in Figure 11-10, the specific possibilities in terms of **size** are normal, large, and small. The main classifications regarding the **shape** of a tissue are normal, intrinsically deformed, and extrinsically compressed. For instance, Figure 11-11, *A*, shows the beak deformity of the quadrigeminal plate in a patient with the Arnold-Chiari malformation. This is an intrinsic deformity, whereas the flattening of the quadrigeminal plate from a pineal tumor seen in Figure 11-11, *B*, is an extrinsic compression. In terms of **position,** the main categories are normal, intrinsically malpositioned, and extrinsically displaced. For instance, the low position of the cerebellar tonsils in the Arnold-Chiari malformation is an intrinsic malposition, usually indicating a congenital anomaly. On

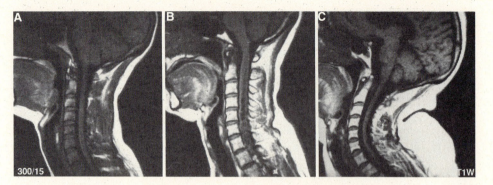

Figure 11-10.   These three spinal cord images demonstrate image evaluation according to object size.   **A,** Normal.   **B,** Large.   **C,** Small.

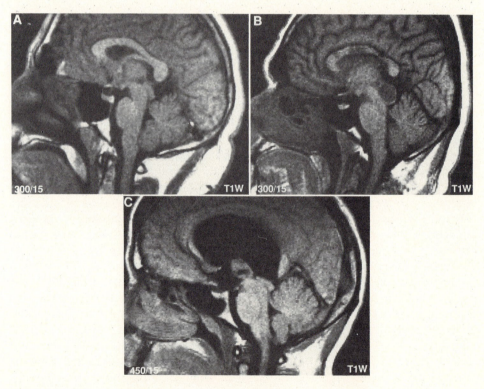

Figure 11-11.   Normal quadrigeminal plate **(A)** as compared with an intrinsic deformity (glioma) **(B)** and an extrinsic deformity (hydrocephalus) **(C).**

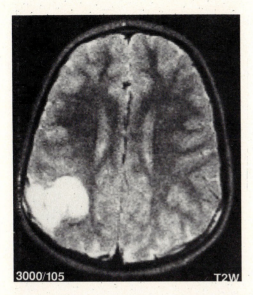

Figure 11-12.   Subjective evaluation of an image easily recognizes brighter regions than expected, as in the case of cerebral glioma.

the other hand, the caudal herniation of the tonsils from a posterior fossa mass is an extrinsic displacement, indicating the presence of a distant mass in addition to the malpositioned tonsil.

Pixel Character

Unexpected pixel brightness indicates abnormal tissue character. The significance of this is entirely dependent on the imaging technique. Pixels that are abnormally bright in the brain on a CT scan suggest either blood or calcium, whereas abnormally bright pixels on T2-weighted MR images suggest multiple sclerosis or tumor, but not blood or calcium.

As with spatial criteria of an image, evaluation of pixel character requires knowledge of what is normal. There are basically two ways to determine such normalcy. The first and most commonly used is the subjective, empirical visual interpretation of the image. In this case, one looks to see if the pixels simply appear to be brighter than expected, as seen in Figure 11-12. This technique works relatively well for experienced individuals looking at focal abnormalities. Here one references the abnormal pixel brightness of the focal lesion to the presumed normal pixel brightness of the adjacent normal tissue. If the organ is symmetric, such as the brain, the normal reference tissue does not have to be adjacent but can be in an equivalent position on the opposite side of the body.

This subjective approach is dependent on appropriate selection of pixel display values, **windowing,** and having appropriate normal reference tissue somewhere on the image. If inappropriate pixel values are chosen for display, the lesion may be excluded or windowed out of the image, as seen in Fig-

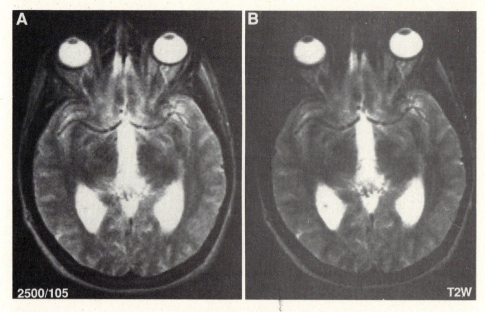

Figure 11-13.   Improper windowing (**A**, width 849, center 469) may obscure an otherwise obvious lesion such as this pinealoma (**B**, width 849, center 757).

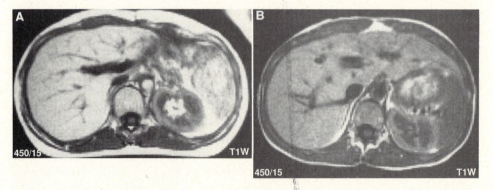

Figure 11-14.   Even with proper windowing diffuse disease may be missed because of lack of adjacent normal tissue.   **A**, Fatty liver.   **B**, Normal liver.

ure 11-13. If an organ is diffusely involved by disease, the abnormality may not be obvious even if appropriately windowed because there is no normal reference density as demonstrated in Figure 11-14.

In general, observers have more difficulty detecting a minor overall change in pixel brightness than detecting focal lesions. Despite the lack of objectivity in the empirical evaluation of images, it is still the primary interpretative skill used. This is because our visual system is extremely well designed for such analysis. It is quick and relatively inexpensive to train, and it requires little or no direct interaction between the observer and the instrument. Furthermore, more detailed, objective, or computer-assisted evaluation of images has generally not improved clinical diagnosis significantly.

Quantitative interpretation of medical images requires knowledge of pixel values. This is an additional analytic step that can slow the interpretive process and increase the complexity of instrumentation. Interpretation of the quantitative data also requires knowledge of the actual normal range of numbers for the particular examining technique. This is not necessarily required in the more subjective approach.

Obtaining quantitative data in a small portion of an image by defining a **region of interest (ROI)** is relatively easy and requires little interaction and instrument complexity. It is the most common type of objective evaluation of an image in the clinical setting.

MR Images

The significance of abnormal pixel brightness in terms of tissue characteristics is directly a function of the imaging technique, which for MR images is the choice of RF pulses and gradient magnetic fields. Therefore, for each imaging technique, the interpreter must know which pathophysiologic processes increase pixel brightness versus those lesions that diminish pixel brightness. At the subjective, empirical level, it often comes down to those lesions that appear very bright versus slightly bright versus slightly dark or very dark. With a quantitative approach, one has to know the disease processes that produce pixel values within specific ranges. In general, **lesions that increase pixel values are distinctly different from those that decrease pixel values.**

There are a number of very practical things one must understand in the day-to-day practice of MRI. Perhaps most important are characteristics of an image and how they are influenced by MRI technique. The location of a pixel is usually well defined. This capability is built into MR imagers in a semiautomatic, nonparticipatory fashion. **The gradient magnetic fields are responsible for pixel location.** Without the gradients there is no spatial definition in MRI. The operator has little or no control over pixel location. However, the operator is directly responsible for determining the character or brightness of pixels. This primarily involves the RF system.

Pixel character can be appreciated in two fashions—black and white or color. In most medical imaging black and white is used, but a color image can provide a great deal more information. In x-ray, gamma-ray, and ultrasound images, the physical information that determines pixel character can be adequately conveyed by a black and white format. An MR image can be displayed in black and white, but a color rendition may potentially convey more information.

MRI CHARACTER

A plane-film radiograph is a flat, gray image with low contrast resolution and, therefore, relatively little detail. The tissue parameter that determines brightness in this image is electron density, which varies by no more than 1% for

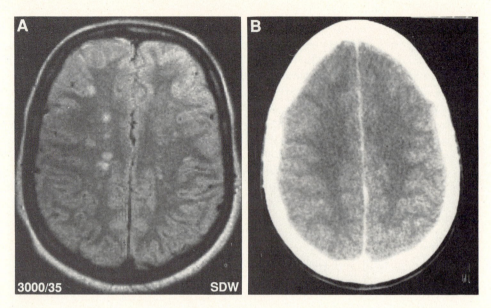

Figure 11-15. These brain images of multiple sclerosis show that the   **(A)** MR image is far superior to the   **(B)** CT image because of better low-contrast resolution.

most soft tissues. Therefore, the inherent subject contrast is very low. Radiographic contrast is improved by using grids, by employing tomographic techniques, and by injecting radiographic contrast medium.

The CT image shown in Figure 11-15, *B*, gives even better contrast resolution than a radiograph because the x-ray beam is highly collimated. This collimation rejects scatter radiation, preventing it from reaching the detectors. In the CT image of the brain, the 0.5% difference between the electron density of gray matter and white matter can just be detected. The principal advantage of the MR image shown in Figure 11-15, *A*, over a CT image is **low contrast resolution.** The anatomic location of the pixels is the same, but the character of the pixels is different. The improved low contrast resolution is due to the intrinsic differences in the tissue values of the MRI parameters. These parameters differ by as much as 30%.

MRI Parameters

The three principal MRI parameters that the MR imager detects and converts into pixel character are spin density (SD), spin-lattice relaxation time (T1), and spin-spin relaxation time (T2). Secondary parameters such as chemical shift, paramagnetic materials, and motion also influence pixel character. A complete MRI examination would include images of all of these parameters. However, such a complete MRI examination is never done. With most current imagers, chemical shift imaging cannot be done, paramagnetic materials are unnecessary, and motion imaging is a special case. This leaves us with three tissue

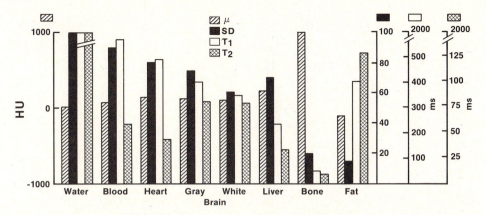

Figure 11-16. This histogram shows that the relative differences in MRI parameters for various tissues are far greater than the range of the linear attenuation coefficients of x-ray imaging as measured by Houndsfield units (HU).

characteristics—SD, T1, and T2—that MRI routinely detects to make an image. One can discuss the MRI parameters in terms of an image without understanding SD, T1, or T2 at all. They are simply MRI characteristics of tissues. With proper technique one can measure each of them as a function of location and create an anatomic map or representational image.

Figure 11-16 is a histogram of x-ray linear attenuation coefficients and the MRI parameters SD, T1, and T2 for various tissues. It is clear that the linear attenuation coefficient of most tissues is about the same. The MRI parameters, however, show a much greater variation. It is this variation of MRI parameters among tissues that results in superior contrast resolution with MRI.

Pure MR Images

Using color as an analogy, one can consider the MRI parameters as being comparable to the three primary colors—blue, yellow, and red. All color images we view consist of a mixture of these primary colors. Depending on the intensity of each primary color in the mix, all of the colors of the spectrum can be obtained. A look at the screen of a color television will confirm this. A magnifying glass may be necessary. The screen actually consists of only three types of dots, or streaks—blue, yellow, or red. Combinations of these dots produce the full-color image that we see from a distance. Regions that appear white have all their dots glowing intensely.

MR images consist of the influences of SD, T1, and T2. Pure MR images are analogous to the primary colors because they represent only a single MRI parameter. Unfortunately, in normal practice pure images cannot be obtained, but reasonably approximate pure images can be obtained by using special RF pulse sequences and sophisticated computer assistance. **Weighted images** are routinely derived, and these are analogous to color images obtained by adding the primary colors in various proportions.

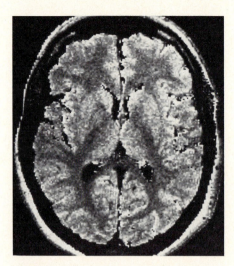

Figure 11-17.   A calculated pure spin density image.

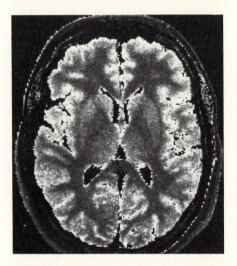

Figure 11-18.   A calculated pure T1 image.

SPIN DENSITY IMAGES.   A pure SD image is shown in Figure 11-17. In this image, pixel brightness is a function only of SD. The higher the SD is, the brighter the pixel. The gray matter has a higher spin density than white matter, and therefore it is brighter. This image shows that one can make a high-contrast MR image of the brain on the basis of spin density alone. There is about a 20% difference between the spin density of gray matter and that of white matter. That is a lot bigger difference than the 0.5% difference in the x-ray linear attenuation coefficient of CT scans.

T1 IMAGES.   Figure 11-18 is a pure T1 image. The character of the pixels is

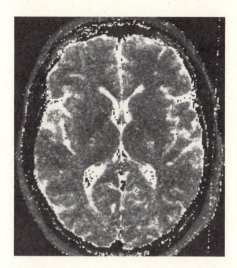

Figure 11-19.   A calculated pure T2 image.

influenced only by the T1 relaxation time of the tissue. One doesn't have to understand anything about T1 to appreciate that there is a big difference in the T1 of gray matter and that of white matter. This is a high-contrast image. The T1 of gray matter is approximately 700 to 800 ms. The T1 of white matter, on the other hand, varies from 500 to 600 ms, resulting in about a 30% difference in the T1 of these two tissues. It is this difference that produces such a high-contrast image of the brain.

T2 IMAGES.   Figure 11-19 shows a pure image of the third primary MRI parameter, T2 relaxation time. This looks significantly different from the other images even though they are all of the same slice from the same patient. You don't have to understand T2 to appreciate that there is not much difference between T2 of gray matter and T2 of white matter because there is very little contrast. The T2 of both gray and white matter is about 100 ms.

These are the three primary MR images that one would like to obtain routinely. Each of these three images is uniquely different from the others; they may only occasionally look similar and happen to have similar contrast.

WEIGHTED IMAGES

One doesn't see many MR images that are pure SD, T1, or T2 because they are not easy or practical to obtain. Such pure images may take several hours to obtain, and one can't spend that much time with each patient.

Clinically, one employs RF pulse sequences to produce images that are a blend of the intrinsic SD, T1, and T2 characteristics of tissue. When the three primary colors are blended, one gets hues that may be very pretty but may obscure original information. Similarly, such an MR image may be practical and aesthetically pleasing but may also obscure inherent tissue contrast. Such **weighted images** have pixel intensity determined more strongly by one of the three MRI parameters.

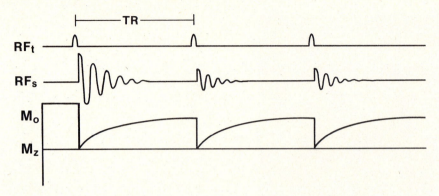

Figure 11-20. A partial-saturation RF pulse sequence is the simplest imaging sequence. FIDs following the first have lower intensity because the proton spins remain partially saturated; that is, they have not all returned to equilibrium, so $M_z = M_o$.

The RF pulse sequences that are routinely used are like color filters over a color photograph; they can hide information. Sometimes that information is not needed for diagnosis, but without it, one is never sure of the diagnosis. Partial saturation, inversion recovery, and spin echo RF pulse sequences result in weighted images. Spin echo will be dealt with more completely because it is most often used.

The following discussion deals only with the RF pulse sequences, since they determine image contrast. It is assumed throughout that the gradient magnetic fields have been pulsed properly to provide spatial localization. In certain situations, gradient magnetic fields may be substituted for RF pulses in spin echo imaging, but this technique will not be discussed here.

Partial Saturation

The partial saturation pulse sequence is the simplest of the three. It consists of a chain of 90-degree RF pulses as shown in Figure 11-20. Prior to the first pulse, net magnetization, M_z, is at its maximum value, M_o, in equilibrium with the external magnetic field, B_o. The 90-degree RF pulse rotates the net magnetization vector onto the XY plane so that M_z is now zero and M_{xy} is at a maximum value determined by M_o. Because M_z equals zero, the nuclear spins are said to be **saturated.** They recover longitudinal magnetization according to the T1 relaxation time. Because M_o is directly proportional to the spin density, the initial amplitude of the FID is dependent on spin density.

For the nuclear spins to recover fully from saturation, a TR equal to at least five times the longest T1 would be required. Clinically, this would require a TR equal to many seconds, which would result in unacceptably long imaging times. However, with a very long TR, the saturated spins would fully recover, resulting in FIDs of equal amplitude each time. Such an RF pulse sequence is called a **saturation recovery** pulse sequence, and **the resulting image would be a completely weighted spin density image.**

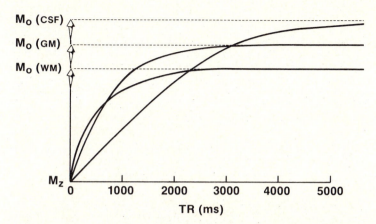

Figure 11-21. Regrowth of longitudinal magnetization, M_z, as encountered in a partial-saturation pulse sequence. More rapid return to equilibrium, M_o, occurs in tissues with short T1, such as white matter (WM). The amplitude of M_o is a function of the spin density, the gyromagnetic ratio, and B_o.

When shorter TRs are employed, as in Figure 11-20, the amplitude of the second FID will be less than that of the first because enough time will not have been allowed for full T1 recovery. The second and subsequent 90-degree RF pulses will excite already **partially saturated** nuclear spins, spins that have not returned to equilibrium, such that they will be of equal amplitude but less than that of the first FID. In a partial-saturation RF pulse sequence, the earliest FIDs are ignored.

A partial-saturation pulse sequence, therefore, is weighted by spin density but will also have a contribution from T1 relaxation time depending on the value of TR. Figure 11-21 is a graph of the return of M_z to equilibrium following a 90-degree RF pulse. Here three tissues are considered—cerebrospinal fluid (CSF), gray matter (GM), and white matter (WM). CSF has the highest spin density of the three; therefore, its relative value of M_o is the highest. It should produce the brightest pixels. CSF also has the longest T1 relaxation time, about 1200 ms. Therefore, CSF nuclear spins will return to equilibrium more slowly than GM or WM nuclear spins. When equilibrium for all tissues is reached, however, M_o will be higher for CSF, resulting in brighter pixels for CFS.

Gray matter has a lower M_o than CSF and a much shorter T1, about 700 ms. Therefore, pixels representative of GM will return to equilibrium more rapidly than CSF, but the equilibrium value will be lower. White matter has the shortest T1 relaxation time of the three, approximately 500 ms, and the lowest spin density. Therefore, WM returns to equilibrium most quickly, but its equilibrium value is least of the three.

Figure 11-21 illustrates the necessity for selecting the proper RF pulse sequence. If a very long TR is selected, the image is totally spin density weighted and CSF will be bright, GM will be gray, and WM will be dark. At a

TABLE 11-1. **Pixel appearance for cerebrospinal fluid, gray matter, and white matter as a function of repetition time in a partial saturation or inversion recovery image**

Tissue	Repetition Time		
	Very Long	Long	Short
CSF	Bright	Dark	Dark
GM	Gray	Bright	Gray
WM	Dark	Gray	Bright

TR of about 2000 ms, CSF and GM will appear equal in intensity, both brighter than WM. If 90-degree RF pulses are applied at 2000-ms intervals, the M_z of both CSF and GM will have recovered to the same value so that the representative FIDs will have the same amplitude and there will be no difference in pixel intensity. Such a TR results in a **crossover** on the time scale of the T1 relaxation curves and an absence of contrast on the image.

Another crossover appears at about 1400 ms between CSF and WM and yet a third crossover at about 600 ms between GM and WM. The crossover at 600 ms is clinically significant because it is within the clinically acceptable TR of about 1000 ms. At this crossover there will be a contrast reversal. Below 600 ms, WM will appear brighter than GM; above 600 ms, GM will appear brighter than WM. Tissue contrast is lost completely at the crossover. Furthermore, at a TR of less than approximately 1000 ms, CSF will appear darker than either GM or WM. This represents another contrast reversal.

Table 11-1 summarizes pixel appearance for various ranges of TR. **A partial saturation image made with a long TR is said to be spin density weighted; with a short TR, say less than 500 ms, it is T1 weighted.**

Figure 11-22 shows a series of partial saturation images in which pixel character is a function of both spin density and T1. There is little contrast between the gray matter and the white matter of the brain in these images. These are not bad images in terms of signal-to-noise ratio and spatial resolution, but they are poor images in terms of contrast resolution and visualization of brain anatomy. This lack of contrast may seem peculiar because the pixel brightness is a function of SD and T1, both of which differ significantly between gray matter and white matter.

This is the problem with RF pulse sequences; initial contrast information can be lost. One can view brain contrast due to SD as making gray matter bright and white matter dark and the tissue contrast due to T1 as making gray matter dark and white matter bright. They are in reverse contrast of each other. Therefore, when one makes an image that puts the two together, it's like doing a subtraction film in angiography. Positive and negative images of the brain together result in a flat image; contrast is lost. That is the case with the partial saturation image obtained with an intermediate TR.

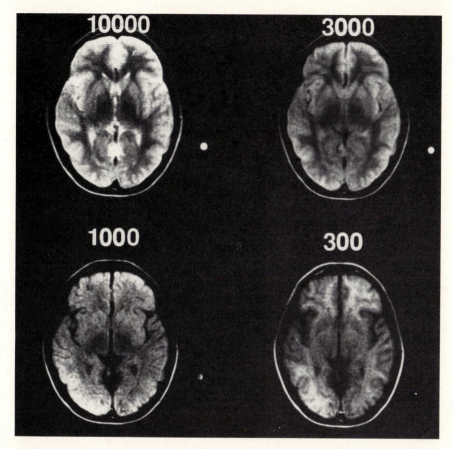

Figure 11-22. This series of partial-saturation images obtained at the indicated repetition times demonstrates contrast reversal owing to changes in SD and T1 influence.

The risk involved in doing routine MRI is that important underlying information may be lost. One must make sure that the information lost is not important. This phenomenon is not a function of the instrument, but a function of the RF pulse sequence, which is under the control of the operator.

Inversion Recovery

To expand the range of longitudinal magnetization, M_z, a 180-degree RF pulse is employed with partially saturated nuclear spins rather than a 90-degree RF pulse. As shown in Figure 11-23, the 180-degree RF pulse inverts the net magnetization vector, which immediately begins to recover to equilibrium according to the T1 relaxation time. This recovery of longitudinal magnetization is not detectable in the presence of the B_o field; therefore, an additional 90-degree pulse is needed to rotate the net magnetization vector onto the XY plane,

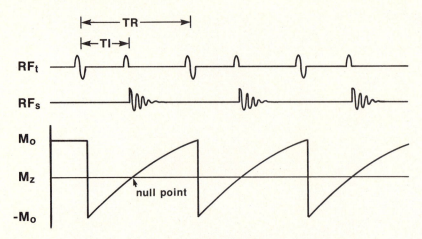

Figure 11-23. An inversion recovery RF pulse sequence consists of a 180-degree RF pulse followed by a 90-degree RF pulse. The T1 can be programmed for any time. Here it is shown occurring at the null point.

where it will be detectable. This two-pulse sequence, a 180-degree RF pulse followed by a 90-degree RF pulse, is called an **inversion recovery** pulse sequence, and it is used to produce predominantly T1-weighted images.

If T1 is very long, M_z will have returned to equilibrium, and FID amplitude will be principally determined by spin density. Such imaging times would be even more objectionable than for the partial saturation sequence. Following shorter inversion times, the FID amplitude will be determined by the SD and T1, since, as in the partial-saturation pulse sequence, the nuclear spins will not have recovered to equilibrium but rather will remain partially saturated. Therefore, pixel brightness will be a function of SD and T1. There is a value of T1 where M_z equals zero. Application of a 90-degree RF pulse at this time will result in no signal because there is no Z magnetization to rotate onto the XY plane. This value of T1 is called a **null point.**

The return to equilibrium magnetization after an inversion recovery pulse sequence follows a similar behavior to that from a partial-saturation pulse sequence, as shown in Figure 11-24. The principal difference is that the dynamic range is twice that for a partial-saturation pulse sequence, resulting in greater image contrast if the T1 is properly chosen. At a T1 of approximately 500 ms, the longitudinal magnetization of the three tissues is more widely separated than in a partial-saturation pulse sequence.

There are some problems with the inversion recovery pulse sequence. If the T1 is chosen at a tissue null point, no signal is generated and the overall signal-to-noise ratio is poor. The negative value of M_z following the 180-degree RF pulse is a problem for some MR imagers. Rather than displaying the full dynamic range of signals, such imagers display the negative magnetization as positive magnetization, as shown in Figure 11-25. This results in more cross-overs for tissues and can confuse image interpretation. To escape this confu-

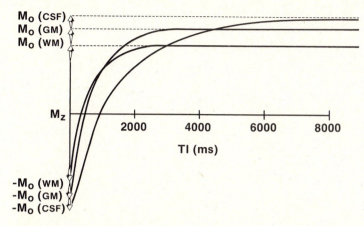

Figure 11-24. Regrowth of longitudinal magnetization, M_z, during an inversion recovery pulse sequence covers twice the range of a partial saturation pulse sequence. The result can be even greater image contrast.

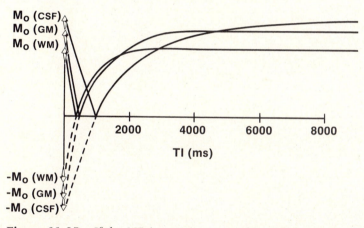

Figure 11-25. If the MR imager is not capable of displaying the negative range of M_z in an inversion recovery, image information may be obscured by reduced dynamic range and confusing crossovers.

sion, the imager must be capable of detecting the phase of the NMR signal as well as its amplitude so that contrast resolution following the scheme of Figure 11-24 is displayed. Most imagers do this.

Inversion recovery images are usually high-contrast images that are T1 weighted. Repetition times in excess of approximately 3000 ms are unacceptable because of low patient throughput. Inversion times of 300 to 600 ms are most often employed. Such long inversion times make multislice techniques more limited.

Several inversion recovery images are shown in Figure 11-26. These im-

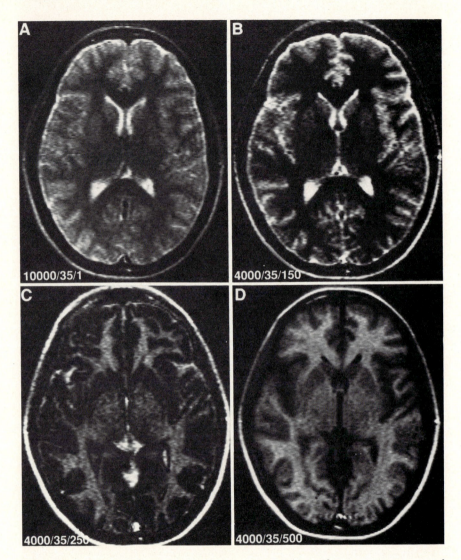

Figure 11-26. This series of inversion recovery images shows contrast reversal and null region as a function of TR and T1.

ages show good contrast between gray matter and white matter. However, a closer look at the relative intensities of CSF, GM, and WM as a function of TR and T1 will demonstrate contrast reversals and null regions. Careful prescription of the RF pulse sequence is also required for inversion recovery images.

Spin Echo

In actuality, the RF pulse sequences just described for partial saturation and inversion recovery imaging are not usually performed. As was noted in Chap-

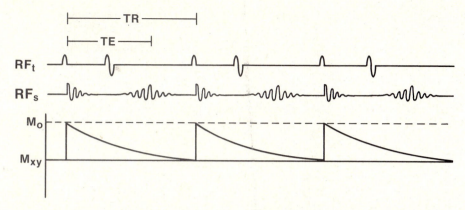

Figure 11-27. A schematic spin echo RF pulse sequence showing the received NMR signals, RFs, and the loss of transverse magnetization, M_{xy}. The actual decrease in M_{xy} is much quicker than shown here because it follows the T2* relaxation time, as discussed in Chapter 6.

ter 10, the NMR signal detected for imaging is usually a spin echo, not an FID. Therefore, a 180-degree RF pulse would follow the 90-degree RF pulses in both sequences so that a spin echo would be formed. This doesn't significantly change the analysis of an image if the time between the 90-degree RF pulse and the spin echo is very short.

The most widely used RF pulse sequence, the **spin echo pulse sequence,** generates spin echoes at various times following the 90-degree RF pulse, as shown in Figure 11-27. The 90-degree RF pulse rotates the net magnetization vector onto the X-Y plane just as in a partial-saturation pulse sequence. The FID that is formed is ignored, and some time later, ½ TE, a 180-degree RF pulse is applied. This RF pulse is called a **refocusing pulse** because it causes the nuclear spins to rephase, as described in Chapter 4. The rephased spins produce a spin echo whose amplitude is less than that of the FID because of spin-spin interactions and the resulting loss of transverse magnetization according to the T2 relaxation time of the tissue.

Multiple spin echoes can be formed by multiple 180-degree RF pulses. Each echo will be reduced in amplitude by T2 relaxation; therefore, the overall signal-to-noise ratio is reduced with later echoes. The decay curves at the bottom of Figure 11-27 plot the loss of M_{xy}, the transverse magnetization.

Whereas partial saturation and inversion recovery images are principally SD and T1 weighted, spin echo images can be SD, T1, or T2 weighted, depending on the values of TR and TE. All images have a contribution from spin density.

Consider the situation shown in Figure 11-28, which describes the T2 relaxation for the three tissues CSF, GM, and WM. As with the other pulse sequences, the initial signal intensity from CNS, GM, and WM is determined by the equilibrium magnetization, M_o, for each. Loss of magnetization in the

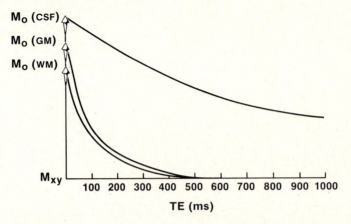

Figure 11-28. T2 decay curves for cerebrospinal fluid, gray matter, and white matter are determined by the amplitude of M_{xy} as a function of TE.

XY plane, M_{xy}, and therefore NMR signal intensity is determined by the T2 relaxation time of each tissue. Cerebrospinal fluid has a relatively long T2, approximately 1500 ms. Gray matter and white matter have shorter T2 relaxation times, both approximately 100 ms. Therefore, the CSF signal will remain intense, resulting in a bright pixel for all echo times.

If repetition times for a spin echo pulse sequence were very long, the relationship between spin echoes for the three tissues would be like that shown in Figure 11-28. Cerebrospinal fluid would always be brightest, and white matter would always be darkest. That is because with TR at least five times the longest T1, all of the proton spins have returned to equilibrium before each new pulse sequence.

Figure 11-29 shows the growth of M_z, longitudinal magnetization, back to equilibrium and the loss of M_{xy}, transverse magnetization, following a 90-degree RF pulse, both plotted on the same scale. It is clear that the loss of M_{xy} is far more rapid than the regrowth of M_z. At a very long TR, say 5000 ms or greater, longitudinal magnetization has returned to equilibrium for nearly all tissues. Subsequent 90-degree RF pulses followed by 180-degree RF refocusing pulses will result in images that are spin density and T2 weighted. At long TR, as the echo time is reduced, the image will become more spin density weighted.

If the TR is shortened, more T1 influence is brought into the image because all tissues will not have recovered to equilibrium magnetization. A review of Figure 11-29 will show how the relationships among these tissues change with reduced TR. Not only is the initial signal amplitude reduced for subsequent 180-degree refocusing pulses, but also the relative amplitudes of the tissue change. Suppose the TR is reduced to 1000 ms; according to Figure 11-29, GM will exhibit a higher initial NMR signal than CNS or WM. Therefore, GM will appear brightest on an early echo, and CNS will appear

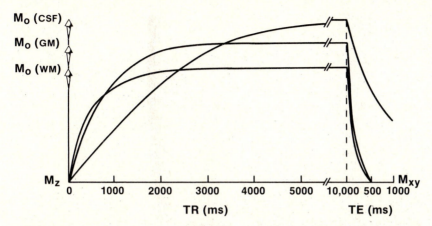

Figure 11-29. Regrowth of longitudinal magnetization and decay of transverse magnetization for a very long TR. If the image is formed after a short TE, it will be weighted by spin density. Use of long TE results in T2-weighted images.

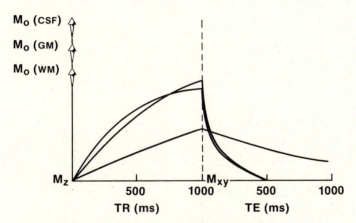

Figure 11-30. Use of an intermediate TR does not allow full regrowth of longitudinal magnetization. Images formed with short TE are SD and T1 weighted, and images formed with long TE are SD, T1, and T2 weighted.

brightest on a late echo. This is a contrast reversal resulting from a crossover, and it is shown graphically in Figure 11-30.

Suppose the TR is made very short, say 300 ms, as in Figure 11-31. Because of such a short TR, there is little growth of longitudinal magnetization, since the T1 relaxation times were too long. White matter now appears brightest on an early echo. CNS is still brightest on a late echo. These contrast reversals result from crossovers of the T2 relaxation curves.

With a long TR, long TE results in T2-weighted images and short TE results in T1-weighted images. At short TR, both long and short TE results in T1-weighted images. Short TE produces early echoes, and long TE produces

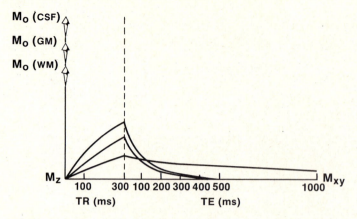

Figure 11-31. With very short TR, little longitudinal magnetization is reformed, which results in more T1-weighted images at all clinically employed echo times.

TABLE 11-2. Weighting of spin echo images as a function of repetition times (TR) and echo times (TE)

	Repetition time (TR)		
	Short (<300 ms)	Intermediate (300–1000 ms)	Long (>2000 ms)
Short TE (<40 ms)	T1 weighted	SD and T1 weighted	SD weighted
Long TE (>80 ms)	T1 and T2 weighted	SD, T1, and T2 weighted	T2 weighted

late echoes. All spin echo images have a spin density contribution. These relationships are shown in Table 11-2. Depending on the T1 and T2 relaxation times of adjacent tissues, there will be many opportunities for obscuring contrast at crossovers.

From these graphs and Table 11-2, a little thought will show that the amplitude of the spin echo from any tissue increases **as the TR is lengthened, as TE is shortened, as T1 decreases, and as T2 increases.** Stated differently, in general, **a long T1 means less signal,** and a **long T2 means more signal.**

The signal intensity of successive spin echoes decreases regardless of TR; therefore, the signal-to-noise ratio also decreases. Long TE results in a dim, noisy image. As a general rule, **short TE (early echoes) results in a T1-weighted image, and long TE (late echoes) results in a T2-weighted image.** Both images, of course, also have some contribution from spin density.

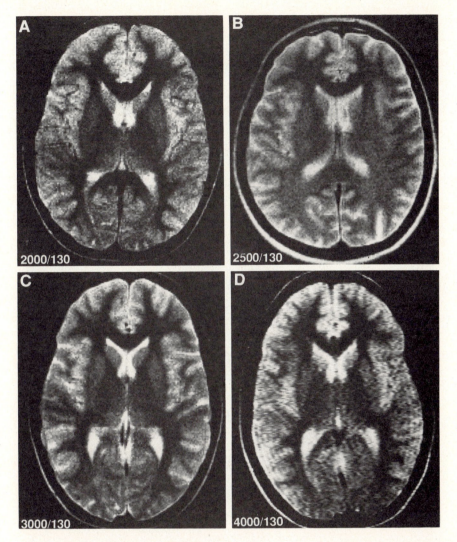

Figure 11-32.   Spin echo images produced at various TR times with a long TE result in T2-weighted images.

The spin echo images shown in Figure 11-32 represent variations of this most common imaging sequence. When considering spin echo imaging, one must specify whether the image is from an "early" echo or a "late" echo. These images were made with four different TR times, ranging from 2000 ms to 4000 ms, at a TE of 130 ms. They are all late spin echo images. Late spin echoes are viewed primarily as providing a T2-weighted image because the character of a pixel is primarily related to the T2 of the tissue. These images, however, are considerably different from the pure T2 images presented earlier. The pure T2 image was dull and had little contrast. On these late spin echo

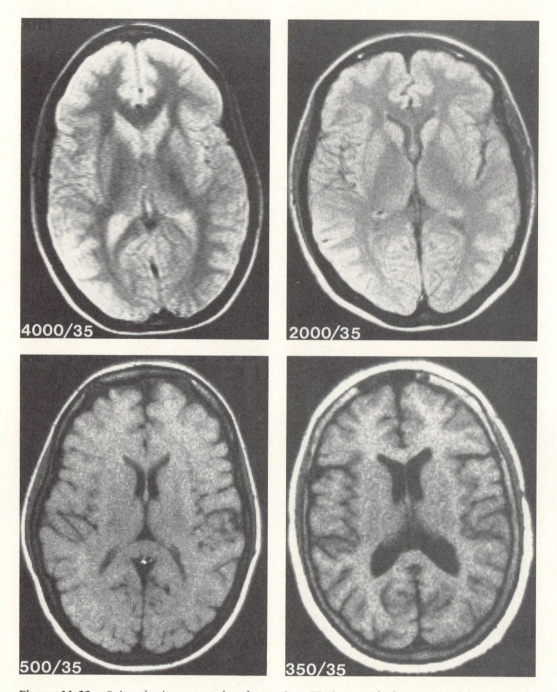

Figure 11-33. Spin echo images produced at various TR times with short TE result in varying SD- and T1-weighted images.

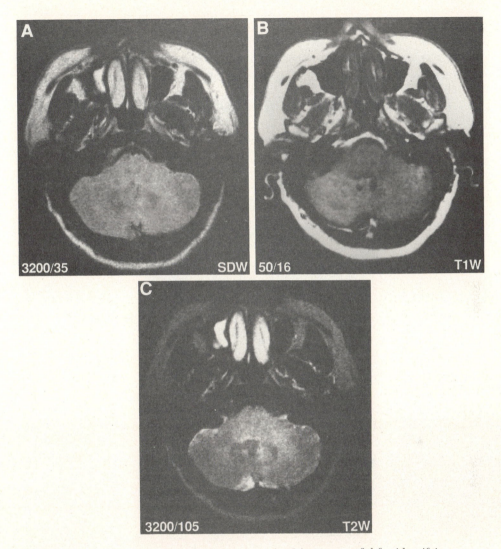

Figure 11-34. The late spin echo image seen in C is most useful for identifying pathology such as this brainstem glioma.

images, there is at least some differentiation between gray matter and white matter. Consequently, there must be some other parameter contributing to contrast. The additional factor is spin density. Spin density always influences pixel intensity. Longer TR images are brighter because of return of all tissues to their equilibrium magnetization.

These images are examples that can be used to begin planning clinically useful spin echo pulse sequences. To view normal anatomy, one would not want to do heavily T2-weighted images. Rather one would produce a spin density or T1-weighted image. Figure 11-33 shows spin echo images produced at various TR times varying from 350 ms to 4000 ms with a short TE of 35 ms. At long TR, in excess of 1000 ms, the image is SD weighted. At very short TR, about 300 ms, the image is principally T1 weighted. If the TE is made very short, say zero time, one has a partial saturation pulse sequence with a 270-degree RF pulse.

Pathology usually differs significantly with T2. Figure 11-34 shows a late SE image that does not have much normal brain contrast, but the lesion is very distinct. The contrast between normal tissues and pathologic tissues of the brain is usually due to differences in T2. Considering clinical pulse sequences, one nearly always wants a heavily SD- or T1-weighted image to show correct anatomy and a heavily T2-weighted image to show pathology.

SUMMARY

Magnetic resonance images are in the category of visual, representational digital images. They represent any one of the three MRI parameters—T1, T2, or SD—or a combination of the three. As a digital image, they are formed by pixels, each of which has location and character. The location is fixed by the gradient magnetic fields and is minimally influenced by operator command. The character refers to pixel brightness, which is due to the relative contribution from T1, T2, and SD. These contributions are determined by the RF pulse sequence, which is under operator control.

Evaluation of an MR image consists of subjective and objective criteria. The subjective criteria are those familiar to the radiologist, such as spatial aspects of size, shape, and position. The objective criteria relate to the use of the digital format of the image by windowing, highlighting, and employing the region of interest mode for quantitative evaluation of MRI values.

MR images acquired for evaluation are based on the three principal RF pulse sequences—partial saturation, inversion recovery, and spin echo. The spin echo pulse sequence is the most commonly used. Early spin echo images are weighted by spin density or T1 and are particularly good for demonstrating normal anatomy. Late spin echo images are weighted by T2 and are good for detecting and identifying pathology.

Chapter
TWELVE

Fast Imaging Techniques

In Chapter 9 the method of choice for obtaining an MR image—the 2DFT technique—was described. To implement 2DFT imaging, one samples the spatial frequency representation of the image produced by the pulsed X and Y gradient magnetic fields. The samples are arrayed on a rectangular grid, and then one converts these abstract numbers from the time domain into concrete images in the frequency domain. An alternative description of converting spatial frequency into spatial location is "inverse space to direct space." Regardless of the words used to describe them, the data sets and the images that have been Fourier transformed from the data sets are identical. Such principles can be extended to sampling in three dimensions.

The minimum time required to obtain a data set for a single two-dimensional slice is shown in Figure 12-1 for a 32 by 32 matrix. Each spin echo can be thought to provide one line of data for the image. Figure 12-1 shows 32 spin echoes; each RF is acquired during 32 incremental, phase-encoded gradients. Each echo, that is, SE1, SE2, and so on, contains sufficient information to reconstruct a 32 by 32 image. The time scale that indicates acquisition of spin echoes by 1-ms intervals is true.

The rectangular grid is formed by digital sampling of a single spin echo along the right to left, or frequency-encoded, direction under the **read gra-**

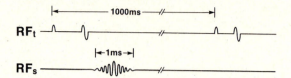

Figure 12-1. A single 32 by 32 matrix image can be obtained from 32 spin echoes acquired at 1 ms intervals with incremental phase-encoding gradients.

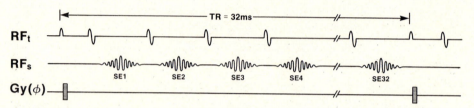

Figure 12-2. Thirty-two complex data samples can be obtained in 1 ms from a single spin echo.

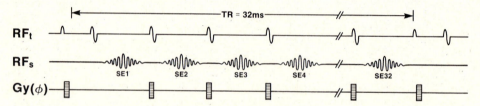

Figure 12-3. Approximately one-half minute is required to sample a single spin echo under 32 stepped phase-encoding gradients.

dient, which is usually the X gradient. During one spin echo, 32 complex data samples are acquired in 1 ms. Thus, as seen in Figure 12-2, the sampling of a spin echo in this read dimension requires very little time, 1 out of 1000 ms, during image formation. The second dimension, the phase-encoding gradient, which is usually the Y gradient magnetic field, is not as forgiving. Lines of data in the rectangular grid are acquired one at a time and in the interval TR. More often than not, TR is chosen to be approximately 1000 ms, and the rectangular grid is sampled for 32 Gy-stepped gradient values. Consequently, as shown in Figure 12-3, the total time for this sampling is 32 × TR, or 32 × 1000 ms, or approximately 0.5 m.

This illustration relates only the properties of SE1 obtained under the 32 Gy gradients. It does not show SE2 through SE32, which would be used to improve the efficiency of data collection.

Thus, one can see that 2DFT MR image formation is somewhat time consuming. How can this process be shortened? Recall the evolution of CT from a first-generation image that required 5 minutes to acquire as opposed to current scan times of less than 5 seconds. MRI is undergoing a similar evolution.

There are several reasons for reducing imaging time. One factor is the inevitable human need to accomplish any chore as quickly as possible. High-speed medical imaging offers several additional advantages for the patient.

1. It is neither convenient nor pleasant to lie motionless for a 1-hour examination.
2. In many instances, trauma patients cannot spare even 10 to 15 minutes for such an examination.
3. Patients with certain conditions such as tremors or nervousness can cooperate for only short periods of time.
4. Even a cooperative patient cannot consciously halt motion effects as a result of cardiovascular functions, peristalsis, and respiration.
5. Faster methods may produce more information in less time.

In summary, many indications for decreased imaging times have led to the invention of very clever MRI techniques.

STRATEGIES

One feature of fast MRI techniques that must be honored requires that **the number of data points must be equal to the number of pixels in the finished image.** That is, a 32 by 32 image will result from a 32 by 32 data set, a 128 by 128 image from a 128 by 128 data set, and so on. **When making a silk purse from a sow's ear, the purse can be no longer than the sow's ear!**

Performance times can be shortened for any given TR by sampling only part of the data set and providing bogus data for the remainder of the data set. Examples of two such methods follow.

Zero Substitution Method

One should sample 256 acquisitions in the frequency-encoded direction and 128 in the phase-encoded direction and then fill out the data set to 256 by 256 with zeros. This data acquisition requires only one half the time. However, as with every benefit, there is a cost. The spatial resolution in the phase-encoded direction is not as good as it is with 256 phase-encoded data acquisitions. This degradation of image quality owing to the reduced sampling usually does not necessarily interfere with the efficacy of the MR image interpretation and diagnosis. The radiologist must rely on his or her medical knowledge to make this determination.

Half Fourier Method

As before, one should sample one half of the 256 phase-encoded acquisitions or 128 data sets and then take advantage of a rigorous mathematical fact that permits us to construct the missing 128 acquisitions from the observed 128 acquisitions. When done correctly, the 256 by 256 data set made up of one half of observed data and one half of simulated data is mathematically equivalent to the full data set that would have been observed. The mathematical rendering of this process, the half Fourier method, is found in more rigorous texts.

Because the data acquisition requirements are cut in half, both methods are twice as fast as the conventional method. The obvious benefit is speed; where is the cost? In the second example, cost is subtle but real. The amount of noise in the processed image is greater because noise in the 128 observed acquisitions is mathematically carried into the 128 simulated acquisitions. In some cases, the degradation in image quality is excessive; therefore, this **half Fourier method** has not achieved great acceptance.

RF PULSE TIMING

The quality of an image is dictated principally by the signal-to-noise ratio of each data acquisition. Performance time is set by the signal-to-noise ratio per unit time. In other words, the more signal that can be gathered in any period of time, the better. Consider the case of 32 by 32 data acquisitions at a TR of 1000 ms. When signal is gathered for 1 ms in the frequency-encoded direction every 1000 ms, only 0.1% of the time is spent on observation and 99.9% of the time is spent waiting, as previously shown in Figure 12-2. Efficiencies can result by using this 99.9% of the time constructively.

One way of using this slack time is to obtain data for other selectively excited slices in the region of interest, as was described in Chapter 10. This interleaving or **multislice** signal acquisition scheme allows up to 20 slices to be collected in a single 1000-ms TR acquisition. This increased efficiency is beneficial, but it does not reduce the total time required. Simultaneous multislice is not considered a fast method, as are the other methods described in this chapter.

Very Short TR Repetition Times

One obvious time efficiency can occur if TR is shortened, say to 10 ms. For example, if a 32 by 32 rectangular grid is sampled in 3.2s, the data are acquired during 10% of this time, which is equivalent to 1 ms per spin echo. Such an obvious temporal savings must have a cost. The penalty is levied by T1 relaxation. For short TR, the nuclear spins become saturated, and the signal level is severely reduced. A 3.2-s image will appear quite dim, noisy, and of low contrast, when the only method of obtaining a 3.2-s image is by shortening TR. However, as developed in Chapter 6, the RF tip angle is an important experimental variable. A low tip angle, as shown in Figure 12-4, say 1 to 5 degrees, produces little saturation and permits the observation of more signal during short TR sequences. Repeated 90-degree tip angles destroy the intensity of subsequent spin echoes, whereas repeated 5-degree tip angles form spin echoes of less intensity, but they remain constant.

Recall that images are made from spin echoes, and spin echoes are generated by 180-degree RF pulses. The effect of the 180-degree RF pulse on a spin system excited by a low-tip-angle RF pulse is a disaster for the spin system. The spin system is inverted with respect to the Z axis after the first 180-degree RF pulse and is **partially phase coherent.** The spin system is then reinverted by the second 180-degree RF pulse and is even less phase coherent, and this process continues. The result is chaos because of the indiscriminate mixing of M_z and M_{xy}, and the image shows it.

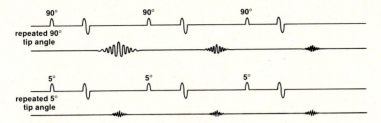

Figure 12-4. Shallow-tip angles result in less intense spin echoes; however, the spin echoes exhibit constant intensity.

Fortunately, there is an alternative strategy for forming a spin echo called **gradient magnetic field refocusing.** In this alternative scheme, a magnetic field gradient is used to refocus the excited-phase coherent spins. The result is similar to that of refocusing with an RF pulse because an echo is formed. However, using a magnetic field gradient creates an effect different from that of refocusing with an RF pulse–**the magnetization M_z is unaltered.** This difference is experimentally important and is the real basis for the low-tip-angle excitations, as seen in Figure 12-4.

The refocusing pulse of the gradient magnetic field can be made fast enough to generate spin echoes at 1 ms and to use TR times of only 10 ms. Thus a 256 by 256 data set can be acquired in only 2.56s.

Multiple Echoes and the Single Image

Still another way to achieve a high density of sampling invokes the properties of a conventional image with multiple spin echoes. When a string of 180-degree RF pulses is applied, it is possible to generate and sample 32 spin echoes in 32 ms. From these 32 echoes, 32 unique T2-weighted images can be constructed, and the imaging time is still 32 × TR. However, when each echo is preceded by a phase-encoding gradient, there is sufficient information to create an image formed in 1/32 of the total time, or only 1 s for a 32 by 32 matrix at a TR of 1000 ms.

Too good to be true! Even the most experienced, highly educated user cannot readily assign pixel intensities to SD, T1, and T2 and then sort their effects. The 32 echoes are modulated not only by the phase-encoding gradient but also by the T2 relaxation time. The result is a confusion of T2 in such a fashion that the familiar image contrast rules described in Chapter 11 may fail.

A Combination of Events

It should now be clear that a refocused spin echo from a gradient magnetic field formed at TE = 1 ms can be refocused every 1 ms thereafter. This gives rise to a possible train of up to 32 echoes in 32 ms. When 32 acquisitions per echo are taken, a data set for a 32 by 32 image can be obtained in 32 ms. The RF pulse sequence diagram is shown as Figure 12-5. Indeed, several investigators have perfected this technique, named it **planar spin echo,** and obtained 32 by 32 pixel images in as little as 30 ms. Not surprisingly, a single 30-ms

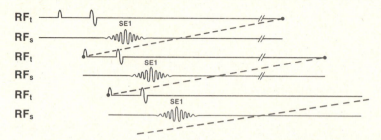

Figure 12-5. Spin echoes can be formed at 1-ms intervals with gradient magnetic field refocusing. In the scheme shown here, data for a 32 by 32 matrix image are acquired in 32 ms.

echo is splotchy, or **pixelated,** and noisy. Still, acquisition of several such echo planar images with summation results in interesting but acceptable images. One especially unusual result is obtained when the 30-ms snapshots of the heart are synchronized with the cardiac cycle and fused into a cine loop. The eye sees past the pixelation and low resolution while viewing the dynamics of a beating heart.

NOMENCLATURE

MR imager manufacturers have been very clever in naming their fast imaging techniques to convince the prospective buyer or user that theirs is the most advanced. General Electric has **GRASS** (Gradient Refocused Acquisition in the Steady State). Phillips terms its technique **FAME** (Fast Acquisition Multiphase Echo). Siemens uses **FLASH** (Fast Low Angle Shot) and **FISP** (Free Induction Steady State Precision) to describe its fast imaging techniques. Picker also has two acronyms—**MAST** (Motion Artifact Suppression Technique) and **STIR** (Short Tau Inversion Recovery). Diasonics uses **PFI** (Partial Flip Imaging) and **AFI** (Advanced Fourier Imaging) for its fast imaging pulse sequence. Each of these fast techniques is a subtle application of small tip angles and gradient refocusing.

The use of acronyms to describe such proprietary imaging sequences is not original. It most likely is an extension of some earlier terms used by NMR spectroscopists. There are Driven Equilibrium Fourier Transformation (**DEFT**) and InterNuclear Excitation Population Transfer (**INEPT**). The forerunner of them all is attributed to John Waugh and Alex Pines and is also an anagram of ''Pines''—**P**roton **E**nhanced **N**uclear **I**nduction **S**pectroscopy.

SUMMARY

MR images can be acquired as fast as 30 ms by application of very clever RF and gradient magnetic field pulsing techniques. The images are noisy but acceptable for some purposes such as cine MRI. The pulsing techniques involve simulation of signal acquisition from a sample of signals and the use of small tip angles of the net magnetization vector. Improvements are being made regularly, and the best is yet to come.

Chapter
THIRTEEN

MRI Anatomy: Central Nervous System

One principal advantage of MRI is its ability to image directly in any orthogonal plane—for example, transaxial, coronal, or sagittal (Figure 13-1). Imaging in any desired oblique plane is likewise possible. Regardless of plane, all MR images are presented as thin slices similar to those of computed tomography without superimposition of overlying and underlying tissues. Unlike CT images, however, MR images are obtained directly from the acquired NMR signals rather than reconstructed from stacked transaxial images.

The purpose of this and the next two chapters is to introduce the diverse planaranatomic views available with MRI. When images in planes other than the transaxial are obtained, a three-dimensional appreciation of normal anatomy is made easier. For example, the transaxial views through the head shown in Figure 13-2 afford excellent visualization of midbrain and brainstem. However, the sagittal images of the same area seen in Figure 13-3 show the anatomy to much better advantage. Generally, anatomic areas or organs that are symmetric about an axis, such as midbrain, are optimally demonstrated by imaging planes either perpendicular or parallel to their long axis.

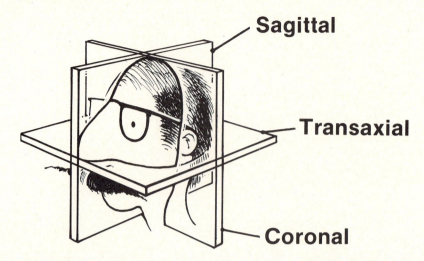

Figure 13-1.   Standard anatomic planes. These planes apply to all body regions.

TABLE 13-1.   RF pulse designation of the American College of Radiology

Pulse Sequence	RF Pulse Times
Partial saturation	TR
Inversion recovery	TR/TE/TI
Spin echo	TR/TE

Each image presented here is annotated in the lower left with RF pulse times according to the convention adopted by the American College of Radiology. This convention is identified in Table 13-1. The images are also annotated in the lower right according to whether they are principally T1 weighted (T1W), T2 weighted (T2W), or spin density weighted (SDW). This nomenclature is continued in the text also.

In these chapters on multiplanar imaging, adult tissue characteristics are reported in tabular form under each specific anatomic area. These tables are somewhat arbitrary in dividing the scale into five subdivisions of signal intensity: white (greatest signal), light gray, gray, dark gray, and black (least signal). At the end of each chapter is an atlas of images designed principally to demonstrate anatomy.

BRAIN

From its outset, MRI has been most useful in examination of the central nervous system (CNS), primarily because of its superior contrast resolution. In-

TABLE 13-2.   MRI tissue appearance of adult brain

Tissues	SDW	T1W	T2W
Fat	Light gray	White	Gray
White matter	Gray	Light gray	Dark gray
Gray matter	Light gray	Gray	Gray
CSF	Gray	Black	White

flammatory reactions, most neoplasms, ischemic changes, degenerative processes of the white matter, hemorrhage after the first 1 to 2 days, and many other conditions are more easily detected and defined by MRI than by any other technique. The normal tissue characteristics of the brain are shown in Table 13-2.

Many anatomic structures previously invisible to other imaging techniques are now easily defined by MRI. Many cranial nerves, for example, can be followed throughout their course (Figures 13-4 and 13-7). Several gray matter nuclei such as the substantia nigra, red nucleus, and dentate nucleus can now be directly visualized. This is accomplished not only by using different imaging planes but also by exploiting the excellent soft-tissue contrast between brain tissues (Figure 13-2).

MRI pulse sequences can be tailored to accentuate specific areas or structures in question. The cerebrospinal fluid (CSF) can be caused to appear white in order to outline various contiguous surfaces or structures within the cisterns and fissures (Figures 13-6 and 13-9). Gray and white matter contrast can be optimized by using tailored inversion recovery or spin-echo RF pulse sequence. Small structures such as the cranial nerves can be seen best by making thin sections at the optimal viewing angle.

With the use of a rapid spin-echo RF pulse sequence, the T1W images seen in Figure 13-7 provide excellent contrast between black CSF spaces and adjacent gray parenchymal tissues. The white matter is considerably brighter than the gray matter. On the T2W images of Figure 13-6, the relative brightness of these three tissues reverses with the CSF signal being bright and the parenchymal tissue a medium to darker gray. The white matter is now darker than the gray matter. With heavily T2W images, the contrast between gray and white matter is minimal. The SDW images of Figure 13-2 show a gray and white matter contrast, but the CSF signal is usually isointense with or slightly brighter than the brain parenchyma. The addition of an SDW image requires little time when it is included in the standard T2W imaging sequence, so the combination is considered a useful imaging protocol.

The flowing blood of the arteries and veins usually produces a signal void within the vessels on both T1W and T2W images (Figures 13-5 and 13-6). This and other flow effects such as the normal signal void within the aqueduct of Sylvius are complicating factors in image interpretation.

Transaxial views are usually best for evaluating abnormal signal or morphology in the telencephalon and diencephalon (Figures 13-2, 13-5, 13-6, and 13-7) Figures 13-8 and 13-9 show that coronal and sagittal views are particularly suitable for evaluating skull base and cranio-vertebral junction. The coronal images allow evaluation of right and left symmetry, whereas midsagittal views show the midline structures to best advantage.

White Matter

Except for the corpus callosum and fornix, the major white matter tracts of the telencephalon and diencephalon are best demonstrated on the transaxial (Figures 13-5 to 13-7) and coronal (Figure 13-8) views. The centrum semiovale is seen in these planes, and the cortical gray matter and the lateral ventricles are on either side of it for contrast. The white matter fibers can be seen coursing inferomedially toward the internal capsule and the corpus callosum on coronal views. The corpus callosum is demonstrated in cross section on coronal views. The internal capsules are bordered by the basal ganglia and thalamic islands of gray matter. They are shown on either the T1W image (Figure 13-2) or the SDW image (Figure 13-5). The corpus callosum and fornix are also visible on sagittal images (Figure 13-9). The white matter tracts within the midbrain and brainstem are better delineated when transaxial views are used.

Gray Matter

The typically gyriform configuration of the cortical gray matter can be seen throughout the brain when various orthogonal planes are used. Figures 13-2 and 13-8 show that the gray matter nuclei within the central portions of the brain are easily distinguished from surrounding white matter. The insula can be demonstrated with great clarity owing to the marked contrast with adjacent cerebral white matter medially and CSF in the sylvian fissure laterally. The substantia nigra, red nucleus of the midbrain, and dentate nucleus of the cerebellum have heretofore been invisible to nonsurgical imaging techniques. With MRI they are outlined by the white matter tracts that surround them.

MIDBRAIN AND BRAINSTEM

Important features of the midbrain and brainstem are demonstrated with all three orthogonal views. Most examinations should include transaxial and sagittal planes. The surrounding CSF affords excellent delineation of various parenchymal contours. The prepontine basilar cisterns delineate the anterior aspect, and the aqueduct, quadrigeminal plate cistern, and fourth ventricle outline the posterior portions. The perimesencephalic cisterns and various posteriorly running vessels provide excellent contrast along the lateral borders. Many of the cranial nerves that originate in this area can be visualized as they pass from the brainstem through the basilar cisterns.

The normal cranial nerves II, III, V, VII, and VIII can be seen routinely and abnormalities in contour or signal characteristics detected with proper planar selection. The optic (II) and trigeminal (V) nerves can be seen in all three orthogonal views. The oculomotor (III) nerve is best delineated with coronal views or on sagittal images near midline. The facial (VII) and acoustic (VIII) nerves are defined on both transaxial and coronal views. They can be followed in their entire length from the cerebellopontine angle cistern into the internal auditory canal of the petrous bone and to the middle ear. Absence of the artifacts from the petrous bones often seen in CT favors use of MRI in this region and throughout the posterior fossa.

The arteries that compose the circle of Willis and their branches are best demonstrated with transaxial imaging and with an SDW or a T2W pulse sequence. These sequences provide the necessary contrast between the signal void of the vessels and the surrounding CSF spaces. These arteries and many of the venous structures can be used for landmarks as in angiography.

The pituitary gland and infundibulum should be imaged with the coronal view (Figure 13-8) and the sagittal view (Figure 13-3). The pituitary gland is surrounded by sphenoid sinus air, clivus high-signal marrow fat, and CSF. The internal carotid arteries also provide a dark lateral border for the pituitary fossa as they traverse the parasellar region. The pituitary infundibulum is routinely seen as a rather bright gray structure in the dark CSF of the suprasellar cistern. This and other small bodies of the midbrain and diencephalon, such as the colliculus, mamillary body, and pineal gland, are shown on T1W images by the dark CSF outlining their contours.

Cerebellum

The various deep fissures and lobulations of the cerebellum are easily shown using either dark CSF or bright CSF contrast to outline their contours. Coronal and sagittal images are frequently best for displaying the cerebellar structures. Transaxial views allow one to follow the white matter tracts from their origin to the brainstem via the cerebellar peduncles. The sagittal plane is optimal for delineating the cerebellar vermis as well as the tonsils and their relationship to the foramen magnum.

Like no prior technique, MRI has shown the variability of the inferior extent of the tonsils. Tonsilar herniations and other abnormalities at the craniovertebral junction are best shown on sagittal view. The high signal from marrow fat within the clivus and inferior occipital bone defines the borders of the foramen magnum.

Cerebrospinal Fluid

The CSF within the various sulci, cisterns, and ventricles provides excellent contrast for outlining many important CNS structures. CSF signal characteristics can be manipulated by use of different RF pulse sequences to produce either positive or negative contrast with adjacent structures. T2W images such as those in Figure 13-6, which produce white CSF, are usually more sensitive to pathologic processes of the brain and are thus frequently used.

The lateral ventricles are best seen on coronal and transaxial images. All three orthogonal planes are useful in evaluating the third ventricle and its surrounding structures. The lateral margins are best demonstrated by transaxial and coronal imaging, whereas the roof and floor are best visualized with sagittal and coronal imaging. The massa intermedia of the thalamus can be seen in Figure 13-3, *B* dividing the third ventricle on sagittal images, which also display the various recesses of the third ventricle.

The aqueduct of Sylvius is routinely visible in its total extent on midline sagittal views, enabling detection of subtle morphologic changes of the tegmentum anteriorly and tectal plate posteriorly and superiorly. The aqueduct and the small amount of gray matter surrounding it can be shown in cross section on transaxial views. One normally sees a signal void within the aqueduct, even on T2W images, when other CSF spaces are white because of rapidly alternating flow of CSF through this narrow channel. Motion artifact from this and other pulsatile CSF flow sometimes produces apparent abnormal signal within the midbrain or upper pons, which can be corrected in part by cardiac gating.

The fourth ventricle is seen as a triangular midline structure in the sagittal plane, and the anatomic relationships of the floor and roof are well depicted. It can also be seen in cross section on transaxial view as on CT images.

ORBIT

The transaxial and coronal planes have become widely accepted as the standard orientations for viewing the orbit. These provide longitudinal and cross-sectional images of most of the important structures. Transaxial images of the optic nerve and chiasm sometimes include high signal from ethmoid mucosa or from the skull base per se as a result of a partial volume effect. This signal can mimic pathologic conditions of the nerve and is usually avoided by use of coronal views, which differentiate these structures better (Figure 13-8, *A*).

Orbital structures can be delineated with tailored RF pulse sequences and appropriate surface coils if the eye is immobilized. The orbits are encased in a bony shell that usually contains little marrow and therefore delimits the bright intraorbital fat with a black cortical border. The various structures of the orbit are gray silhouettes within the background of bright fat on T1W images (Figure 13-7).

The vitreous and aqueous humors of the globe are similar to other fluids and are thus dark on T1W images but very bright on heavily T2W images. The choroid and retina have a higher signal intensity than the more fibrous sclera and can usually be defined if the patient can avoid eye movement. The lens is brighter than the humors on T1W images and darker on T2W images. The lacrimal gland is also visible.

HEAD AND NECK

The head and neck comprise many tissues, whose characteristics are shown in Table 13-3. The transaxial plane, as seen in Figures 13-10 and 13-11, is excellent for MRI of the head and neck. Direct sagittal and coronal views are also helpful.

TABLE 13-3. MRI tissue appearance of head and neck

Tissues	SDW	T1W	T2W
Fat	Light gray	White	Gray
Muscles	Gray	Gray	Dark gray
Thyroid	Gray	Gray	Dark gray
Cartilage	Light gray	Light gray	White

The scalp with its subcutaneous fat exhibits a bright signal on both T1W and T2W images. Cortical bone, the next layer, appears black. The thickness of the diploic spaces is quite variable. It usually shows as a bright curvilinear strip because of the contained fatty marrow and the slowly flowing blood located between the black cortical bone of the outer and inner tables.

The neck muscles are usually outlined by high signal intensity of the fat that lies between muscle groups. The low-intensity signal of airways and vessels is surrounded by these medium-intensity soft tissues. The mucosa of the pharynx is usually slightly brighter than the muscular tissue, especially in young individuals. The adenoids are initially bright in children and with age become more isointense with the surrounding mucosa.

Most anatomic features of the neck are better demonstrated on T1W images (Figures 13-10 and 13-11). The soft-tissue structures of the larynx appear gray like muscle. The cartilaginous structures produce a bright signal, outlining the true cords and vestibule. The epiglottis and sinuses can usually be seen, although motion may degrade anatomic detail. A deposit of fat frequently marks the location of the pre-epiglottic space, which is posterior to the hyoid bone. The thyroid gland surrounding the trachea is somewhat brighter than the muscles but of less signal intensity than the nearby fat.

Normal and enlarged lymph nodes are frequently isointense or only slightly darker than muscle on T1W images but are easily distinguished from adjacent dark vessels. The parotid and submandibular glands are of a higher signal intensity than surrounding muscles but somewhat less bright than adjacent fat.

Teeth are visible as focal areas without signal. Changes in the normal pattern may indicate local pathologic conditions, but various dental materials may also produce aberrant signals that can be confusing. Typical is the metallic dropout artifact seen if fillings contain ferromagnetic material (see Chapter 16).

Skull Base

The petrous bone and mastoid air cells are black as a result of lack of signal from dense bone and air, respectively. Any signal from the mastoid region will usually be due to sterile or infected fluid. Deposits of fat within the petrous apex are sometimes present asymmetrically and must not be confused with pathologic conditions.

The superior and inferior extent of pathologic processes and the normal longitudinal anatomic relationships are better demonstrated with sagittal and coronal images. This is particularly important in evaluating tumor extension at the skull base. Transaxial planes are tangential to the area of interest and are thus less helpful. The coronal view of Figure 13-11, for example, allows one to appreciate abnormal assymmetries, which may be the first and only sign of a lesion.

The sagittal views are helpful in evaluating the anatomy at the skull base. The depiction of the pharynx and larynx at midline in the sagittal plane allows easier evaluation of anatomy and pathologic processes.

SPINE

With time, MRI of the spine may replace myelography and metrizamide CT. In addition to providing excellent anatomic information, it has no associated discomfort or known harmful effects. The normal tissue characteristics of the spine are shown in Table 13-4. Most regions of the spine are imaged best with transaxial and sagittal views (Figure 13-12).

Figures 13-13 and 13-14 show that the spinal cord, spinal nerves, CSF, and disk material can be accentuated through MRI for excellent anatomic detail. The nervous tissue is generally gray, and CSF density can be operator controlled to appear anywhere from black, as in Figure 13-13, *A*, to white, as in Figure 13-13, *B*.

Making CSF appear black to outline the cord usually gives the best image, but the vertebral body cortical bone, degenerative osseous and fibrous spurs, and disk materials will also be dark and will blend with the CSF. This problem can be overcome by using a T2W image in which the white CSF defines the thecal sac, revealing any indentations from osteophytes or other causes of narrowing.

The intervertebral disks are dark gray on T1W images and become relatively bright on T2W images, probably because of the fluid and protein content of the nuclear and annular structures. The degenerated disk can be seen as darker than any surrounding normal disk even before bulging or herniation occurs. This is not necessarily true with traumatic herniated disks, in which the disk material usually has a normal signal intensity.

Vertebral bodies are fairly bright in most images because of the high signal from bone marrow. Fractures or replacement of bone marrow by infection

TABLE 13-4.   MRI tissue appearance of spine

Tissues	SDW	T1W	T2W
Bone marrow	Light gray	Light gray	Light gray
Disk	Light gray	Gray	White
Fat	Light gray	White	Gray
CSF	Gray	Black	White
Cord	Light gray	Light gray	Gray

or neoplasm usually changes this appearance, causing a less intense signal. Figure 13-14 shows that high-signal fat is easily demonstrated within the neural foramina and usually outlines the nerves as they leave the spinal canal.

The cord and other neural tissues are usually gray on both T1W and T2W images. With optimal technique, even the contrast between central gray matter sensory and motor neurons can be differentiated from the outer white matter tracts (Figure 13-14).

The conus medullaris, which is the caudal end of the spinal cord, is usually near the level of the L1 vertebral body. The individual nerve roots leaving the conus become the cauda equina. Occasionally these nerves remain close to the filum terminale (posteriorly) for an extended distance below the conus, giving the appearance of a low conus (Figure 13-18, *A*). The individual nerves can almost always be seen adjacent to and within the fat of the recesses along the anterolateral aspects of the spinal canal.

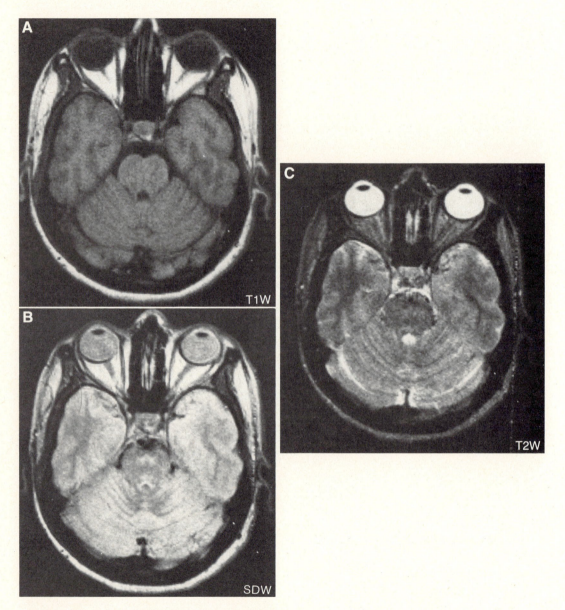

Figure 13-2.   CNS, transaxial. Changes in pulse sequence parameters produce marked differences in relative signal strength of normal structures. These differences are evident if one compares the standard T1W   (**A**), SDW   (**B**), and T2W (**C**) images at the same level within the brain.

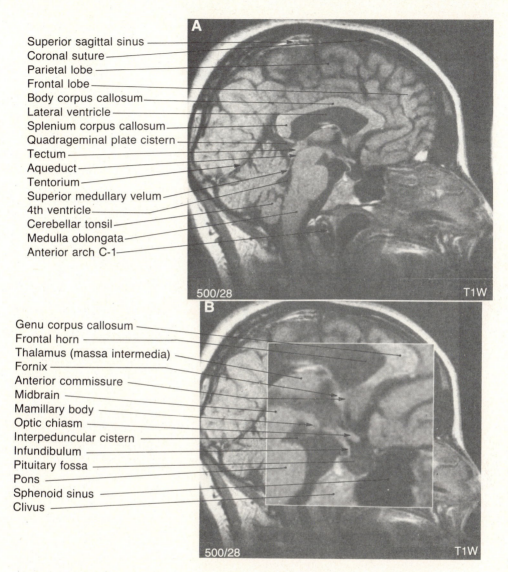

Superior sagittal sinus
Coronal suture
Parietal lobe
Frontal lobe
Body corpus callosum
Lateral ventricle
Splenium corpus callosum
Quadrageminal plate cistern
Tectum
Aqueduct
Tentorium
Superior medullary velum
4th ventricle
Cerebellar tonsil
Medulla oblongata
Anterior arch C-1

500/28   T1W

Genu corpus callosum
Frontal horn
Thalamus (massa intermedia)
Fornix
Anterior commissure
Midbrain
Mamillary body
Optic chiasm
Interpeduncular cistern
Infundibulum
Pituitary fossa
Pons
Sphenoid sinus
Clivus

500/28   T1W

Figure 13-3. CNS, sagittal. **A,** The sagittal view demonstrates conventional relationships of brain, face, and skull base. **B,** A magnification view of the parasellar region shows the structures well defined and the sella mostly filled with CSF, a normal variant. (Courtesy Thompson-CGR).

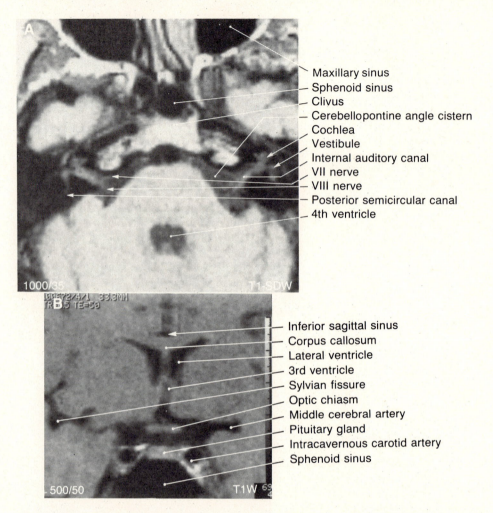

Maxillary sinus
Sphenoid sinus
Clivus
Cerebellopontine angle cistern
Cochlea
Vestibule
Internal auditory canal
VII nerve
VIII nerve
Posterior semicircular canal
4th ventricle

Inferior sagittal sinus
Corpus callosum
Lateral ventricle
3rd ventricle
Sylvian fissure
Optic chiasm
Middle cerebral artery
Pituitary gland
Intracavernous carotid artery
Sphenoid sinus

Figure 13-4.   Brain base.   **A,** This 3-mm-thick transaxial section through the internal auditory canal shows a branch of the posteriorly located eighth (auditory) nerve and the more anterior seventh (facial) nerve.   **B,** The pituitary fossa and its relationship to the cavernous sinuses and suprasellar cistern is ideally demonstrated in the coronal plane.

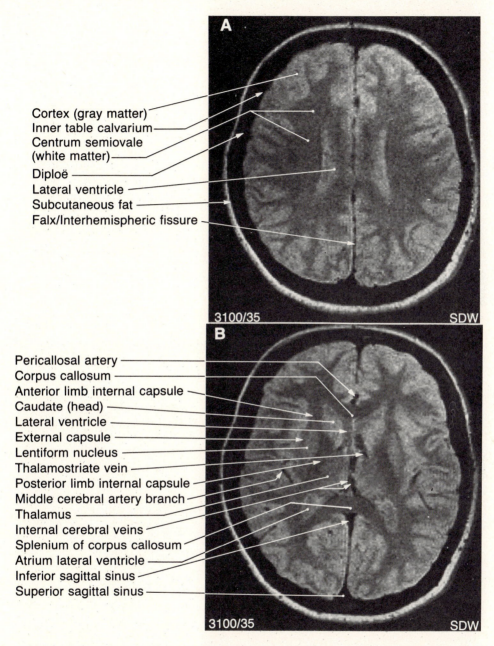

Cortex (gray matter)
Inner table calvarium
Centrum semiovale
(white matter)
Diploë
Lateral ventricle
Subcutaneous fat
Falx/Interhemispheric fissure

Pericallosal artery
Corpus callosum
Anterior limb internal capsule
Caudate (head)
Lateral ventricle
External capsule
Lentiform nucleus
Thalamostriate vein
Posterior limb internal capsule
Middle cerebral artery branch
Thalamus
Internal cerebral veins
Splenium of corpus callosum
Atrium lateral ventricle
Inferior sagittal sinus
Superior sagittal sinus

Figure 13-5. Brain, transaxial. These SDW images are taken sequentially from vertex to base through the brain. **A,** The white matter, called the centrum semiovale at this level, is darker than the more peripheral cortical gray matter. **B,** The basal ganglia, internal capsule, anterior cerebral artery branches, and internal cerebral veins are seen.

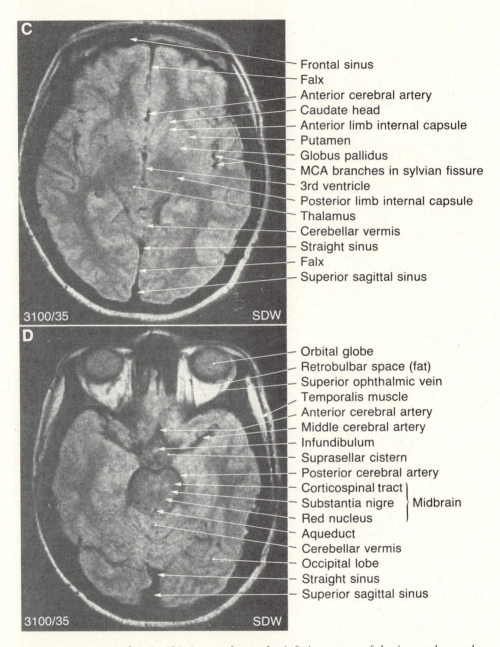

C

3100/35   SDW

- Frontal sinus
- Falx
- Anterior cerebral artery
- Caudate head
- Anterior limb internal capsule
- Putamen
- Globus pallidus
- MCA branches in sylvian fissure
- 3rd ventricle
- Posterior limb internal capsule
- Thalamus
- Cerebellar vermis
- Straight sinus
- Falx
- Superior sagittal sinus

D

3100/35   SDW

- Orbital globe
- Retrobulbar space (fat)
- Superior ophthalmic vein
- Temporalis muscle
- Anterior cerebral artery
- Middle cerebral artery
- Infundibulum
- Suprasellar cistern
- Posterior cerebral artery
- Corticospinal tract ⎫
- Substantia nigre ⎬ Midbrain
- Red nucleus   ⎭
- Aqueduct
- Cerebellar vermis
- Occipital lobe
- Straight sinus
- Superior sagittal sinus

Figure 13-5, cont'd.   C, This image shows the inferior extent of the internal capsule separating the lentiform nuclei from caudate anteriorly and thalamus posteriorly. D, This midbrain section includes the region of the circle of Willis, orbital contents, and a portion of the cerebellum. The posterior cerebellar arteries are seen sweeping around the midbrain.

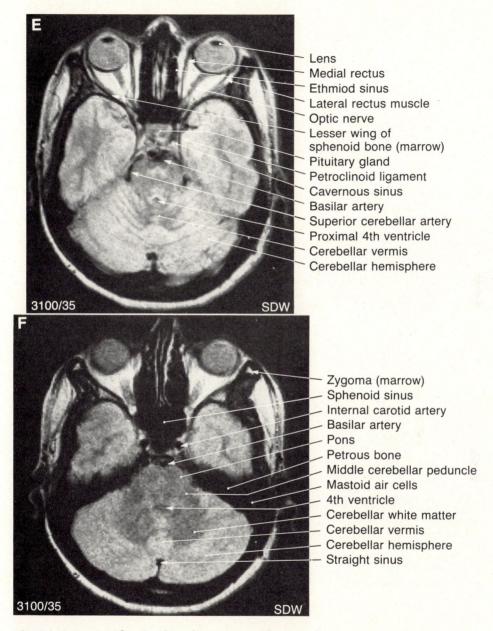

Figure 13-5, cont'd.   **E,** The orbits, pituitary fossa, and cavernous sinus region are seen at the junction of the pons and midbrain.   **F,** At the level of the pons, the fourth ventricle is surrounded by low-intensity broad bands of white matter connecting the pons and the cerebellum.

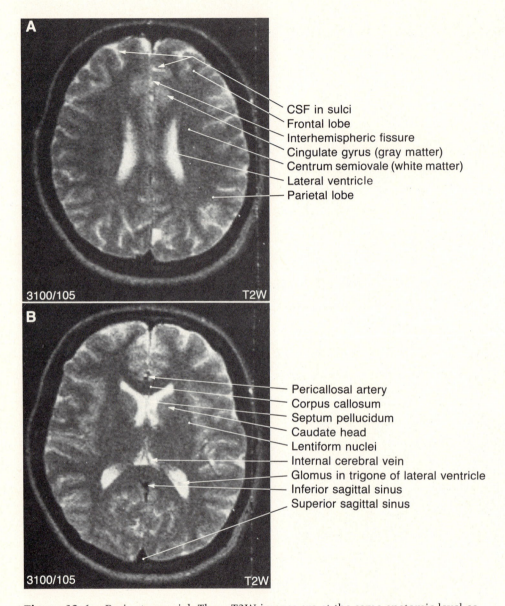

Figure 13-6. Brain, transaxial. These T2W images are at the same anatomic level as the images shown in Figure 13-4. **A,** In this cardiac-gated image, there is little gray and white matter signal difference compared with that in the SDW image. **B,** With the exception of the caudate head, the basal ganglia are barely distinguishable on this image.

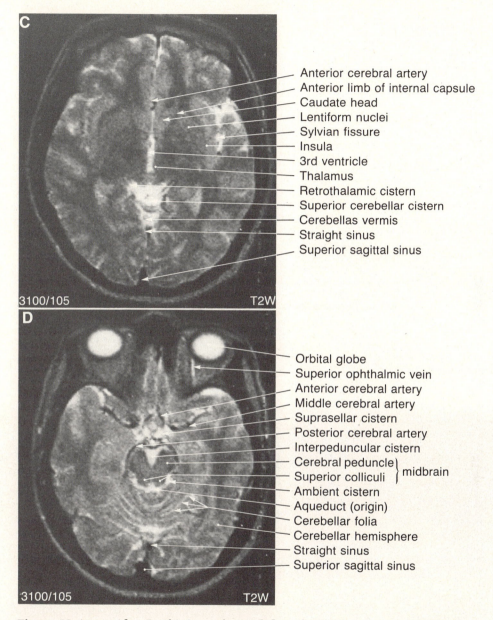

C, 3100/105   T2W

- Anterior cerebral artery
- Anterior limb of internal capsule
- Caudate head
- Lentiform nuclei
- Sylvian fissure
- Insula
- 3rd ventricle
- Thalamus
- Retrothalamic cistern
- Superior cerebellar cistern
- Cerebellas vermis
- Straight sinus
- Superior sagittal sinus

D, 3100/105   T2W

- Orbital globe
- Superior ophthalmic vein
- Anterior cerebral artery
- Middle cerebral artery
- Suprasellar cistern
- Posterior cerebral artery
- Interpeduncular cistern
- Cerebral peduncle } midbrain
- Superior colliculi
- Ambient cistern
- Aqueduct (origin)
- Cerebellar folia
- Cerebellar hemisphere
- Straight sinus
- Superior sagittal sinus

Figure 13-6, cont'd.   C, This image better defines the CSF spaces, since the CSF is now white. The third ventricle is more visible, as are the sylvian fissures and cisterns. D, The sulci of the cerebellar vermis become prominent. The bright CSF outlines the dark signal voids from the vascular structures.

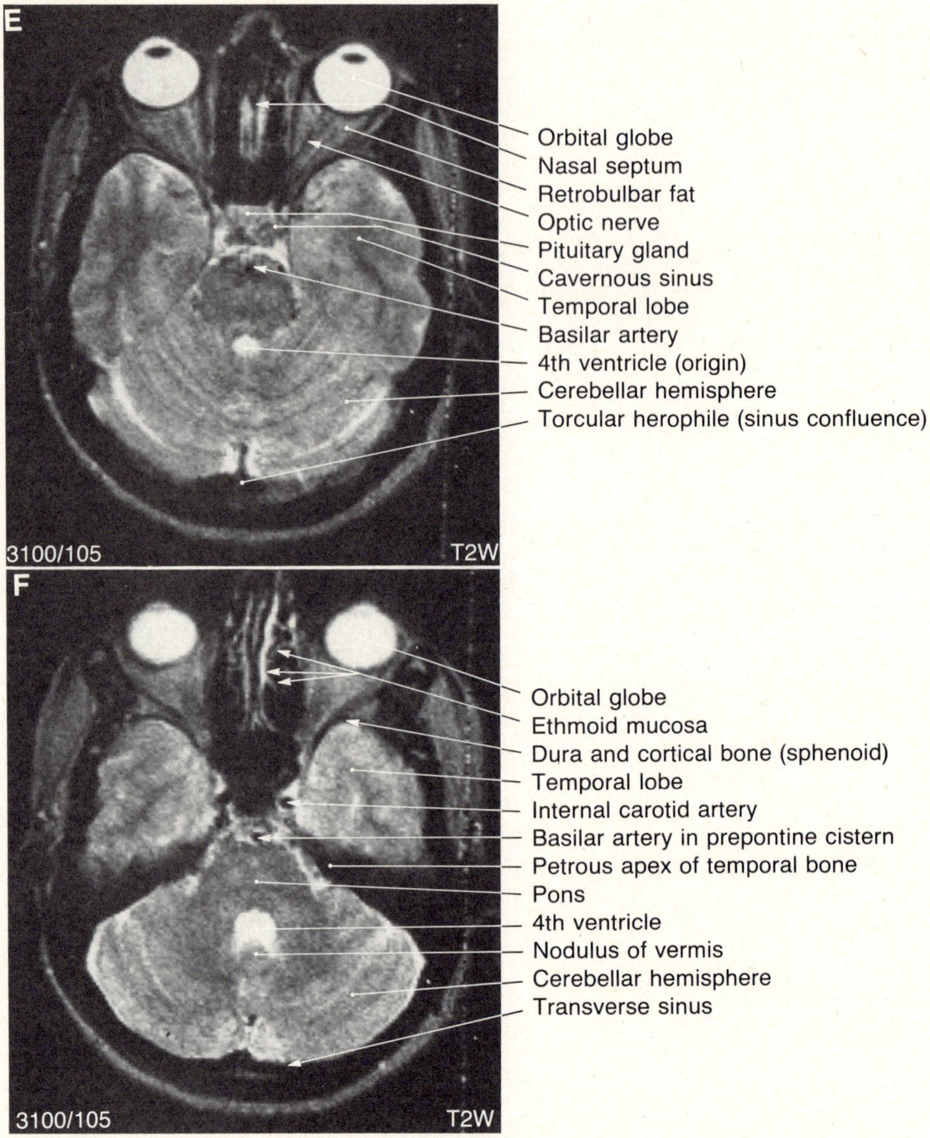
E
Orbital globe
Nasal septum
Retrobulbar fat
Optic nerve
Pituitary gland
Cavernous sinus
Temporal lobe
Basilar artery
4th ventricle (origin)
Cerebellar hemisphere
Torcular herophile (sinus confluence)
3100/105
T2W
F
Orbital globe
Ethmoid mucosa
Dura and cortical bone (sphenoid)
Temporal lobe
Internal carotid artery
Basilar artery in prepontine cistern
Petrous apex of temporal bone
Pons
4th ventricle
Nodulus of vermis
Cerebellar hemisphere
Transverse sinus
3100/105
T2W

Figure 13-6, cont'd. E, The orbital fluids are now white, as is the visible CSF, including the previously dark proximal end of the fourth ventricle. **F,** The carotid and basilar arteries are outlined by white CSF. The nasal and ethmoidal mucosa has become fairly bright in an asymmetric fashion, probably secondary to mild subclinical inflammation.

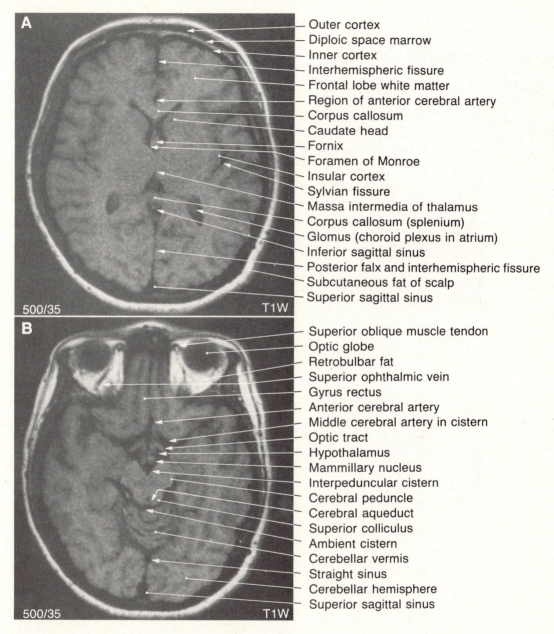

A
- Outer cortex
- Diploic space marrow
- Inner cortex
- Interhemispheric fissure
- Frontal lobe white matter
- Region of anterior cerebral artery
- Corpus callosum
- Caudate head
- Fornix
- Foramen of Monroe
- Insular cortex
- Sylvian fissure
- Massa intermedia of thalamus
- Corpus callosum (splenium)
- Glomus (choroid plexus in atrium)
- Inferior sagittal sinus
- Posterior falx and interhemispheric fissure
- Subcutaneous fat of scalp
- Superior sagittal sinus

500/35   T1W

B
- Superior oblique muscle tendon
- Optic globe
- Retrobulbar fat
- Superior ophthalmic vein
- Gyrus rectus
- Anterior cerebral artery
- Middle cerebral artery in cistern
- Optic tract
- Hypothalamus
- Mammillary nucleus
- Interpeduncular cistern
- Cerebral peduncle
- Cerebral aqueduct
- Superior colliculus
- Ambient cistern
- Cerebellar vermis
- Straight sinus
- Cerebellar hemisphere
- Superior sagittal sinus

500/35   T1W

Figure 13-7. Brain, transaxial. These T1W images are taken at four levels from top to base. The CSF is black. The white matter is brighter than the gray matter but with less contrast than in SDW images. This type of image may prevent visualization of the many vessels within or adjacent to the CSF spaces. A and B, At the basal ganglia and midbrain levels, the interface between brain and CSF space is sharp.

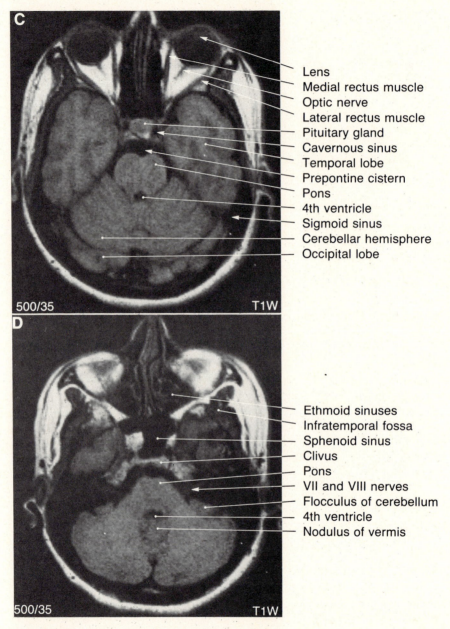

C

Lens
Medial rectus muscle
Optic nerve
Lateral rectus muscle
Pituitary gland
Cavernous sinus
Temporal lobe
Prepontine cistern
Pons
4th ventricle
Sigmoid sinus
Cerebellar hemisphere
Occipital lobe

500/35   T1W

D

Ethmoid sinuses
Infratemporal fossa
Sphenoid sinus
Clivus
Pons
VII and VIII nerves
Flocculus of cerebellum
4th ventricle
Nodulus of vermis

500/35   T1W

Figure 13-7, cont'd.   C, The retroorbital anatomy and region of the pituitary gland
are well displayed with the use of T1W images. Many signal averages of the same slice
can be obtained in a short time with the use of T1W imaging parameters, providing
better detail.   **D,** The high signal from marrow within the clivus and other skull
bones defines these structures well. The seventh and eighth cranial nerves can be
visualized from their origin in the pons to the middle ear within the cerebellar pontine
angle cistern and internal auditory canal.

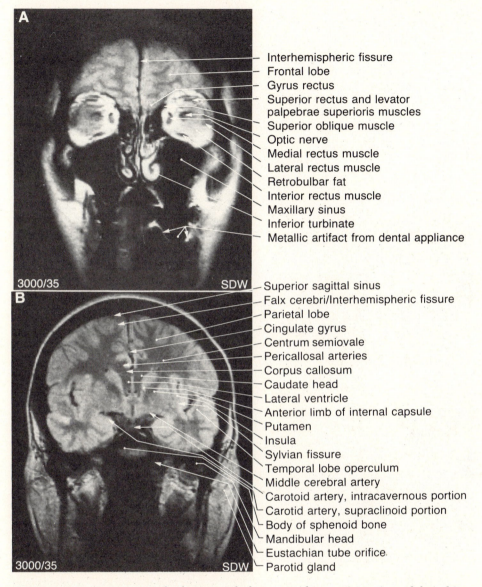

A

- Interhemispheric fissure
- Frontal lobe
- Gyrus rectus
- Superior rectus and levator palpebrae superioris muscles
- Superior oblique muscle
- Optic nerve
- Medial rectus muscle
- Lateral rectus muscle
- Retrobulbar fat
- Interior rectus muscle
- Maxillary sinus
- Inferior turbinate
- Metallic artifact from dental appliance

3000/35　　　　SDW

B

- Superior sagittal sinus
- Falx cerebri/Interhemispheric fissure
- Parietal lobe
- Cingulate gyrus
- Centrum semiovale
- Pericallosal arteries
- Corpus callosum
- Caudate head
- Lateral ventricle
- Anterior limb of internal capsule
- Putamen
- Insula
- Sylvian fissure
- Temporal lobe operculum
- Middle cerebral artery
- Carotoid artery, intracavernous portion
- Carotid artery, supraclinoid portion
- Body of sphenoid bone
- Mandibular head
- Eustachian tube orifice
- Parotid gland

3000/35　　　　SDW

Figure 13-8. Brain, coronal. The coronal plane provides a unique view of the white matter tracts and midline relationships of the brain. **A,** This view shows the interhemispheric fissure, adjacent brain, orbital muscles, and optic nerves. **B,** The white matter tracts of the centrum semiovale can be seen extending across midline via the corpus callosum and forming the internal capsule inferiorly, which separates the caudate and lentiform nuclei. Middle cerebral artery branches are visible in the sylvian fissures.

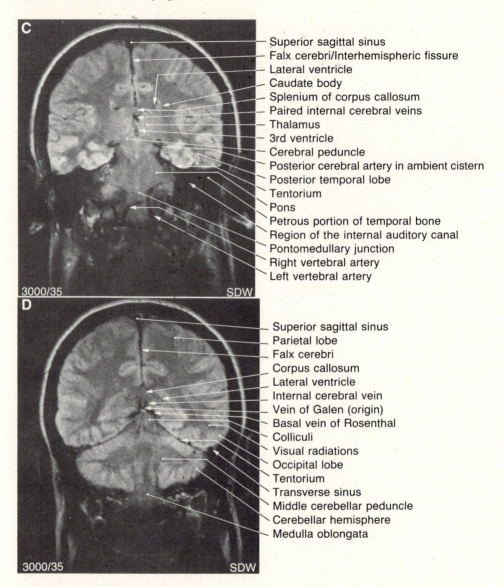

C
- Superior sagittal sinus
- Falx cerebri/Interhemispheric fissure
- Lateral ventricle
- Caudate body
- Splenium of corpus callosum
- Paired internal cerebral veins
- Thalamus
- 3rd ventricle
- Cerebral peduncle
- Posterior cerebral artery in ambient cistern
- Posterior temporal lobe
- Tentorium
- Pons
- Petrous portion of temporal bone
- Region of the internal auditory canal
- Pontomedullary junction
- Right vertebral artery
- Left vertebral artery

3000/35   SDW

D
- Superior sagittal sinus
- Parietal lobe
- Falx cerebri
- Corpus callosum
- Lateral ventricle
- Internal cerebral vein
- Vein of Galen (origin)
- Basal vein of Rosenthal
- Colliculi
- Visual radiations
- Occipital lobe
- Tentorium
- Transverse sinus
- Middle cerebellar peduncle
- Cerebellar hemisphere
- Medulla oblongata

3000/35   SDW

Figure 13-8, cont'd.   C, The brainstem and structures around the craniovertebral junction are seen in this projection.   D, The tentorium and its relationship to the cerebrum and cerebellum are illustrated.

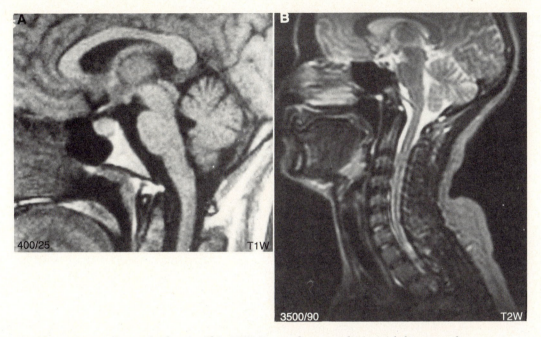

Figure 13-9. Brain, sagittal. **A,** This T1W image does not distinguish between the dark CSF, the black cortical bone, air, or any other dark structure. **B,** This image is cardiac gated to every fifth heartbeat, producing a white CSF cisternogram effect. The linear artifacts along the midcervical spine and cord are probably due to CSF pulsation despite the gating.

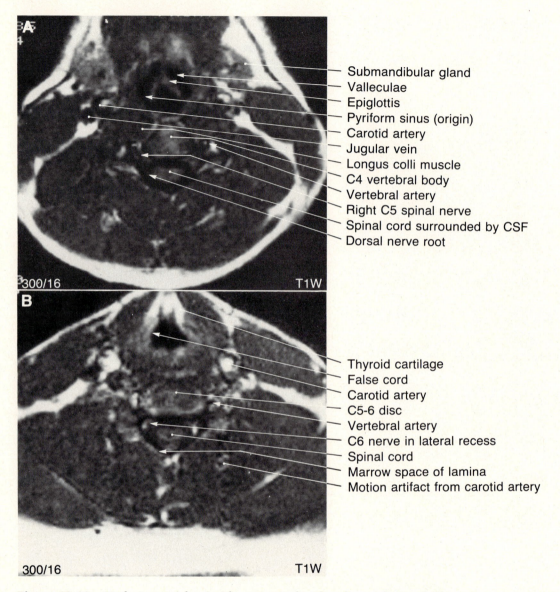

Submandibular gland
Valleculae
Epiglottis
Pyriform sinus (origin)
Carotid artery
Jugular vein
Longus colli muscle
C4 vertebral body
Vertebral artery
Right C5 spinal nerve
Spinal cord surrounded by CSF
Dorsal nerve root

300/16   T1W

Thyroid cartilage
False cord
Carotid artery
C5-6 disc
Vertebral artery
C6 nerve in lateral recess
Spinal cord
Marrow space of lamina
Motion artifact from carotid artery

300/16   T1W

Figure 13-10.   Neck, transaxial.   **A,** The paraspinal and neck muscles are delineated by the fat within the soft-tissue planes. The epiglottis protrudes up into the pharynx, with the valleculae forming anterior to it. The submandibular glands are a higher signal intensity than nearby muscle but a lower signal intensity than fat.   **B,** The anterior thyroid cartilage gives a bright signal identifying the level of the larynx. Artifact from motion of the carotid artery degrades the image quality in the phase-encoding direction (anteroposterior in this image).

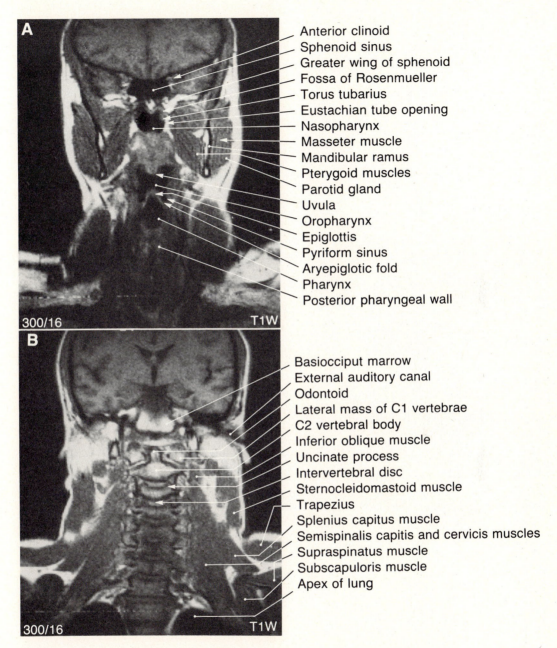

Figure 13-11. Neck, coronal. **A,** The pharynx, oropharynx, nasal cavities, and ethmoid sinuses are well defined using coronal planes and can be combined with the standard axial views to provide better localization of abnormalities. **B,** The soft tissues of the neck, base of the brain, skull, and spine are seen well on coronal views. The vertical extent of lesions can be demonstrated best in this and the sagittal planes.

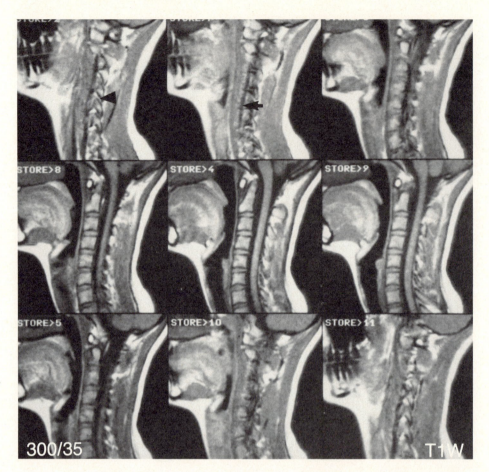

Figure 13-12.   Spine, cervical. Parallel sequential sagittal images of the cervical spine show the side-to-side relationships of the spine and paraspinal soft tissues. Cortical bone remains black outlining the disks and the anterior prevertebral soft tissues, but it blends with the dark CSF. (Courtesy Steve Sax, M.D., The Methodist Hospital, Houston, TX.)

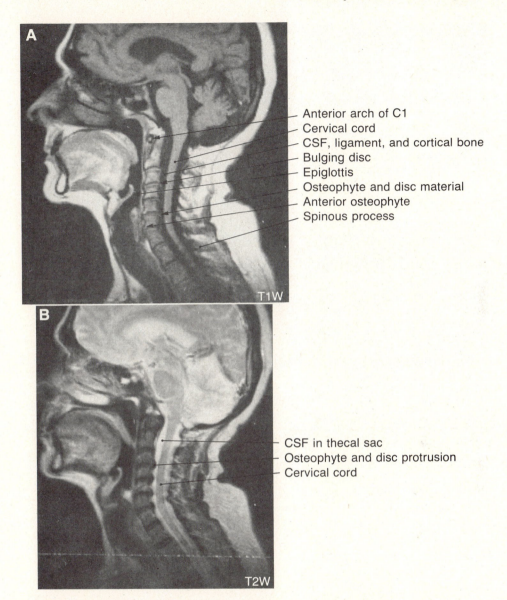

Figure 13-13. Spine, cervical, sagittal. These images were obtained with cardiac gating and show the relative change in the CSF from nearly black **(A)** to very bright **(B)**. The spinal cord is outlined best with the T1W image. The patient illustrated in **(B)** has degenerative disks that are darker than normal. The impressions of degenerative osteophytes and/or bulging disks into the anterior thecal sac are seen easily when the CSF is white.

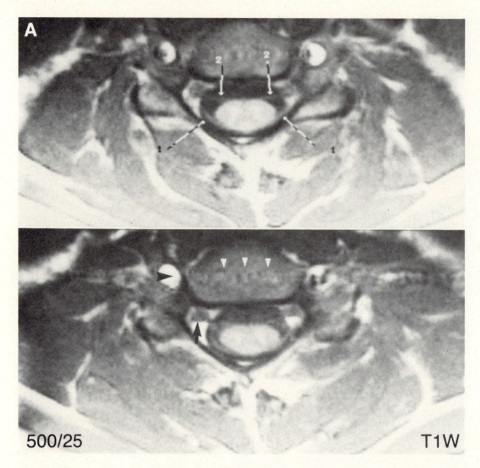

Figure 13-14.   Spine, cervical, paraxial. The nerve roots, cord, paraspinal soft tissues, and vessels are easily seen on these surface coil images. The dorsal and ventral nerve roots, numbers 1 and 2 respectively (in **A**) *(arrow)* in the anterolateral recesses before exiting. The gray matter dorsal and ventral horns (2 and 1 in **B**) are surrounded by

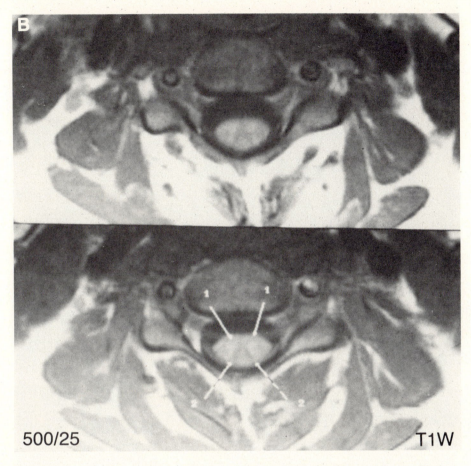

500/25   T1W

the brighter white matter tracts of the cord. The motion artifact *(small arrowheads)* produced by the arterial pulsations obscures anatomic detail in the plane of the phase-encoding gradient. The right vertebral artery *(large arrowhead)* is bright owing to an entry slice flow phenomenon. (Courtesy Siemens Medical Systems.)

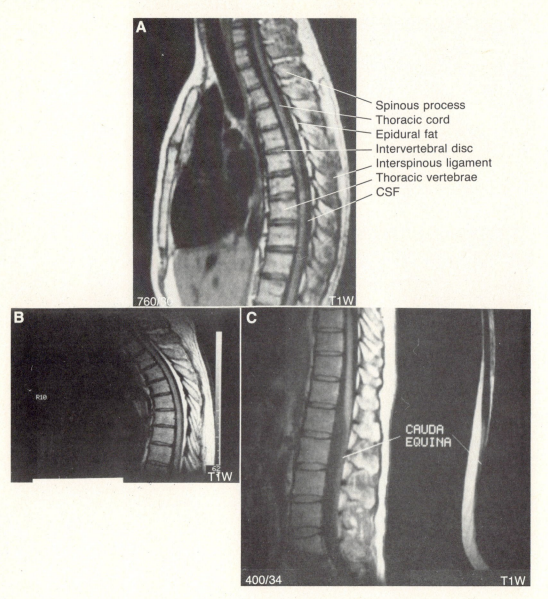

Labels on image A:
- Spinous process
- Thoracic cord
- Epidural fat
- Intervertebral disc
- Interspinous ligament
- Thoracic vertebrae
- CSF

CAUDA EQUINA

Figure 13-15. Spine, thoracic and lumbar, sagittal. **A,** The entire thoracic cord can be seen when a body coil is used, but the spatial resolution may be reduced because a larger area is viewed. **B,** With the use of a posterior surface coil, the kyphosis of this patient's spine brings the superior and inferior extents farther away from the coil, and there is an associated loss of detail. **C,** The left image illustrates the thoracolumbar junction containing the cord and cauda equina. The right image shows an MR myelography effect (Courtesy Bruker Medical Instruments, Inc.)

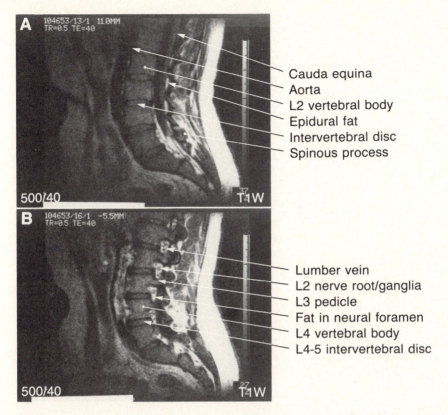

Figure 13-16.   Spine, lumbar, sagittal. Midline **(A)** and lateral recess and foramina **(B)** images illustrates the spinal confines and lateral structures.

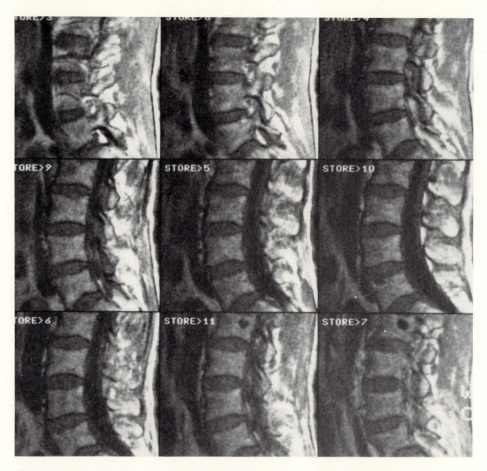

Figure 13-17. Multisagittal views through the lumbar spine allow for evaluation of disk and other disease at all levels. (Courtesy Steve Sax, M.D., The Methodist Hospital, Houston, TX.)

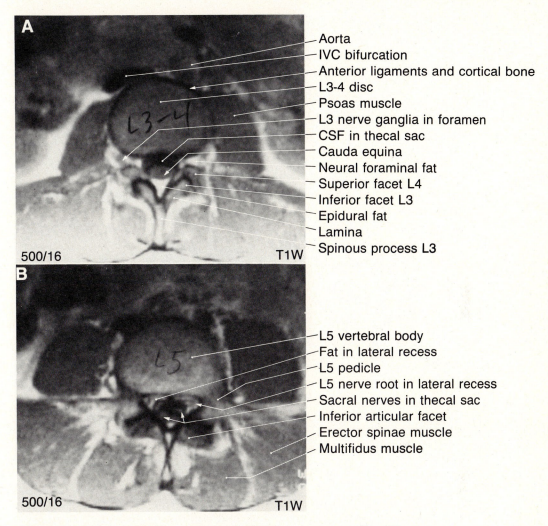

Figure 13-18. Spine, lumbar, transaxial. The nerve roots, ganglia, CSF space, paraspinal muscles, and bone are shown. Ganglia are surrounded by fat in the neural foramina.

Chapter
FOURTEEN

MRI Anatomy: Thorax and Abdomen

THORAX

The unique abilities of MRI in the thorax stem mainly from the display of blood vessels as black structures. This stark contrast of the vessels from other mediastinal tissues allows easy discrimination of those structures that are difficult to image by other noninvasive techniques. The pulmonary vessels and bronchi beyond the hila usually blend with the lung tissue, also black, although vessels in the peripheral lung field can be seen if an RF pulse sequence is used that shows flowing blood as white (Figure 14-3, *B*). The normal tissue characteristics of the thorax are shown in Table 14-1. Cardiac gating should be used to reduce motion artifacts. Fast imaging techniques are being introduced that also decrease motion artifacts.

The transaxial plane (Figure 14-1) will probably remain the standard view for routine thoracic MRI. Most major vessels and the airways are seen in cross section. This is also a familiar orientation for technologists and radiologists with prior experience in CT.

The coronal plane (Figure 14-2) also has several advantages and is used

TABLE 14-1.   MRI tissue characteristics of the thorax

Tissues	SDW	T1W	T2W
Fat	Light gray	White	Gray
Blood, flowing	Black	Black	Black
Lungs	Black	Black	Black
Adult thymus	Light gray	White	Gray
Vessel walls	Gray	Gray	Dark gray

routinely by some. Most of these same tubular structures are visualized well in their longitudinal axis when the coronal planes are used. The trachea can be followed on several contiguous slices from its anterior entrance into the thoracic cage down to the more posterior carinal region.

The sagittal plane (Figures 14-4 and 14-5) is usually applied only to the mediastinal portion of the thorax unless apical or diaphragmatic disease is suspected. However, it has considerable utility in demonstrating pathologic processes in the anterior, middle, and posterior compartments of the mediastinum. Substernal and pretracheal lesions are probably best delineated with this view. Oblique projections are particularly useful in cardiac imaging.

Thoracic Wall

The thoracic wall is bright on both T1W and T2W images because of signal from subcutaneous fat. It is easily visualized because of the adjacent dark lung tissue and external air. Some loss of detail occurs in the lower thorax because of the greater respiratory motion and cardiac activity. The internal mammary arteries and other blood vessels are visible as signal voids within the relatively bright fat. The ribs show the bright marrow signal surrounded by the black cortical bone. None of the orthogonal views are ideally suited for demonstration of ribs; however, rib abnormalities can be detected easily by loss or distortion of marrow signal.

Breasts

The breasts have a variable signal appearance depending on the amount of parenchymal fatty replacement. As in other places, fat has an intense signal on T1W images and a moderate signal on T2W images. The central parenchymal tissue is usually gray on both T1W and T2W images. The cysts of mammary fibrocystic disease are easily identified on the T2W images as a characteristic fluid collection with an intense signal. The breasts are ideally visualized by using surrounding surface coils because of the increased signal-to-noise ratio (Figure 14-6). A damping mechanism for the surface coils is needed to avoid receiving too much signal from the subcutaneous fat. Transaxial and sagittal views are best, although coronal views may be helpful if the view is coplanar with the lesion.

Pleura

The pleura is not routinely seen with MRI, unless outlined by pleural air or fluid. Most pathologic processes of the pleura are dark or gray on T1W images and brighter on T2W images. The ability to use multiple imaging planes may be an indication for MRI in evaluating such areas as the apices and diaphragmatic surfaces, especially with faster imaging techniques that allow scanning during a single breath hold.

Mediastinum

The mediastinal structures are extremely well imaged by MRI because the major components have widely different signal intensities (see Figures 14-1, 14-2, 14-4, and 14-5). T1W images of the mediastinal fat produce a bright signal, whereas other soft tissues give various shades of gray. The airways and vessels are usually black and differentiated by their anatomic locations. On T2W images, the fatty tissues remain brighter than the normal mediastinal soft tissues. Normal-sized or enlarged lymph nodes may occasionally be brighter than fat on the T2W image, particularly if they are draining an active infectious process. The esophagus is usually not differentiated from the adjacent mediastinal connective tissue and aortic wall, unless air or fluid remains within it.

The trachea and first- and second-order bronchi are seen because of their black lumen contrasted with the gray signal of their walls and the bright signal from adjacent fat and other tissues. On most T1W and T2W images, only the vessel walls have any significant signal. This is one of the great advantages of mediastinal MRI because the signal void within vessels prevents their confusion with nonvascular pathologic lesions. All three orthogonal planes and several specific oblique views have been useful in mediastinal imaging.

Cardiovasculature

The anatomic definition of cardiovascular structures (Figures 14-1 to 14-7) are currently best imaged by MRI, and its use for obtaining functional data shows great potential. Multiple consecutive slices may be acquired throughout a cardiac cycle, or multiple images of the same slice may be used to accummulate functional information about blood flow and myocardial activity. The ability of MRI to obtain these various functional data and to define the anatomic features exquisitely in a single examination may make it the study of choice in many cardiac patients.

The MR signal from heart muscle is similar to that from skeletal muscle except that it is usually slightly more intense on both T1W and T2W images. The heart is surrounded by the darker-gray intensity of the pericardial membrane, which can be seen anterior to the heart between the epicardial and anterior mediastinal fat.

The coronary arteries can usually be seen at their origin near the aortic root. The left circumflex and right coronary arteries are seen more distally in the grooves, where they are surrounded by epicardial fat. Surface coils can help obtain the spatial resolution needed to determine coronary artery and graft patency, where a gray signal may indicate occlusion.

All of the orthogonal planes and several specific oblique views are useful in cardiac imaging. As with CT, the transaxial plane demonstrates the heart chambers. All four chambers are seen clearly in cross section, and the interventricular septum is adequately visualized. Septal defects, thinning of the myocardial wall, and intraluminal abnormalities can all be identified in this plane. The coronal view offers a more familiar anatomic representation of the heart and vessels, as seen on a typical posteroanterior chest radiograph. The sagittal plane demonstrates the anteroposterior relationships of the heart chambers to the adjacent organs.

Oblique planes are used in cardiac imaging to obtain long- and short-axis views of the ventricles. This allows for optimal observation of wall thickness and motion, which is otherwise slightly misrepresented. More accurate data can be derived from these oblique images obtained throughout the cardiac cycle.

Great Vessels

Unlike any other imaging modality, MRI has the ability to readily visualize the great vessels (Figures 14-1 to 14-7) in any orientation, sometimes in their entirety. The vessel walls can be seen as dark to gray lines, whereas the intraluminal flowing blood usually produces little if any signal.

The coronal plane demonstrates most of the vessels and heart chambers in a useful orientation. The brachiocephalic vessels angle slightly obliquely through the various coronal planes. Long segments of the superior and inferior vena cava can be seen, and their entry into the right atrium is well visualized. The descending aorta and even the azygos vein are routinely visualized and well defined. The main, left, and right pulmonary arteries are routinely followed throughout their mediastinal course. The pulmonary veins can intermittently be seen inserting into the left atrium; the superior veins are more frequently seen than the inferior ones.

The sagittal plane demonstrates the aortic and pulmonary arterial outflow tracts and roots. It also is perhaps ideal for imaging the aorta, especially when off-axis parasagittal angulation is used.

Off-axis views may be particularly helpful in imaging mediastinal vessels. The parasagittal angle corresponding to the angle between ascending and descending aorta may be used to view the entire thoracic aorta on a single section in the absence of tortuosity.

Blood

Blood is a complex tissue that has a variable appearance on MR images, depending on the selected RF pulse sequence and orientation of the blood flow to the image plane. It is usually best to select the plane of the vessel for imaging. Current computer imaging programs do not account for the blood motion characteristics, and thus many artifacts may result. Usually, rapidly flowing blood is black, whereas low-velocity blood flow occasionally has a low to moderately high signal intensity. Exceptions exist when a very short TR and TE are used (Figure 14-3, *B*). The proximal end of a flowing column will often have varying degrees of bright intraluminal signal with multislice imaging techniques. In-plane flowing blood usually results in medium to bright signal intensity.

During late diastole, slow or even retrograde flow occurs in the large arteries. This produces a bright signal (Figure 14-5) from intraluminal blood, and that is normal on these images. When using most of the fast imaging techniques, the flowing blood usually returns a bright signal, giving an angiogram appearance.

ABDOMEN

Most abdominal organs (Figures 14-8 to 14-12) are of intermediate signal and, therefore, are easily seen when contrasted with the intense signal of surrounding fat. Flowing blood within vascular structures of the kidneys, spleen, liver, periportal, and retroperitoneal regions is easily demonstrated in transaxial, sagittal, and coronal views. The organs in the upper abdomen have more degradation of image quality than those in the lower abdomen or retroperitoneum because of respiratory motion. This is especially noticeable if long imaging times are employed. Many new techniques using shorter acquisition times are available to decrease motion artifacts.

The most common MRI protocols used in the abdomen involve spin echo and gradient echo images, with images acquired from all orthogonal planes depending on the clinical question. The normal tissue characteristics of abdominal organs are shown in Table 14-2. Their appearances, characteristics, and anatomic relationships are described as follows.

Liver

The liver is a bright gray intensity on T1W images and a relatively dark gray intensity on T2W images. It can be compared with the spleen, which is seen on many of the same transaxial and coronal images. It is normally brighter than the spleen on T1W images and darker on T2W images.

The lobes of the liver and their segments are demarcated by the hepatic

TABLE 14-2. MRI tissue characteristics of the abdomen

Tissues	SDW	T1W	T2W
Fat	Light gray	White	Gray
Adrenal	Gray	Gray	Dark gray
Kidney cortex	Gray	Light gray	Gray
Kidney medulla	Gray	Gray	Gray
Liver	Gray	Light gray	Dark gray
Muscle	Gray	Gray	Dark gray
Pancreas	Gray	Gray	Dark gray
Spleen	Gray	Gray	Gray

veins and the various fat-containing fissures, both of which are easily visualized with MRI. The portal veins are demonstrated as a signal void on most standard pulse sequences. Transaxial views (Figure 14-8) of the liver are usually the most informative because the anatomic landmarks and relationships to other organs are well demonstrated. Occasionally sagittal (Figure 14-10) and coronal (Figure 14-12) views are useful in defining the inferior extent or diaphragmatic relationship of an abdominal lesion or in looking at specific structures such as the inferior vena cava.

Spleen

The spleen is readily visible along the posterolateral aspect of the left upper quadrant immediately below the diaphragm. The signal intensity is gray on T1W images and relatively bright gray on T2W images. The splenic signal is usually homogeneous, as no blood vessels or other internal structures are readily visible within its parenchyma. As with the liver, the transaxial and coronal planes usually show it to best advantage.

Gallbladder

The gallbladder is usually seen as dark on a heavily T1W image and bright on T2W images (Figure 14-9). On moderately T1W images it may be a surprisingly bright gray because of the cholesterol content, which has a short T1 relaxation time. The gallbladder is well visualized in the transaxial plane within the interlobar fissure, and additional planes of view are usually not needed to define it. Its relationship to the inferior liver edge is well demonstrated on the coronal view.

Pancreas

The pancreas usually appears gray relative to other nearby organs (Figure 14-8). It is similar to the liver signal, usually slightly darker on T1W images and relatively brighter on T2W images.

It is the most difficult abdominal organ to image consistently because of its close relationship anteriorly with the stomach and small bowel. Peristalsis of these organs produces motion and partial-volume artifacts. This, along with respiratory motion and a frequent lack of fat at its anatomic border, make this margin difficult to visualize. The posterior border is well demarcated by the signal void of the splenic vein. The head and neck region is usually well defined by the superior mesenteric vein. The pancreas is usually best demonstrated in the transaxial plane.

Adrenal Glands

Normal adrenal glands maintain a signal intensity almost identical to that of the liver when most RF pulse sequences are used. They are readily demonstrated (Figure 14-8), as they are usually surrounded by high signal from fat and in predictable locations. The adrenals are seen best in transaxial planes. Coronal and sagittal views demonstrate the adrenal gland relationships to kidneys and liver, although optimal visualization is less frequently obtained in these planes. A T2W image is helpful because malignant primary or metastatic neoplasms generally have a higher signal intensity compared with that of the liver and normal adrenal tissue when this RF pulse sequence is used.

Kidney

Being outlined by the high signal of perirenal fat, the kidneys have a medium signal intensity on T1W and SDW images (Figure 14-11). They tend to blend with the fat on heavily T2W images. Prominent contrast between the higher signal cortex and lower signal medullary portion is observed on heavily T1W images. This characteristic can be used to identify the degree of T1W. The corticomedullary contrast is lost on SDW and T2W images as a result of the increased signal in the medullary space.

High signal from peripelvic fat is frequently seen surrounding the collecting systems in adults. Like other fluids, the urine is usually dark on T1W and bright on T2W images, although partial volume averaging may cause it to appear gray on T1W images. Urine in the collecting systems may not always be well visualized because of normal variation in size. Simple kidney cysts are well defined and have the same morphologic features as demonstrated on CT except they have the MRI characteristics of other simple fluids. They are black to dark gray on heavily T1W images. The relationship of the kidneys to adjacent organs above and below can best be demonstrated on a coronal image.

Gastrointestinal Tract

At present, MRI of the bowel is generally unsatisfactory because considerable motion occurs during the relatively long imaging times required. However, this is expected to change with the development of faster imaging techniques and oral MR contrast agents. Transaxial and coronal planes usually provide the most diagnostic views.

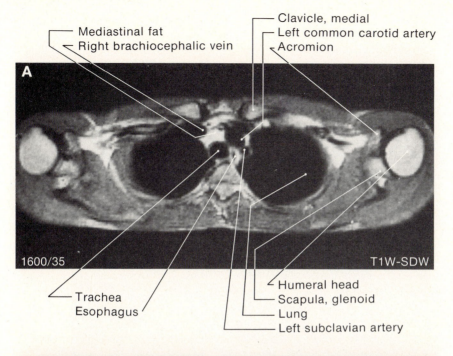

Mediastinal fat
Right brachiocephalic vein

Clavicle, medial
Left common carotid artery
Acromion

1600/35

T1W-SDW

Trachea
Esophagus

Humeral head
Scapula, glenoid
Lung
Left subclavian artery

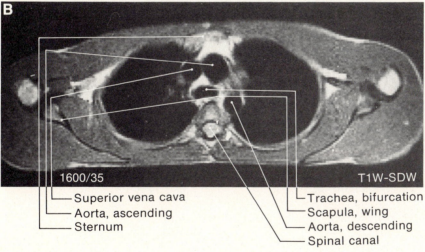

1600/35

T1W-SDW

Superior vena cava
Aorta, ascending
Sternum

Trachea, bifurcation
Scapula, wing
Aorta, descending
Spinal canal

Figure 14-1. Thorax (mediastinum), transaxial, T1W–SDW mixed and cardiac gated. These images (**A–F**) are taken sequentially from superior mediastinum to the inferior portions of the heart. **A,** At the supraortic level, blood vessels have a black lumen, outlined by the gray vessel walls and high signal from mediastinal fat. An exception is the right subclavian vein, which has internal signal due to in-plane flow. The black tracheobronchial tree is distinguished from vessels only by its characteristic position. **B,** The aortopulmonary window level shows several areas that are of less intensity than fat, representing small, normal lymph nodes.

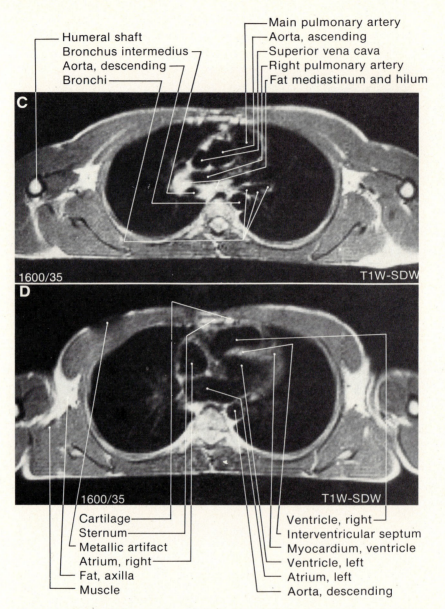

Humeral shaft
Bronchus intermedius
Aorta, descending
Bronchi

Main pulmonary artery
Aorta, ascending
Superior vena cava
Right pulmonary artery
Fat mediastinum and hilum

1600/35   T1W-SDW

Cartilage
Sternum
Metallic artifact
Atrium, right
Fat, axilla
Muscle

Ventricle, right
Interventricular septum
Myocardium, ventricle
Ventricle, left
Atrium, left
Aorta, descending

1600/35   T1W-SDW

Figure 14-1, cont'd. **C,** The subcarinal level displays the aorta and pulmonary artery roots well, with the right pulmonary artery crossing posterior to the aorta and superior vena cava. After the initial main-stem bronchial branching, the bronchial tree cannot be readily differentiated from the rest of the lung. **D,** The heart chambers are outlined in the region of the base of the heart. A small metal artifact with signal void from an electrocardiographic lead is noted on the right chest.

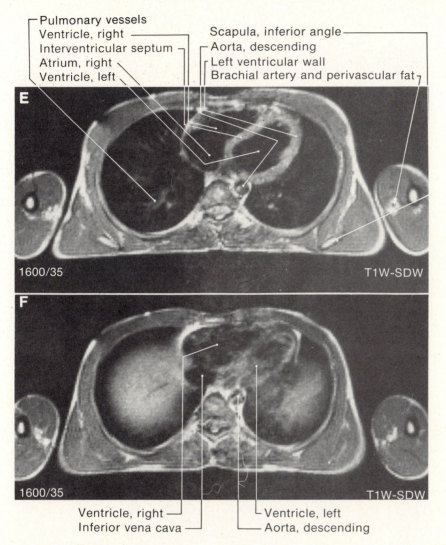

Pulmonary vessels
Ventricle, right
Interventricular septum
Atrium, right
Ventricle, left

Scapula, inferior angle
Aorta, descending
Left ventricular wall
Brachial artery and perivascular fat

E

1600/35   T1W-SDW

F

1600/35   T1W-SDW

Ventricle, right
Inferior vena cava

Ventricle, left
Aorta, descending

Figure 14-1, cont'd.   E, At the ventricular level, the wall of the left ventricle is normally much thicker than that of the right ventricle. Pathologic thinning or thickening is readily evaluated. The signal intensity within the descending aorta in this figure and Figure 14-1 is probably due to slow flow, as these images were obtained during diastole with a time delay of 742 msec after the R wave.   F, At the level of the heart apex and the diaphragm there is frequently respiratory and heart motion, which degrades the image. MRI signal within the ventricles is due to slow and turbulent flow at the apices during late diastole, with a time delay of 865 ms after the R wave.

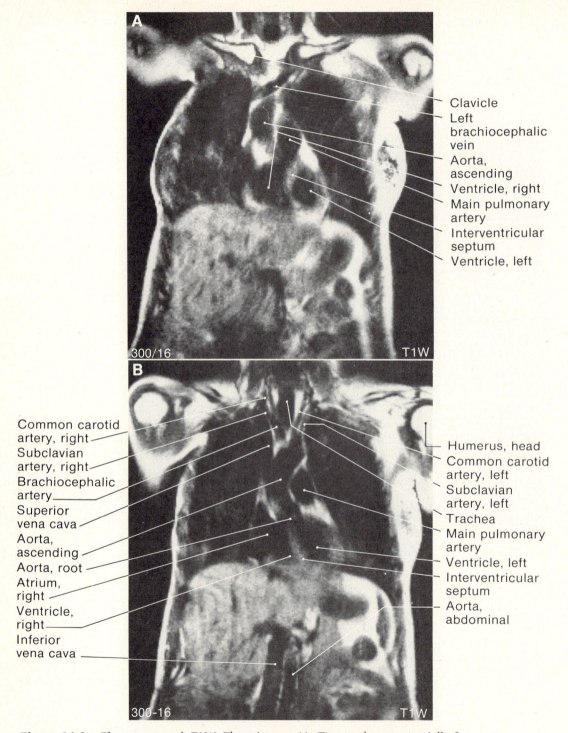

Clavicle
Left brachiocephalic vein
Aorta, ascending
Ventricle, right
Main pulmonary artery
Interventricular septum
Ventricle, left

300/16

T1W

Common carotid artery, right
Subclavian artery, right
Brachiocephalic artery
Superior vena cava
Aorta, ascending
Aorta, root
Atrium, right
Ventricle, right
Inferior vena cava

Humerus, head
Common carotid artery, left
Subclavian artery, left
Trachea
Main pulmonary artery
Ventricle, left
Interventricular septum
Aorta, abdominal

300-16

T1W

Figure 14-2. Thorax, coronal, T1W. These images (A–F) are taken sequentially from anterior to posterior. **A,** At the level of the anterior ascending aorta, the right ventricle outflow tract and main pulmonary artery are seen. **B,** The aortic arch and great vessels are shown superiorly. Bilateral malignant pleural effusions account for the diffuse low signal seen in the lower lungs.

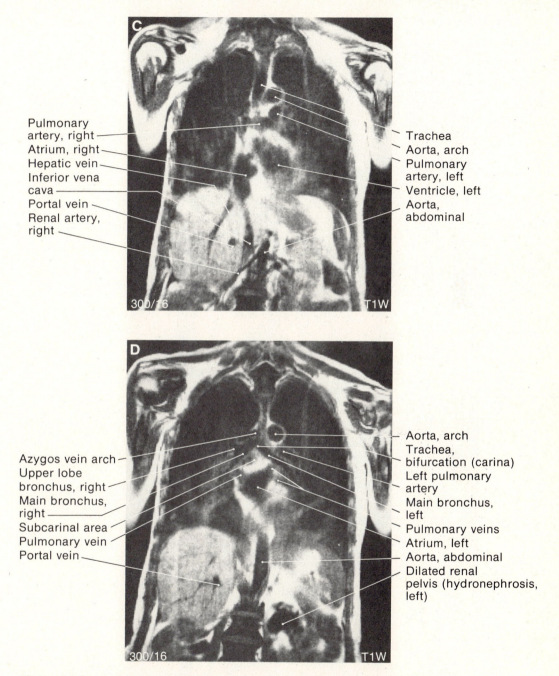

Pulmonary
artery, right

Atrium, right

Hepatic vein

Inferior vena
cava

Portal vein

Renal artery,
right

Trachea

Aorta, arch

Pulmonary
artery, left

Ventricle, left

Aorta,
abdominal

300/16   T1W

Azygos vein arch

Upper lobe
bronchus, right

Main bronchus,
right

Subcarinal area

Pulmonary vein

Portal vein

Aorta, arch

Trachea,
bifurcation (carina)

Left pulmonary
artery

Main bronchus,
left

Pulmonary veins

Atrium, left

Aorta, abdominal

Dilated renal
pelvis (hydronephrosis,
left)

300/16   T1W

Figure 14-2, cont'd. **C,** The inferior vena cava is shown entering the right atrium.
The trachea can be differentiated from vasculature by its position. A relatively bright
signal from the humoral head is normal, especially in young patients. **D,** Pulmonary
veins entering the left atrium, tracheal bifurcation, and subcarinal region are imaged.

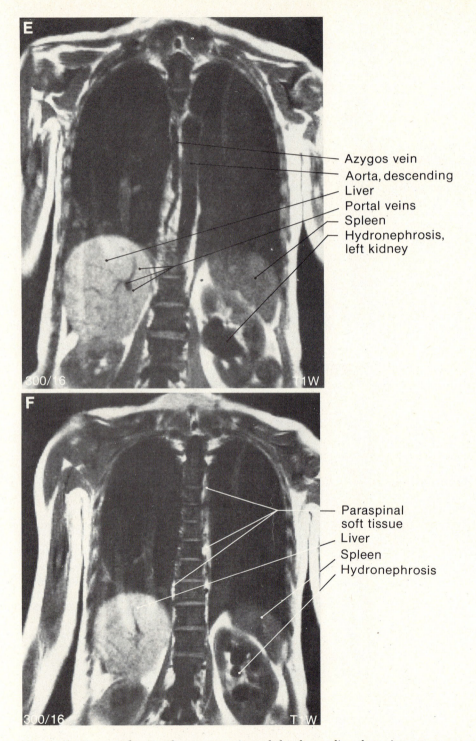

Figure 14-2, cont'd.   E, The azygos vein and the descending thoracic aorta are seen nearly in their entirety on this coronal view. Hydronephrosis of the left kidney is present.   F, Paraspinal relationships are well demonstrated in the coronal plane.

Flow artifact,
left ventricle
Main pulmonary
artery
Atrium, right
Ventricle, right

Brachiochephalic
artery (flow artifact)
Aorta, ascending
Wall left ventricle
Ventricle, left
Atrium, right

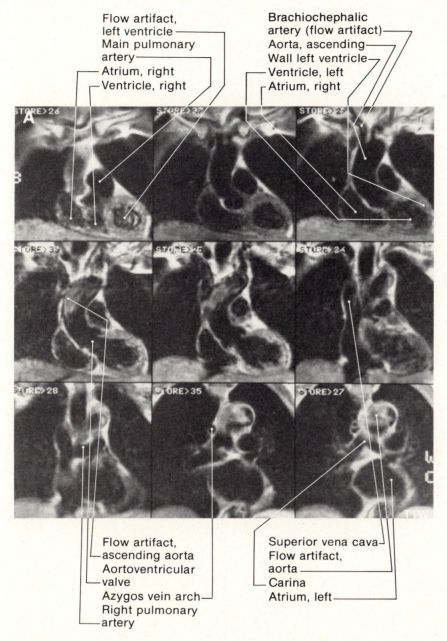

Flow artifact,
ascending aorta
Aortoventricular
valve
Azygos vein arch
Right pulmonary
artery

Superior vena cava
Flow artifact,
aorta
Carina
Atrium, left

Figure 14-3.   Thorax (heart).   A, Sequential anterior to posterior coronal T1W images show the cardiac chambers and great vessels. The intraluminal NMR signal in the left ventricle and aorta, as seen here, is usually due to in-plane turbulent and/or slow blood flow. If it is seen along the wall throughout the cardiac cycle, atherosclerotic plaques or clots should be considered.

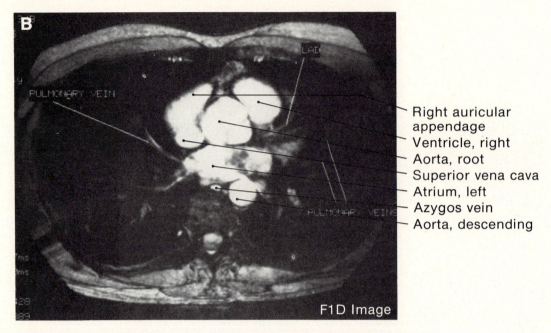

Figure 14-3, cont'd.   B, This transaxial free induction decay (FID) image of the heart demonstrates flowing blood as a high signal. Note the visualization of the left anterior descending (LAD) coronary artery. (Courtesy Picker International.)

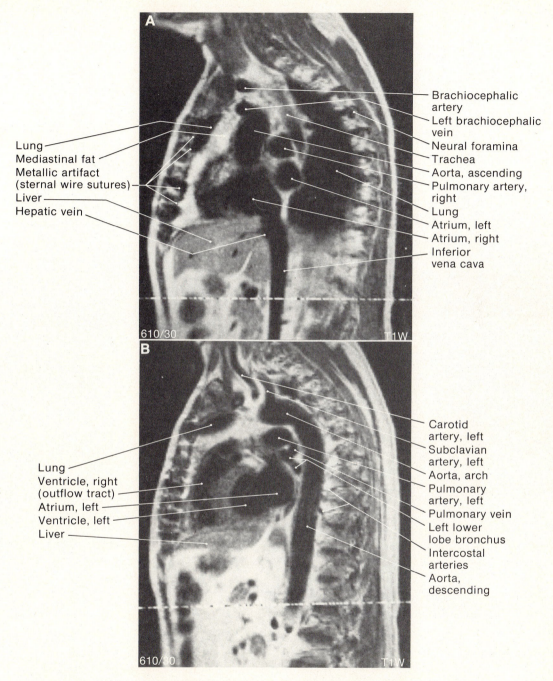

Figure 14-4. Thorax (heart), parasagittal, T1W. **A** and **B,** The thoracic aorta can be seen almost always on two or three contiguous or slightly overlapping parasagittal sections. This allows identification of the branching vessels of the aortic arch. The entry of the inferior vena cava into the right atrium, all cardiac chambers, and the pulmonary vasculature are usually well demonstrated in the sagittal plane. Metallic artifacts are present around sternal wires.

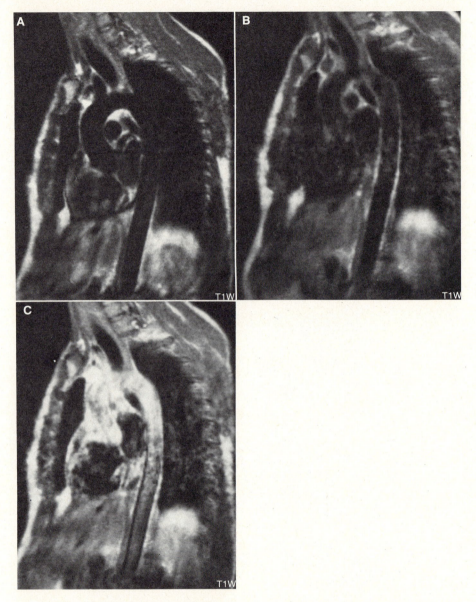

Figure 14-5. Thorax (heart), parasagittal, T1W.   **A,** A parasagittal view of the entire thoracic aorta can be obtained after measuring the angle between the ascending and descending aorta on a transaxial view to determine the parasagittal plane angle.   **B,** This parasagittal section was obtained during systole.   **C,** The increased aortic signal is an excellent example of slow flow producing increased signal during diastole. Aortic flow may actually revert to a retrograde direction in late diastole.

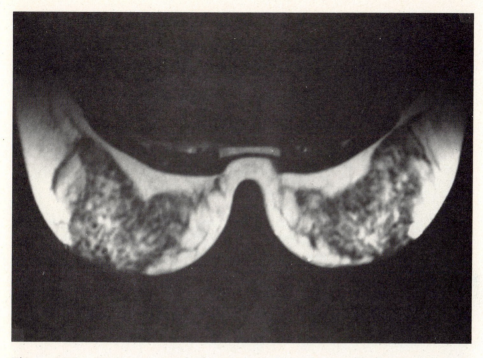

Figure 14-6.   Breasts, transaxial. This image is obtained using double circumferential surface coils that partially surround the breasts. The central stromal tissue has a lower signal than the surrounding adipose tissue. Cystic and fibrous components will both be dark on T1W scans, with the cysts becoming bright on T2W studies. (Courtesy Bruker Instruments.)

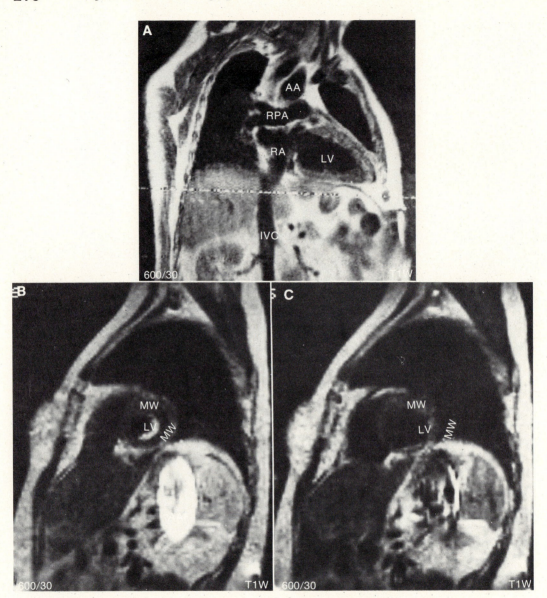

Figure 14-7.   Thorax (heart), T1W.   **A,** This paracoronal view demonstrates the left ventricle (LV) in its long axis, right pulmonary artery (RPA), aortic arch (AA), right atrium (RA), and inferior vena cava (IVC).   **B,** Parasagittal view through the left ventricle in systole show myocardial wall (MW) thickening and reduction of the chamber size. There is a very bright complex aliasing artifact (AAF) overlying the upper abdomen.   **C,** Parasagittal view during diastole shows left ventricular distention.

Gallbladder
Portal veins
Caudate lobe liver
Inferior vena cava
Azygos vein
Liver

Stomach
Crus of diaphragm
Aorta, descending
Hemiazygos vein
Spleen

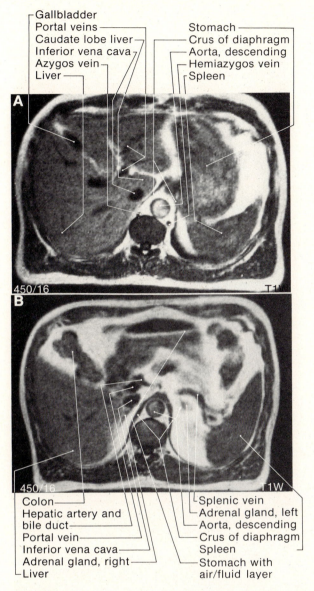

450/16   T1W

Colon
Hepatic artery and
bile duct
Portal vein
Inferior vena cava
Adrenal gland, right
Liver

Splenic vein
Adrenal gland, left
Aorta, descending
Crus of diaphragm
Spleen
Stomach with
air/fluid layer

Figure 14-8.   Abdomen, transaxial, T1W. These images **(A to F)** provide excellent
anatomic display of the abdominal organs and vascular structures. They are taken
sequentially from the upper to the lower abdomen.   **A,** The liver fissures are easily
seen because of the high signal from fat within them. Liver is brighter than muscle
and spleen on these T1W images. Low signal from bile is present in a partially
contracted gallbladder. Inhomogeneous signal from the stomach is seen because of
fluid and other material.   **B,** The vessels, with their lack of signal, are easily seen
when outlined by bright fat. The adrenals are of medium intensity and also outlined
by fat.

Celiac artery axis
Left gastric artery
Stomach with
air/fluid layer
Colon
Portal vein
Inferior vena cava
Adrenal gland, right
Liver

Spleen
Adrenal gland, left
Aorta, descending
Crus, diaphragm
Splenic vein
Pancreas, tail
Kidney, left, top
Pancreas, body

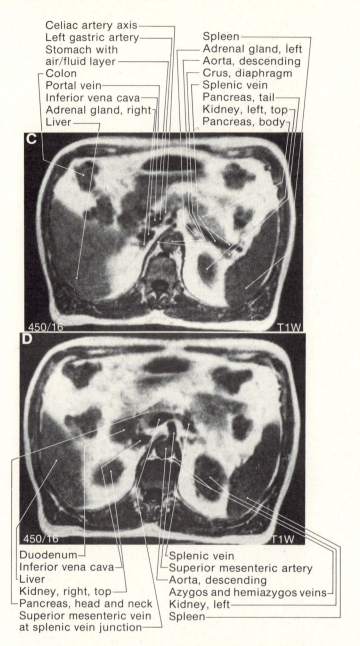

Duodenum
Inferior vena cava
Liver
Kidney, right, top
Pancreas, head and neck
Superior mesenteric vein
at splenic vein junction

Splenic vein
Superior mesenteric artery
Aorta, descending
Azygos and hemiazygos veins
Kidney, left
Spleen

Figure 14-8, cont'd.   **C,** The splenic vein is seen adjacent to the pancreas. The characteristic left adrenal **Y** shape is partially seen.   **D,** The dark superior mesenteric vein marks the location of the pancreatic neck. Azygos and hemiazygos veins are visible in the retrocrural area.

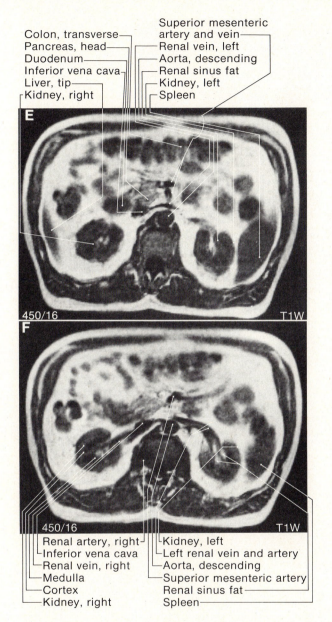

Colon, transverse
Pancreas, head
Duodenum
Inferior vena cava
Liver, tip
Kidney, right

Superior mesenteric
artery and vein
Renal vein, left
Aorta, descending
Renal sinus fat
Kidney, left
Spleen

E
450/16   T1W

F
450/16   T1W

Renal artery, right
Inferior vena cava
Renal vein, right
Medulla
Cortex
Kidney, right

Kidney, left
Left renal vein and artery
Aorta, descending
Superior mesenteric artery
Renal sinus fat
Spleen

Figure 14-8, cont'd.   E, The left renal vein crosses anterior to the aorta to join the inferior vena cava.   F, The renal medulla and cortex have different signal intensities, which are visible only on T1W scans. The right renal vein is seen entering the inferior vena cava. The origin of the left renal artery from the aorta is shown.

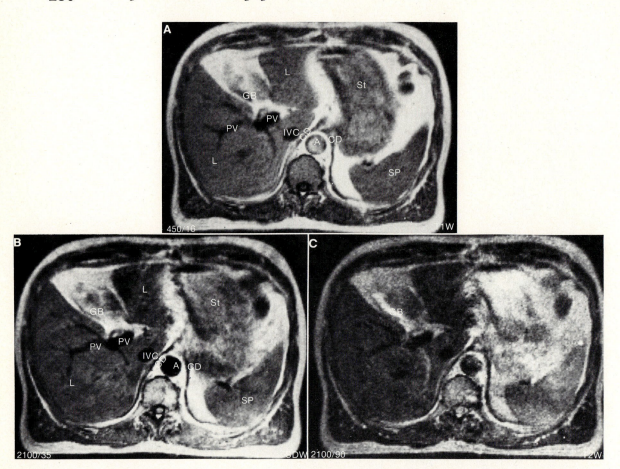

Figure 14-9. Three transaxial abdominal images at the same level demonstrate the different appearances seen with different RF pulse sequences. A large fissure anteriorly within the liver contains a small gallbladder (GB) and abundant fat. The liver (L), portal veins (PV), inferior vena cava (IVC), aorta (A), crura of the diaphragm (CD), spleen (Sp), and stomach (St) are demonstrated.   **A,** The signal of the crus of the diaphragm is lower on T1W and T2W images than that of other muscle because they are fiberlike and highly organized, similar to ligaments and tendons.   **B,** Fat remains relatively bright. Gallbladder bile becomes isointense with fat. Simple fluid would be less intense than fat on this SDW image. Liver is isointense with spleen. There is an air-fluid level in the stomach.   **C,** All tissues have lost considerable signal, producing decreased image quality secondary to the lower signal-to-noise ratio. Gallbladder and stomach fluid signals are now brighter than fat. The intensity of the spleen is greater than that of the liver on T2W images because greater water content in the spleen increases the signal with this pulse sequence.

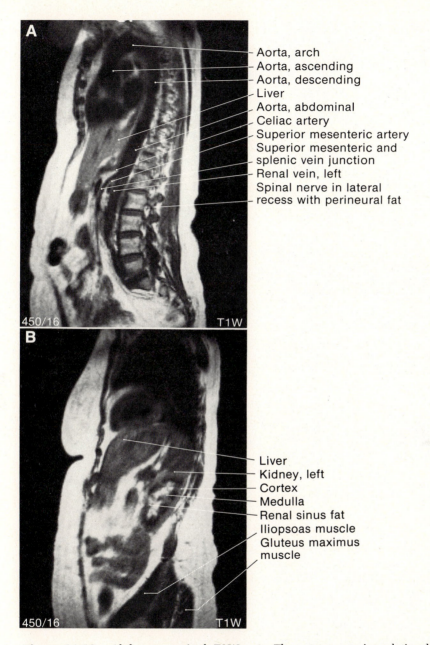

A

Aorta, arch
Aorta, ascending
Aorta, descending
Liver
Aorta, abdominal
Celiac artery
Superior mesenteric artery
Superior mesenteric and
splenic vein junction
Renal vein, left
Spinal nerve in lateral
recess with perineural fat

450/16   T1W

B

Liver
Kidney, left
Cortex
Medulla
Renal sinus fat
Iliopsoas muscle
Gluteus maximus
muscle

450/16   T1W

Figure 14-10.   Abdomen, sagittal, T1W.   **A,** The anteroposterior relationships of the vessels and the surrounding organs are well demonstrated, particularly the aorta and its anterior branches. The spinal nerves can be seen exiting the neural foramina because they are surrounded by fat. This image is 1.5 cm left of midline.   **B,** The renal peripelvic fat is bright (signal intensity similar to other fat), and corticomedullary signal difference is well seen. This image is 7.5 cm left of midline.

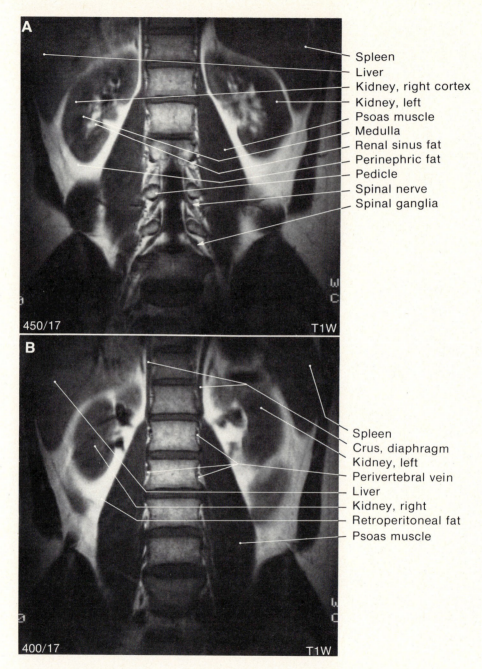

Figure 14-11. Abdomen, coronal, T1W. These images (**A** and **B**) demonstrate the relationship of the kidneys to adjacent abdominal organs. The spinal nerves are seen exiting beneath the pedicles. The retroperitoneal fat, psoas muscles, paravertebral veins, and diaphragmatic crura are well shown. (Courtesy Siemens Medical Systems, Inc.)

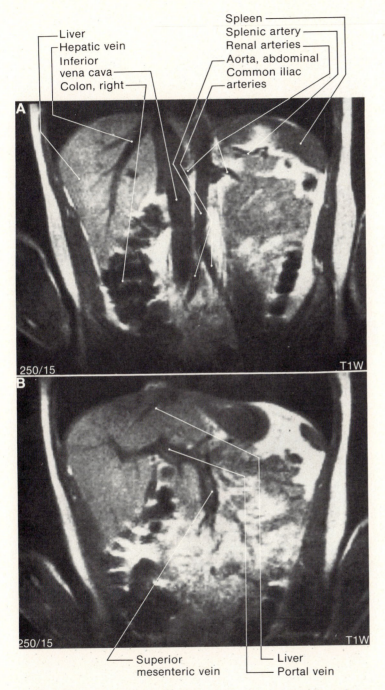

Figure 14-12. Abdomen, coronal, T1W. **A** and **B,** The inferior vena cava, aorta, and relationship of abdominal organs (including the retroperitoneal portions of bowel such as the colon) are well defined. Major abdominal vessels, including the portal vein, hepatic veins, and renal arteries, are seen.

CHAPTER
FIFTEEN

MRI Anatomy: Pelvis and Extremities

PELVIS

MRI of the pelvis can display the normal anatomic planes of the soft tissue and adjacent pelvic viscera with excellent detail because there is very little motion in this region. An understanding of the pelvic anatomy and the relationships of the pelvic viscera is important in the evaluation of the multiplanar magnetic resonance images. The symmetric muscular walls of the pelvis provide landmarks for imaging the other structures. The pelvic vascular structures are well demonstrated and also helpful as landmarks. Because the major organs of the pelvis are near the midline, they are easier to image. Tissue characteristics of the male pelvis and female pelvis are given in Tables 15-1 and 15-2, respectively.

BLADDER

The bladder must be well distended for optimal examination. The urine provides an ideal contrast material on either T1W or T2W images, allowing visualization of the inner surface of the bladder. The bladder wall is demonstrated

Table 15-1   MRI tissue characteristics of the male pelvis

Tissues	SDW	T1W	T2W
Fat	Light gray	Gray	Gray
Penis	Gray	Dark gray	Light gray
Prostate	Light gray	Gray	Gray
Seminal vesicles	Gray	Gray	Light gray
Testes	Gray	Dark gray	Gray

Table 15-2   MRI tissue characteristics of the female pelvis

Tissues	SDW	T1W	T2W
Fat	Light gray	White	Gray
Bladder wall	Dark gray	Gray	Dark gray
Cervix	Dark gray	Gray	Gray
Ovary	Light gray	Gray	Light gray
Uterus*			
Endometrium	Light gray	Gray	White
Junction zone	Dark gray	Gray	Dark gray
Myometrium	Gray	Gray	Light gray
Vagina	Gray	Dark gray	Dark gray

*Highly variable depending on time of menstrual cycle, birth control pills, and pre- and postmenopausal states.

best with T2W images by the moderately bright surrounding pelvic fat and the high signal of urine from the inside. The relationship of the bladder to other pelvic organs is seen best on T1W images when the urine is dark. Transaxial, coronal, and sagittal images can be used to good advantage. The transaxial view is tangential to the bladder's interface with most of the midline pelvic organs, except the seminal vesicles. The ureters can be identified, but the points of insertion are not always seen.

MALE ORGANS

PROSTATE.   The prostate is a gray structure immediately inferior to the bladder. It can be divided into central and peripheral zones that are best seen on the T2W images. The central zone is usually darker, presumably because of the presence of striated muscle. High signal fat usually separates the prostate from the seminal vesicles. This makes spread of prostate disease to the seminal vesicles easier to detect, particularly when the transaxial view is used. Coronal and sagittal planes are better for viewing the bladder base and its relationship to the prostate. Oblique planes perpendicular to the long axis of the prostate have been used to optimally view the prostate's relationship to the other regional tissue.

SEMINAL VESICLES.   The seminal vesicles have an intermediate signal intensity on T1W and SDW sequences but becomes moderately bright on T2W images. They are outlined by the bright signal from fat and best demonstrated on transaxial view. Invasive cancers from the bladder, prostate, or rectum may infiltrate the seminal vesicles and intervening fat and disrupt their visualization.

PENIS AND URETHRA.   The urethra is dark gray on most pulse sequences. The corpus spongiosum and corpora cavernosa are moderately bright, whereas the bulbospongiosus muscles at the base are darker. The three compartments are divided by dark bands of connective tissue. The urethra may occasionally be followed in its entirety with a single sagittal view. However, the cross-sectional views of the coronal and transaxial planes are usually more helpful.

SCROTUM AND TESTES.   The spermatic cord can be followed from the inguinal canal to the epididymis in the transaxial plane. The course through the anterior abdominal wall and into the scrotum can occasionally be visualized on a single coronal slice. The cord contains the ductus deferens and spermatic artery and vein. The artery and vein usually produce signal voids. The testicles and epididymides are moderately bright and maintain similar signal characteristics throughout most spin-echo pulse sequences. Masses and architectural derangement can be appreciated best when surface coils are used.

FEMALE ORGANS

OVARIES.   The ovaries are gray on T1W images and relatively bright on T2W images. They are easily differentiated from the high signal of fat, but they exhibit an intensity similar to that of the uterus. On heavily T2W images the ovaries become even brighter than fat. The normal peripherally located follicles and the larger corpus luteum are seen with typical features of small cysts. The dominant follicles can be followed to the point of rupture during the normal menstrual cycle.

Differentiating the ovaries from bowel loops and adjacent foci of mesenteric fat is sometimes difficult, especially if T2W images or contiguous coronal views are not part of the imaging protocol. A paraxial plane perpendicular to the uterine body can be employed to allow optimal visualization of the uterus and localization of the ovaries within the broad ligament.

UTERUS.   The premenopausal and postmenopausal uterus is gray and shows much less zonal contrast than the active uterus. The zonal contrast consists of the bright endometrium, the dark junctional zone, and the medium signal from myometrium. The greatest contrast between these zones is generally during the late proliferative stage and is seen best on T2W images.

The vagina lies between the urethra, bladder, and rectum, all of which provide good contrast, even if the bladder is not distended or the rectum filled with air. Optimal imaging of the vagina is obtained in the proliferative stage.

The transaxial plane demonstrates the cervical uterus and vagina well, although the corpus is not usually seen in cross section. Sagittal views of the uterus, which show the entire uterine length, can supplement the transaxial images. Coronal views can be helpful if pelvic sidewall invasion is questioned in patients with uterine or cervical carcinoma. Uterine fibroids, the extent of pelvic endometriosis, and certain ovarian neoplasms such as teratomas are shown particularly well with MRI.

PELVIC VESSELS

The pelvic arteries and veins are identified by their dark circular or tubular appearance, which is in contrast to the strong signal from surrounding fat and muscle. An intraluminal signal is occasionally seen on some pulse sequences. This may produce a confusing image because the intraluminal signal changes are not always symmetric; that is, one iliac vein may have more intraluminal signal because of focal slower flow. Most major vessels are oriented vertically, and their course can be followed on contiguous transaxial images. The locations of the associated nerves can be inferred once these vessels are identified. The vessels are readily distinguishable from adjacent normal and enlarged lymph nodes.

PELVIC GIRDLE

The skeletal and muscular components of the pelvis are well demonstrated on T1W images where the high-signal fat outlines the various muscle groups. Cortical bone is outlined by the bright signal from marrow along the internal surface and the gray signal from muscle along the external surface. The normal bright signal from marrow on both T1W and T2W images is secondary to the signal from both fat and water. This property allows MRI techniques to be very sensitive to any pathologic changes within the marrow.

The signals from the sacroiliac joints and the symphysis pubis are predominently dark in adults. Medium-intensity signal can be seen from the cartilage components of the sacroiliac joints in children and occasionally until the start of the fourth decade. The fibrous material that develops in these joints remains dark on all pulse sequences.

MRI of the iliopsoas and other muscle groups of the pelvis is unsurpassed by any other modality. This is accomplished by obtaining a T1W or SDW image because the signal from muscle and surrounding tissues decreases on T2W images.

Coronal and transaxial views are best suited for imaging of the pelvic musculoskeletal region. Normal symmetry and most of the major muscle groups and bones are seen in cross section and longitudinal orientation with these imaging planes. The sagittal view can be useful in sacral and acetabular evaluation.

EXTREMITIES

MRI of the musculoskeletal system gives excellent anatomic and pathologic information, much of which is unobtainable with other noninvasive imaging techniques. Because of the exquisite soft-tissue contrast present with the high-

Table 15-3   MRI tissue characteristics of the musculoskeletal system

Tissues	SDW	T1W	T2W
Fat	Light gray	White	Gray
Bone Marrow	Light gray	White	Light gray
Cartilage	Light gray	Light gray	Gray
Cortical Bone, meniscus, ligament, and tendon	Black	Black	Black
Muscle, skeletal	Gray	Gray	Dark gray

signal intensity of the marrow space and adjacent soft tissues about the cortical bones, one can demonstrate exquisite detail of intraskeletal, paraskeletal, and intraarticular anatomy. Even though cortical bone does not contribute to the signal, a very readable image of the bony structures can be obtained. Tissue characteristics of the musculoskeletal system are listed in Table 15-3.

HIPS

The hips are ideally imaged with MRI in all age groups, although the normal signal from various components changes with age. The unossified epiphysis and apophysis of the infant are moderately bright on both T1W and T2W images and the growth plates are darker. On T1W images there is a slow increase in signal intensity from the femoral head and neck up to approximately age 30. This is probably secondary to increasing marrow fat that replaces the cellular hematopoietic marrow. The ossified epiphyseal regions remain the area of highest signal intensity within the normal femur throughout life.

The hyaline cartilage appears as a moderately bright signal covering the cortical surfaces of the acetabula and femoral head. Its thickness and signal strength decrease with increasing age. Focal thinning or decrease in signal can suggest degeneration.

The transaxial and coronal planes are the most useful for evaluation of the hips as these planes intersect the skeletal structures in parallel and cross-sectional orientation. The transaxial plane is better for evaluating the long bone marrow involvement, as it avoids most partial volume artifacts. The coronal orientation is suited for determining the extent of pathologic processes along the vertically oriented muscle planes and with the femoral heads.

KNEES

The knee cartilage, ligaments, menisci, and regional bone marrow can be imaged with great ease and definition. Sagittal views provide excellent visibility of the anterior and posterior cruciate ligaments, menisci, popliteal vessels, and surrounding tissues. Coronal views allow visualization of the collateral ligaments and lateral aspects of the menisci. The identification of muscle groups, tendons, patellae, collateral ligaments, and diaphyseal bone marrow spaces is shown best on transaxial views.

ANKLES

The anatomy of the ankle and foot produces excellent contrast between all of the major structures. T1W images are primarily used for anatomic resolution, with the bone marrow spaces being bright, muscle groups gray, and the various ligamentous structures black. The hyaline cartilage of the tibiotalar joint is visible as a bright curvilinear structure between the corresponding cortices of the tibia and talus. T2W images are used to detect areas of inflammation, edema, and other pathologic states.

Direct sagittal imaging is probably the most useful orientation to view the foot, as the relationship beween the various tarsal and metatarsal bones can be appreciated. Coronal and, to a lesser extent, transaxial planes, are valuable in examination of the ankle, as this provides longitudinal and cross-sectional views of the deltoid and medial ligaments.

SHOULDER

Evaluation of the shoulder by MRI is of similar utility and appearance as for the hips. The regional skeleton is best seen on T1W images where the marrow is brightest. The normal long head of the biceps is dark on all pulse sequences, as are all tendons and ligamentous structures. The coronal and transaxial views are most often used for viewing the muscles and tendons of the rotator cuff. For ideal image quality, a surface coil is necessary because the shoulder is near the edge of the field of view in the standard body coil.

WRIST AND HAND

The contrast between the black cortices and bright bone marrow components of the carpal and tubular bones, along with the ability to use multiple planes of view, allows for precise definition of the anatomic structures of the wrist and hand. The nerves, blood vessels, and tendons can be followed through the carpal tunnel, which is difficult by other imaging techniques.

A T1W image is usually used for imaging of the hand. T2W images can reliably detect edema or other inflammatory changes. The transaxial views are suited for examination of the structures within the carpal tunnel and the tubular bones in cross section. The sagittal and particularly the coronal views are helpful in examination of the radiocarpal joint.

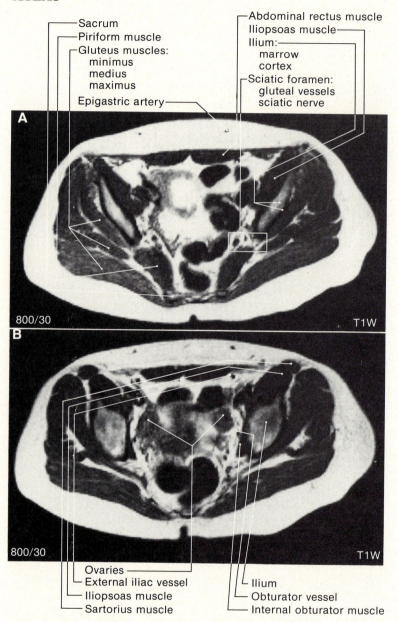

Sacrum
Piriform muscle
Gluteus muscles:
    minimus
    medius
    maximus
Epigastric artery

Abdominal rectus muscle
Iliopsoas muscle
Ilium:
    marrow
    cortex
Sciatic foramen:
    gluteal vessels
    sciatic nerve

A

800/30   T1W

B

800/30   T1W

Ovaries
External iliac vessel
Iliopsoas muscle
Sartorius muscle

Ilium
Obturator vessel
Internal obturator muscle

Figure 15-1. Pelvis (female), transaxial. These images (**A-D**) provide excellent soft-tissue contrast and differentiation of pelvic structures. They are taken sequentially from the ileum superiorly to the femoral neck inferiorly. **A,** High-signal fat between muscles helps define the muscle groups. Gluteal vessels and the associated sciatic nerve are nearing their exit through sciatic foramen. Fat of the anterior abdominal wall outlines the epigastric arteries. **B,** The ovaries are of lower signal intensity than fat on T1W and SDW images.

Muscles:
gluteus minimus
iliopsoas
femoral rectus
tensor fascia lata
sartorius

Bladder
Femoral artery and vein
Femur, head
Femur, greater trochanter
Gluteus maximus muscle
Ischium

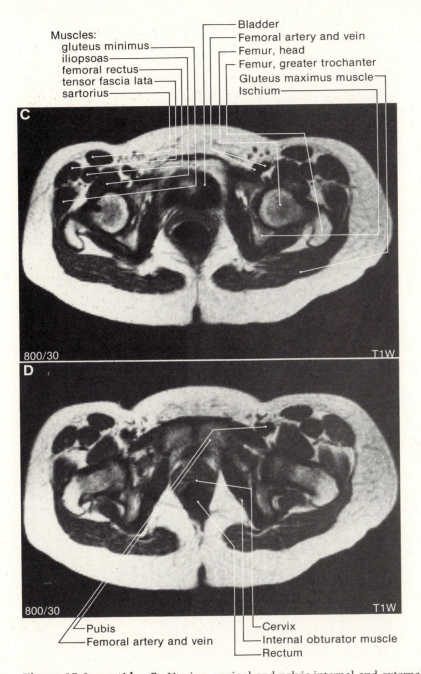

C

800/30   T1W

D

800/30   T1W

Pubis
Femoral artery and vein

Cervix
Internal obturator muscle
Rectum

Figure 15-1, cont'd.   C, Uterine, vaginal and pelvic internal and external tissue planes are imaged better on T2W images. The uterine body blends with the urine in the partially filled bladder because of partial volume effects on this T1W image.
D, The cervix is seen very close to the rectum. Because the use of this pulse sequence does not allow differentiation of the cervix and rectal wall, pathologic thickening could be missed.

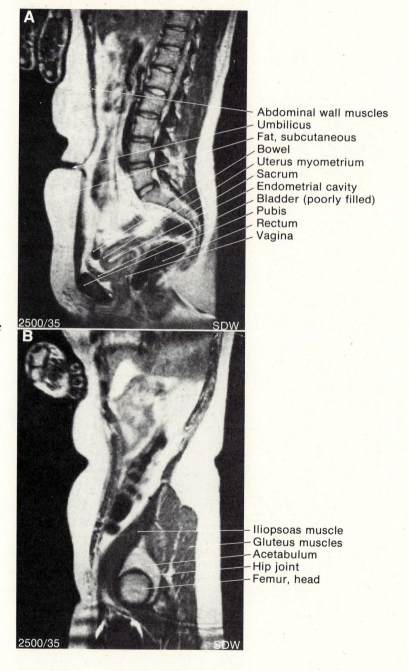

Figure 15-2. Pelvis (female), sagittal. These images (**A** and **B**) demonstrate the vertical and anteroposterior relationships of pelvic structures. **A,** This midline saggital view is ideal for demonstrating the uterus and its relationship to the bladder, rectum, and lower abdomen. Bowel motion artifact occasionally obscures the uterine fundus with this projection. **B,** The iliopsoas muscles and acetabular regions are demonstrated on this parasagittal image. The structures extending into or from these areas can be easily detected. The rim of high signal inferior to the femoral head is an artifact resulting from aliasing and diaphragm motion.

Abdominal wall muscles
Umbilicus
Fat, subcutaneous
Bowel
Uterus myometrium
Sacrum
Endometrial cavity
Bladder (poorly filled)
Pubis
Rectum
Vagina

Iliopsoas muscle
Gluteus muscles
Acetabulum
Hip joint
Femur, head

2500/35   SDW

2500/35   SDW

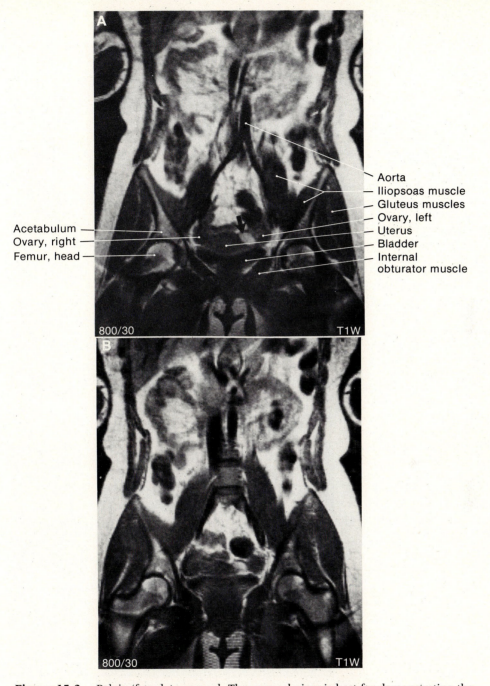

Acetabulum —
Ovary, right —
Femur, head —

Aorta
Iliopsoas muscle
Gluteus muscles
Ovary, left
Uterus
Bladder
Internal
obturator muscle

800/30   T1W

800/30   T1W

Figure 15-3. Pelvis (female), coronal. The coronal view is best for demonstrating the adnexa. These images are taken from anterior to posterior. **A,** Both ovaries are seen with the right visibly connected to the uterus and the left separated from the uterus by a "knuckle" of fat *(arrow)* in the bowel mesentery. The uterus and adnexa are isointense on T1W images, and the ovaries become relatively brighter on T2W images. **B,** The soft-tissue planes between the cervix and pelvic sidewalls are demonstrated. The left adnexa can be seen better on this more posterior slice.

Figure 15-4. Localization.
A, Localization with a transaxial image allows one to determine if a particular sequence's range of coverage will include the areas of interest. It also allows the radiologist to confirm whether a specific organ or lesion is seen on another orientation view covering the same area. **B,** The right ovary *(arrow)* is nearly isointense with fat, making it difficult to identify, but its location can be confirmed by noting that its position on the transaxial image is at "grid" number −4.8 c.m. on the right. The right ovary can be localized on the sagittal image by taking the corresponding plane at the numer SP −48 (slice position). **C,** The right ovary *(arrow)* shows a characteristic bright periphery because of the many small follicles, which have a very long T2 relaxation time.

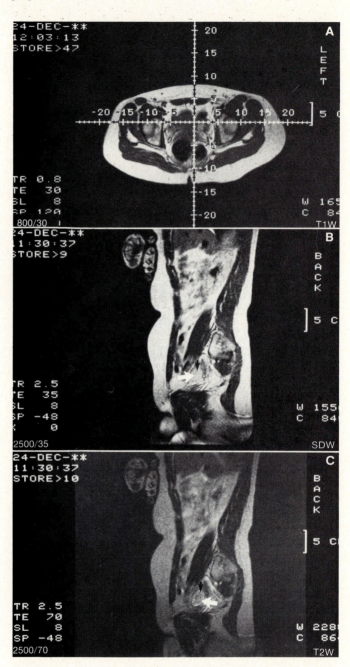

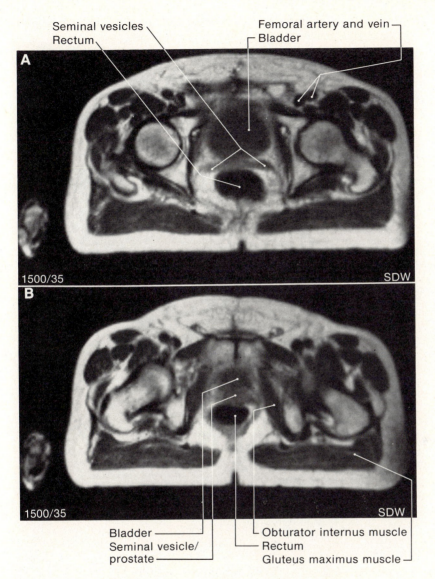

Seminal vesicles
Rectum

Femoral artery and vein
Bladder

A

1500/35   SDW

B

1500/35   SDW

Bladder
Seminal vesicle/
prostate

Obturator internus muscle
Rectum
Gluteus maximus muscle

Figure 15-5. Pelvis (male), transaxial. **A,** Seminal vesicles are outlined and separated from the bladder by fat. The urine in the bladder is of medium signal intensity, neary equal to that of the seminal vesicles and prostate on this sequence. **B,** The neck of the bladder and the prostate are in contact with each other normally. The anterior rectal wall is also directly adjacent to the prostate. The prostate shows medium signal intensity and remains that way relative to other tissues on most pulse sequences. Obturator internus muscles outline the lateral pelvic wall.

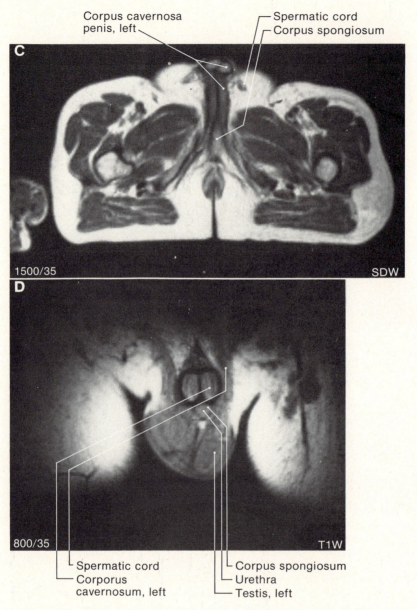

Figure 15-5, cont'd. **C,** The proximal urethra is seen almost in its entirety. The spermatic cords are anterior and outlined by abdominal wall fat as they descend into the scrotum. **D,** The scrotum and three compartments of the penis are seen in cross section on this coronal view. The intensity of the testicles and epididymides remains approximately the same on most spin-echo sequences.

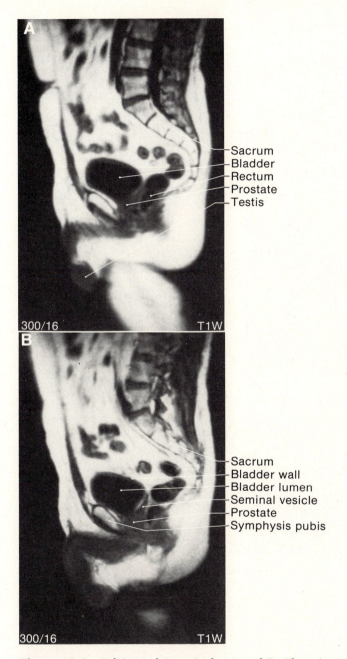

Sacrum
Bladder
Rectum
Prostate
Testis

300/16   T1W

Sacrum
Bladder wall
Bladder lumen
Seminal vesicle
Prostate
Symphysis pubis

300/16   T1W

Figure 15-6. Pelvis (male); sagittal. **A** and **B,** These images show the relationship of the prostate, bladder, rectum, and seminal vesicles. The internal surface of the bladder can be adequately evaluated if full. A seminal vesicle is outlined by fat between the bladder and rectum.

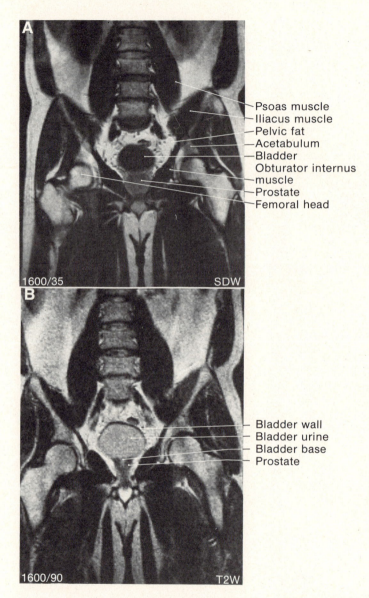

Figure 15-7. Pelvis (male), coronal. **A,** This image shows the relationship of the prostate to the lateral pelvic walls (obturator internus muscles) and the base and neck of the bladder. **B,** The bladder urine in this image is brighter when a longer TE is used, allowing the bladder wall to be seen as a dark structure between urine and pelvic fat.

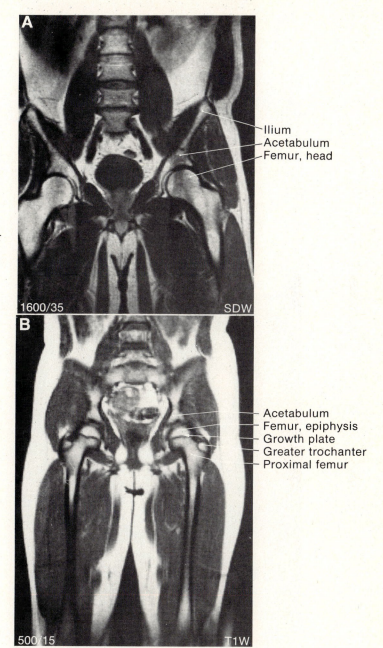

Figure 15-8. Hips, coronal. **A,** Within the proximal femur, a slight decrease in intensity from marrow fat is seen diagonally from the superior femoral head to the inferior neck. This is secondary to the normally thicker trabecular bone in this region displacing the marrow fat. **B,** This image of a 9-year-old girl shows the epiphysis and apophysis with a normal, brighter signal, which is secondary to the greater amount of fat. The epiphyseal portion of the femoral head frequently remains relatively bright well into the fourth decade and sometimes beyond. The growth plate is thicker than that seen in adults.

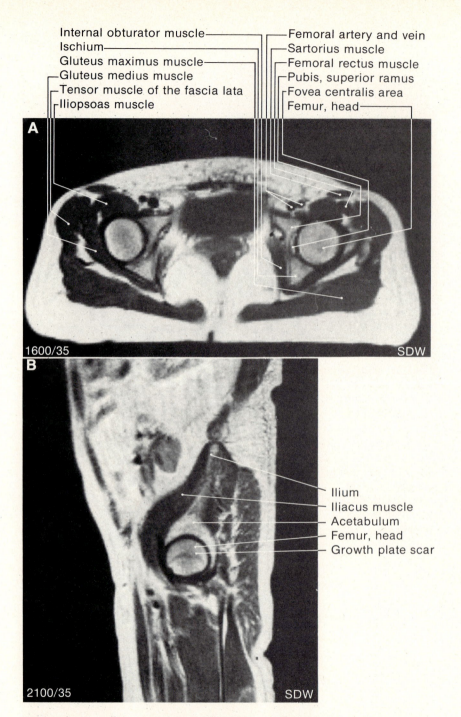

Internal obturator muscle ──────────
Ischium ───────
Gluteus maximus muscle ────────
Gluteus medius muscle ──────
Tensor muscle of the fascia lata ──
Iliopsoas muscle ──

Femoral artery and vein
Sartorius muscle
Femoral rectus muscle
Pubis, superior ramus
Fovea centralis area
Femur, head ──────

A

1600/35   SDW

B

Ilium
Iliacus muscle
Acetabulum
Femur, head
Growth plate scar

2100/35   SDW

Figure 15-9. Hips. **A,** The transaxial image shows the bilateral, relatively symmetric areas of low intensity in the femoral heads. These are normal and secondary to the increased thickness of stress-bearing trabecular bone. **B,** The sagittal image shows the acetabular hips, which are particularly useful for evaluating dislocation fractures in patients with prior trauma or chronic hip dislocation.

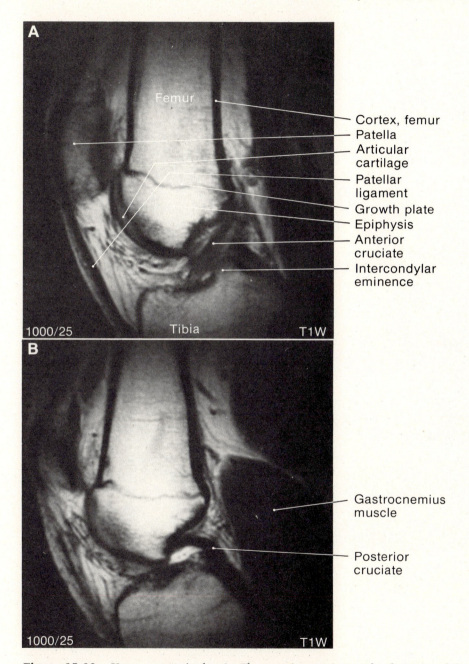

A

Femur

Cortex, femur
Patella
Articular
cartilage
Patellar
ligament
Growth plate
Epiphysis
Anterior
cruciate
Intercondylar
eminence

1000/25   Tibia   T1W

B

Gastrocnemius
muscle

Posterior
cruciate

1000/25   T1W

Figure 15-10. Knee, parasagittal. **A,** The anterior cruciate and soft tissues of the intracondylar notch are shown. **B,** The posterior cruciate is seen as a black curvilinear band near midline. It stretches between the posterior tibia and the inferior femoral surface and is easily seen because it is fairly thick and surrounded by fat.

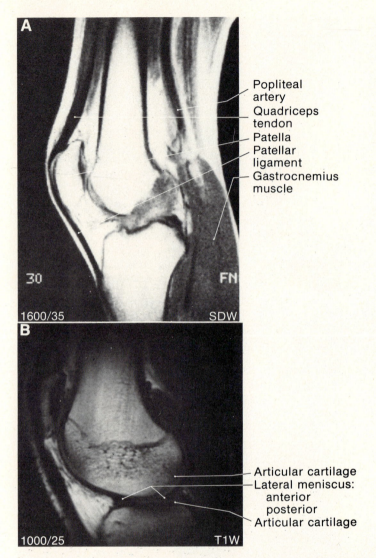

Figure 15-11.   Knee, sagittal.   **A,** This midline sagittal image of the knee shows the relationship of the joint to the structure of the popliteal space, including the vessels and musculature.   **B,** This sagittal knee image shows the "bowtie" of the lateral meniscus. The normal menisci are black and outlined by bright strips of cartilage in the vertical directions and by high signal fat in the anteroposterior directions.

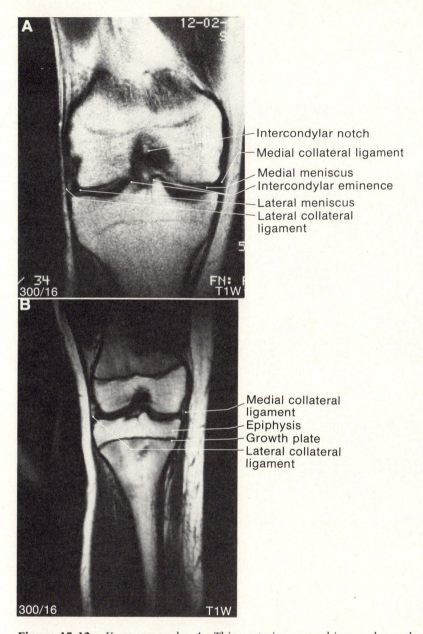

Figure 15-12.   Knee, coronal.   **A,** This posterior coronal image shows the medial and lateral collateral ligaments and menisci. The anterior and posterior cruciates are seen in cross section as dark circles entering the intercondylar notch. The epiphyses in this 15-year-old boy are normally bright.   **B,** The collateral ligaments are better seen in this more anterior view as compared with **A.** The inhomogeneity with associated dark areas in the proximal tibia is secondary to a chondrosarcoma, which has not disrupted the growth plate in this case.

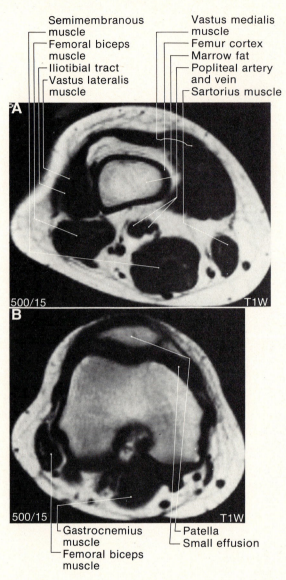

Semimembranous muscle
Femoral biceps muscle
Iliotibial tract
Vastus lateralis muscle

Vastus medialis muscle
Femur cortex
Marrow fat
Popliteal artery and vein
Sartorius muscle

A

500/15   T1W

B

500/15   T1W

Gastrocnemius muscle
Femoral biceps muscle

Patella
Small effusion

Figure 15-13. Knee, transaxial. **A,** This cross-sectional image through the distal femoral shaft shows the various muscle groups, vessels, and neurovascular bundles. **B,** This view is at the level of the femoral condyles. A small effusion is seen anterior to the medial condyle. This same effusion is seen to increase in intensity in **D** and **E,** which are SDW and T2W images, respectively.

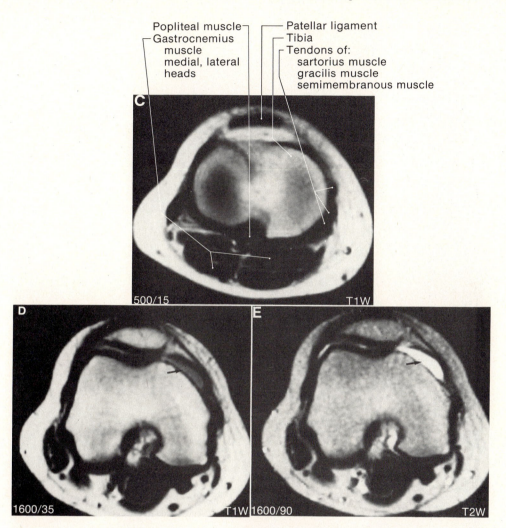

Popliteal muscle
Gastrocnemius
muscle
medial, lateral
heads

Patellar ligament
Tibia
Tendons of:
sartorius muscle
gracilis muscle
semimembranous muscle

Figure 15-13, cont'd. C, This view through the proximal tibia at the joint surface shows the normal structure of the upper calf. The infrapatellar portion of the quadriceps muscle tendons appears as a wide dark band prior to its insertion into the anterior tibia tubercle. D and E, These images show a small effusion *(arrow)* increasing the signal intensity with the increasing TE. Also, an alteration in the TE causes a change in some of the peripheral veins, which become brighter on T2W images.

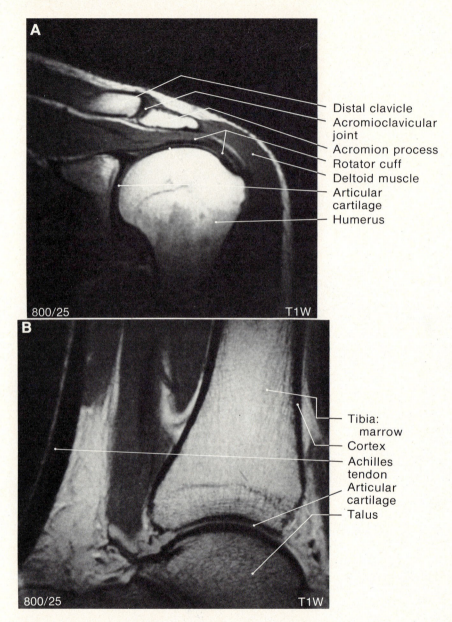

A

800/25   T1W

Distal clavicle
Acromioclavicular joint
Acromion process
Rotator cuff
Deltoid muscle
Articular cartilage
Humerus

B

800/25   T1W

Tibia: marrow
Cortex
Achilles tendon
Articular cartilage
Talus

Figure 15-14.   **A,** The coronal image of the shoulder well demonstrates the rotator cuff and its component muscle groups. (Courtesy Medical Advances, Inc., and Medical College of Wisconsin.)   **B,** This sagittal surface coil view of the ankle shows the high contrast and image quality obtainable with surface coil MRI of the joint. The Achilles tendon is beautifully demonstrated as a black strip outlined by fat. (Courtesy Siemens Medical Systems, Inc.)

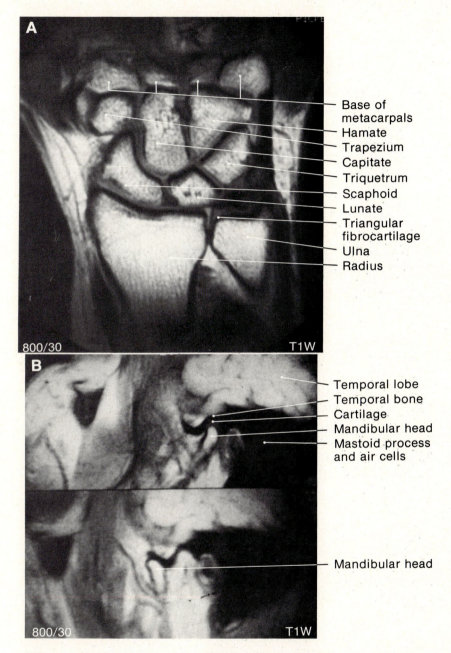

Base of
metacarpals
Hamate
Trapezium
Capitate
Triquetrum
Scaphoid
Lunate
Triangular
fibrocartilage
Ulna
Radius

Temporal lobe
Temporal bone
Cartilage
Mandibular head
Mastoid process
and air cells

Mandibular head

Figure 15-15.   A, The soft tissues, bony detail, and cartilage structures of the wrist are demonstrated with this surface coil technique. (Courtesy Picker International.) B, The fibrocartilage of the menisci of the temporomandibular joint are dark, lying between the bright marrow of the mandibular condyle and the temporal lobe. Top view is with mouth closed, and bottom view is with mouth open. (Courtesy Siemens Medical Systems, Inc.)

CHAPTER
SIXTEEN

MRI Artifacts

The complexity of MRI has unfortunately brought with it a plethora of new imaging artifacts. Luckily, many can be interpreted easily and do not interfere with diagnosis. However, the addition of each new imaging technique or RF pulse sequence brings the possibility of new artifacts. The MRI artifacts illustrated here fall into several categories. The outline following summarizes the scheme of artifact classification used here.

Classification of MRI artifacts

I. Magnetic and RF Field Distortion Artifacts
   A. Patient-related
      1. ferromagnetic materials
      2. body shape and conductivity assymmetry
      3. extension of body outside magnetic field
      4. chemical shift
   B. System-related
      1. main magnetic field inhomogeneity
      2. magnetic gradient field inhomogeneity
      3. RF coil of transmission and reception inhomogeneity
      4. gradient coil switching/timing inaccuracy
II. Reconstruction Artifacts
   A. Patient-related
      1. aliasing (wraparound)
      2. partial volume averaging

MAGNETIC AND RF FIELD DISTORTION ARTIFACTS

Metals have different effects on the local magnetic field, depending on the type and quantity of ferromagnetic components they contain. Metallic artifacts may range from almost none, as with titanium, to a rather severe effect, as with iron. **Ferromagnetic materials** can produce not only a local signal loss but also a warping distortion of the surrounding areas. An example of such field distortion is provided by the friendly "cone-head" seen in Figure 16-1.

The typical metallic artifact has a partial or complete loss of signal at the site of the metal. Additionally, a partial rim of high-signal intensity may be seen at the periphery of the signal void, which allows differentiation of metal from other causes of focal signal loss. With few exceptions, the degree of anatomic information loss owing to such an artifact is less than seen on CT images because the loss is local in nature.

Exceptions to this are usually caused by the screws in some metallic orthopedic devices, but occasionally distortion is produced by small metallic objects such as buttons, snaps, zippers, or barrettes (Figure 16-2). The distortion of the surrounding tissue is due to the metal-induced change in the local magnetic field. The magnetic field lines are distorted, resulting in a change in the local Larmor frequency (Figures 16-3 to 16-5).

More mundane but relatively common metallic materials that may be encountered include belt buckles, keys, mascara and other makeup, foreign bodies in the eye or elsewhere, and even certain types of nylon found in clothing such as gym shorts or warm-up suits (Figures 16-6 to 16-9).

Text continued on page 315.

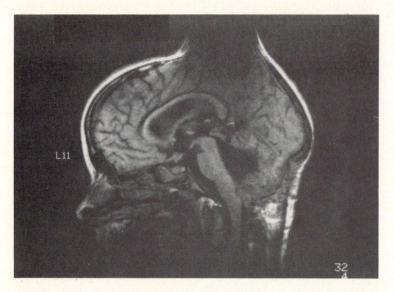

Figure 16-1.   A small band of metal in this patient's ponytail produced this other-world appearance of the head—the cone-head artifact. Although the region of interest was not affected by the artifact, the images were incinerated to avoid publicity about unanticipated adverse bioeffects of MRI.

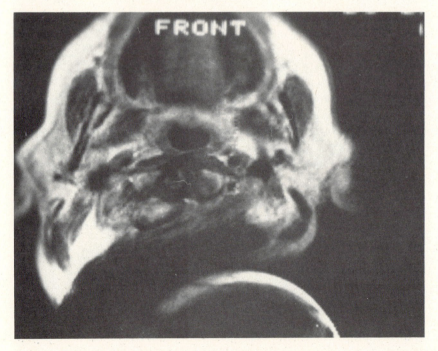

Figure 16-2.   The metallic zipper in this patient's shirt produced the marked loss of signal seen on this image. The high-signal rim at the edges of the void is typical.

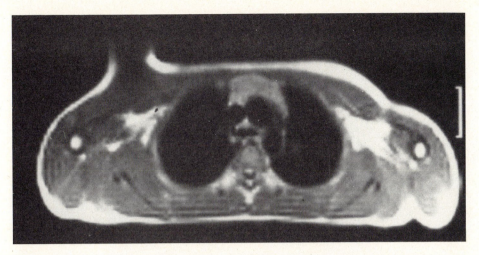

Figure 16-3. An electrocardiographic lead makes a small localized distortion of the anterior chest wall.

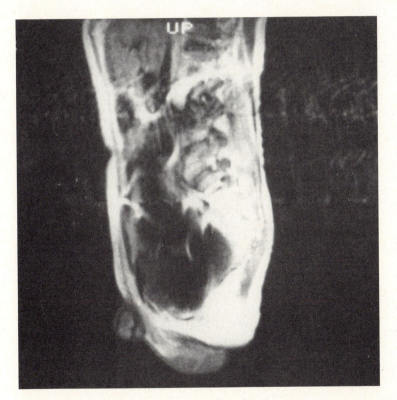

Figure 16-4. A metallic stent temporarily placed in this patient's ureter caused image degradation along the entire path from the kidney to the bladder.

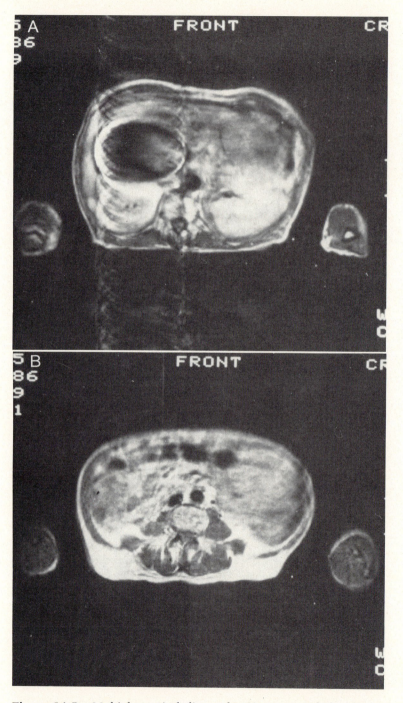

Figure 16-5.   Multiple surgical clips and a Gianturco embolization coil were in place at the time of this examination.   A, The embolization coil causes a relatively large signal void within the liver.   B, Some clips show only small amounts of signal dropout, as seen in the lower abdomen of the same patient. The effect differs depending on the specific alloy used in the clip and the imaging technique.

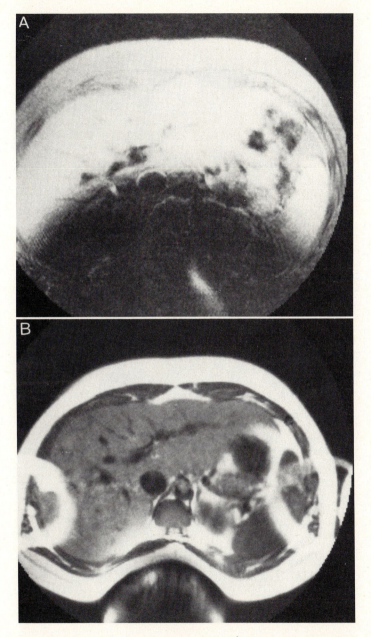

Figure 16-6. The use of gradient echo techniques in most fast scanning methods causes accentuation of local magnetic field inhomogeneities produced by ferromagnetic materials. The large area of signal dropout in **A** is due to two small metallic bra clips that were pulled up between this patient's scapulae. This spin echo image (**B**) was obtained through the same level, showing a more typical and less prominent metallic artifact. A wraparound aliasing artifact of the arms onto the abdomen is also present.

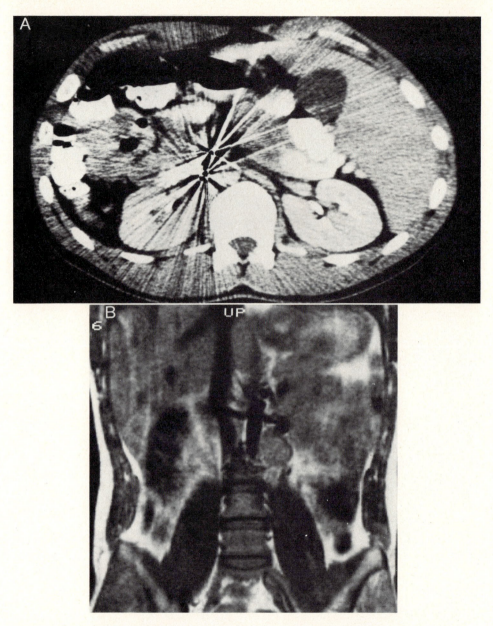

Figure 16-7.   This CT scan of the abdomen (A) was nondiagnostic as a result of the artifacts produced by surgical clips in the postoperative bed. The MRI of this same patient (B) revealed the recurrent pheochromocytoma. A small signal void immediately above the mass was due to one of the clips.

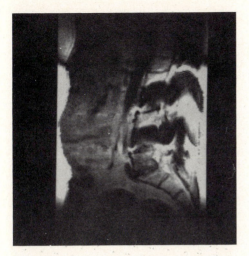

Figure 16-8. Metallic orthopedic devices can produce severe distortion and signal loss. The screws in the Harrington rods caused the image to be nondiagnostic.

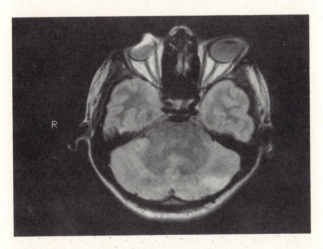

Figure 16-9. Ferrometallic material may cause significant artifacts, such as distortion of the orbital globes produced by eyeshadow.

The patient shape, conductivity, and filling of the RF coil all become factors in creating inhomogeneity of both the magnetic field and the transmitted RF pulse. Extension of the body part outside the area of maximum field homogeneity will frequently cause a metallic-like artifact at the edges of this area. This curvilinear artifact conforms to the shape of the magnetic field at the edges and may have a characteristic pattern for an individual magnet system.

There are also many system-related causes of RF and magnetic field in-

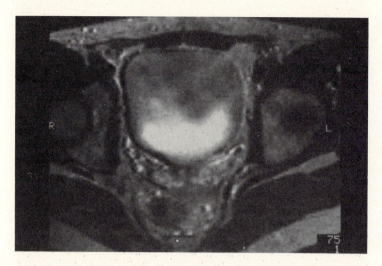

Figure 16-10.   The dark rim of signal along the right bladder wall is due to chemical-shift artifact at the interface between pelvic fat and bladder urine and wall. The left side of the bladder is brighter, which could occasionally be mistaken for edema or tumor infiltration of the normally darker bladder wall. The bright signal within the posterior urine-filled bladder is an entry slice flow phenomenon more commonly seen in blood vessels.

homogeneity. The main magnetic field can never maintain perfect stability and will vary regionally from day to day. In a similar manner, each of the hardware components used to transmit and receive RF signals and manipulate the magnetic field will be able to do so with limited consistency. **The images produced by surface coils and with magnetic gradient refocusing techniques are especially sensitive to field inhomogeneities.**

Chemical-shift artifacts are present wherever contiguous tissues have considerably different molecular organization. The artifact is seen as a bright rim of signal at one interface and a dark rim on the opposite side of the particular organ, oriented in the frequency-encoding direction. The most prominent examples seen are at interfaces of fat and the other body tissues.

The molecular environment within fat causes hydrogen nuclei to process at a slightly different frequency than those in other tissues. Fat will therefore be slightly displaced because spatial localization is based on the hydrogen spin frequency of water. The artifact is seen only at interfaces where the bright signal of fat is shifted into or away from signal of the darker, water-based tissues. The prominence of the artifact intensifies with increasing magnetic field. Therefore, stronger gradient magnetic fields are required for high field strength systems to reduce the visibility of this artifact. The chemical-shift artifact is most prominent at the border of the kidneys and perirenal fat around the bladder and at the interface of retroorbital fat with the optic nerve and muscles (Figure 16-10).

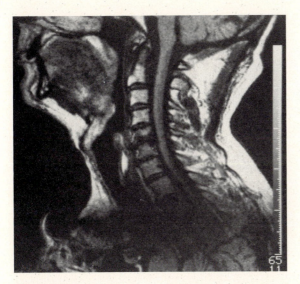

Figure 16-11.   The top of the head overlaps the lower neck in this image obtained with a circumferential neck coil. When a portion of the body is outside the coil, it can wrap around to the bottom of the image, creating an aliasing artifact.

RECONSTRUCTION ARTIFACTS

Frequently observed MRI artifacts relate to pulse sequence techniques used and computer reconstruction algorithms. They include aliasing, partial volume averaging, truncation, and quadrature artifacts.

The **aliasing artifact** is one of the most commonly encountered of this group. It occurs when portions of the patient's body are outside the field of view but within the area of RF excitation. RF signals that cannot be properly interpreted are produced. When hydrogen nuclei outside the area of interest are excited, the signal they return is interpreted to have originated from within the imaging field of view. It is then projected over the real portion of the image on the opposite side of its actual location.

The aliasing artifact occurs because the phase angles of the external nuclei are essentially equal to the nuclei in the imaging volume but on the opposite side of the image. The reconstruction algorithm dutifully places these signals where they should be (Figure 16-6). This "wraparound" artifact is always in the phase-encoding direction; however, manufacturers have solved this problem with the use of reconstruction filters. An example is seen in Figure 16-11, where the top of the head, which was outside the RF coil, projects over the upper thorax and lower neck.

Partial volume averaging is an artifact familiar to those engaged in CT imaging. It results whenever the particular structure of interest is contained within two contiguous slices. The artifact is worse with thick slices and large voxels. The use of thin slices reduces this artifact. However, thin-slice imaging

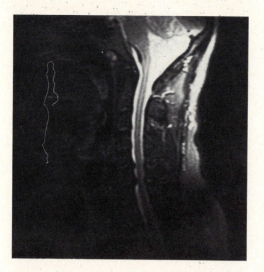

Figure 16-12. This truncation artifact has multiple evenly spaced curvilinear lines of bright and dark signal that follow the contour of the back of the head. When the lines project in both the phase and frequency encoding directions, one knows the artifact is not due to motion. (Courtesy R. Mark Henkelman, Ontario Cancer Institute, Toronto.)

requires more time for signal averaging because it must attain adequate signal to noise ratios and because more slices will be necessary. Furthermore, the adequacy of the manufacturer's magnetic gradient coils may not be equal to the task of precisely defining such thin slices.

The **truncation** or "ringing" artifact seen in Figure 16-12 appears as multiple well-defined curved lines regularly conforming to the anatomic boundary. The truncation artifact is more pronounced when the number of phase-encoding acquisitions is small and when the reconstruction matrix is assymetric, that is, 128 by 256. It occurs in areas where there is a great difference in signal intensity, such as interfaces of fat and air or fat and cortical bone. The sharp contrast boundaries of these interfaces consist of high spatial frequencies. With a small matrix there are not enough data to represent such high frequencies accurately. The orientation of the artifact can be along both frequency and phase-encoding axes.

A zero line or **zipper artifact** is caused by RF feed through from the RF transmitter along the frequency encoding direction at the central or reference frequency of the imaging sequence. It is typically seen on images on which only one average is acquired because in some systems no signal is obtained in the center line of the matrix. The result is a segmented line extending across the middle of the field of view in the frequency-encoding direction and having a zipperlike appearance, as seen in Figure 16-13**A**. Occasionally a single point, either bright as in Figure 16-13**B** or dark as in Figure 16-13**C**, is the only manifestation of this artifact.

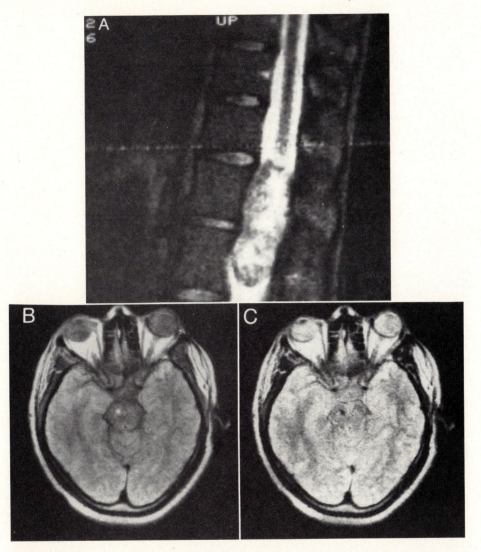

Figure 16-13.   **A,** The "zipper" artifact is always at the center of the field of view but not necessarily through the center of the patient as seen here.   **B,** A central point of brightness, as illustrated here over the right midbrain, could potentially cause a misdiagnosis.   **C,** The central point artifact can also be dark, as seen here on the second echo image.

NOISE INDUCED ARTIFACTS

A similar-appearing line artifact, as shown in Figure 16-14, can be produced by RF noise from extraneous sources and is sometimes called an **FID line.** The source of such RF emissions can be any electrical appliance or broadcast authorized by the Federal Communications Commission (Figure 8-12) op-

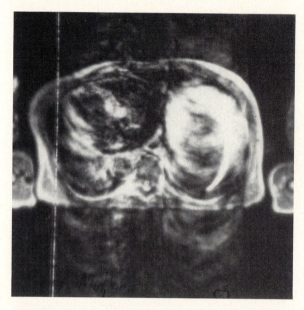

Figure 16-14.   Lines produced by random RF noise can occur whenever RF shielding of the room is inadequate. Extraneous RF noise at two frequencies shows up on this image.

erating at the magnet's frequency. This artifact will not normally be located on the center line.

The **off-resonance artifact** is simply the degradation of the image as a result of inexact tuning of the RF transmitter and/or receiver to the Larmor frequency, resulting in overall noisy images. A "bleeding" artifact, as seen in Figure 16-15, results when inexact duplication of the RF pulses occurs or when the magnetic gradients between each acquisition are incorrectly formed. This produces slight inaccuracies in the placement of signals into the appropriate pixel. The result is a smeared image of wavelike patterns similar to ghosting from motion. The off-resonance artifact can also appear similar to the truncation artifact, but not as regular and well defined.

An additional group of artifacts is caused by voluntary, involuntary, and even microscopic physiologic motion. As with photography, one cannot easily take a picture of a moving target. An MR image is severely degraded if motion occurs during the imaging time. This is especially true if the motion occurs near the middle of the acquisition. Physiologic motion of the blood, heart, larynx (swallowing), diaphragm, bowel, and cerebrospinal fluid (CSF) in the brain and spinal canal causes various types of motion artifacts.

Most motion artifacts result in a poorly defined, smeared appearance of the image in the area of motion. Repetitive motion of a linear or curvilinear surface, such as the diaphragm or heart, can produce the typical "ghosting," or irregular wavelike lines of increased and decreased signal.

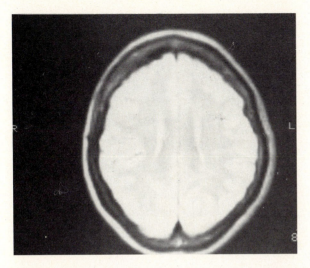

Figure 16-15. The "bleeding" artifact can be mistaken for a displacement of signal as a result of motion; however, this artifact is a more diffuse smearing of signal both within and outside the body.

Techniques for decreasing motion artifacts without increasing imaging time have been developed for abdominal imaging. These include various corrective algorithms, physically restricting the motion of the anterior abdomen, and rapid imaging techniques (Chapter 12) that can be performed during breath holding (Figure 16-16). Use of short TR and TE with multiple acquisitions produces good images by averaging the motion artifacts (Figure 16-17).

The problems with artifacts produced by swallowing and bowel peristalsis are less easily handled but are generally not as severe as those caused by vascular and respiratory motion. Rapid imaging techniques appear to provide a partial if not complete solution to such artifacts. Furthermore, the direction of the phase-encoding gradient can be changed with most systems, rendering the artifact less bothersome.

The CSF flow in the region of the foramen of Monro and Magendie can produce bright foci in the region of the midbrain and brainstem. This signal occurs in the phase-encoding direction and may mimic various lesions, such as infarcts, MS plaques, and gliosis. The flow of CSF in the cervical thecal sac can also produce high-signal artifacts overlying the cord that can obscure this area or be mistaken for pathologic conditions. This artifact is relatively easy to recognize, as it is more linear and parallel with the spine on sagittal images, projecting in the phase-encoding direction (Figure 16-18).

Blood flow artifacts can be extremely useful because most vessels are seen as black on standard spin-echo pulse sequences. The blood would return a relatively strong signal on SDW and T2W images if it were stationary or flow-

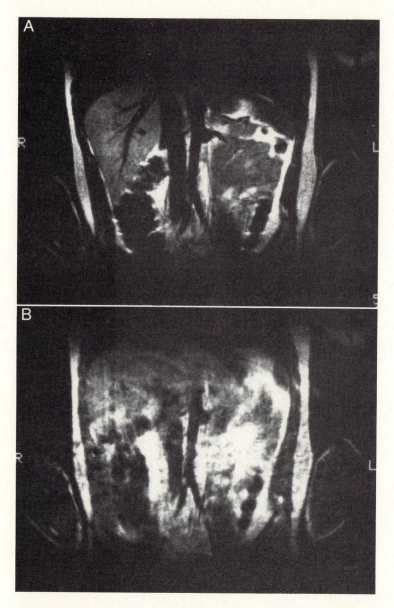

Figure 16-16.   **A,** This coronal image of the abdomen was obtained during breath holding. Notice the complete absence of blurring that is usually seen near the diaphragm.   **B,** A similar image obtained in an equal amount of time but during quiet respiration shows poor definition of the subdiaphragmatic structures.

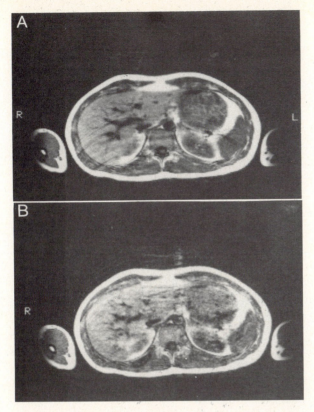

Figure 16-17. A, The motion artifact can be masked because it is, for the most part, a random signal that will subtract out in multiple average images. B, A comparison on the same patient with only two averages shows a considerable amount of distortion from respiratory motion.

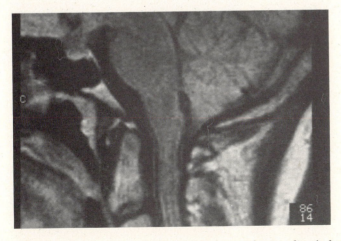

Figure 16-18. The loss of CSF signal at and immediately below the aqueduct and foramen of Magendie is mostly due to the rapid dephasing of spins caused by turbulent flow.

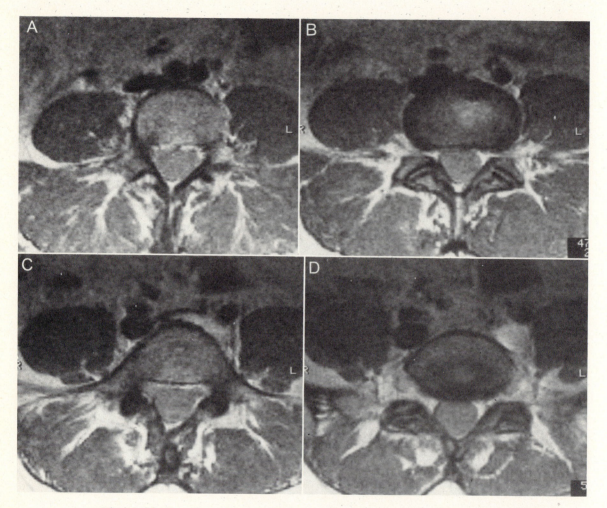

Figure 16-19. These four contiguous images from **A** superior to **D** inferior, show the normal black signal void in the inferior vena cava and right iliac vein resulting from rapidly flowing blood. The left iliac vein is compressed as it passes beneath the left iliac artery and has a relatively bright intraluminal signal in the more slowly flowing portion distal to the point of compression.

ing very slowly (Figure 16-19), but the artifact created by its motion produces the typical signal void instead. A problem can occur when flowing blood is oriented diagonally within the imaging plane. The nuclei in this case remain in the imaging field of view so that the emitted RF signal is received even though there may be rapid flow. The resultant displaced blood signal parallels the dark blood vessel and appears as an adjacent bright line (Figure 16-20).

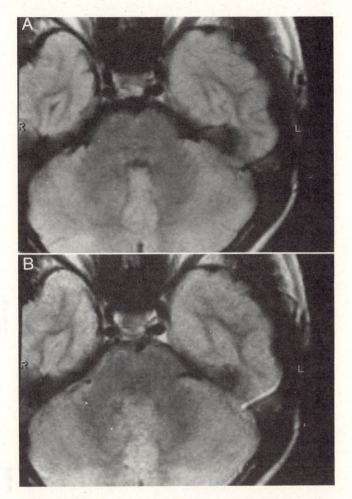

Figure 16-20.   A, A petrosal vein is seen traveling obliquely through this transaxial image of the brain. A normal signal void is demonstrated.   **B,** The second, even echo of this four-echo sequence shows a double linear track at the site of the vein. Even echo rephasing of the blood signal has occurred, accounting for the bright line, but it has been displaced laterally.

SUMMARY

There are three principal categories of MRI artifacts: magnetic and RF field distortion artifacts, reconstruction artifacts, and noise-induced artifacts. Each type of artifact can further be identified as patient related or system related.

Although a complete understanding of the many MRI artifacts is not necessary for accurate image interpretation, a certain level of familiarity is required. Knowledge of common system-specific artifacts will help avoid misdiagnosis and repeat examinations. Some artifacts may even provide additional specificity to the diagnosis if the radiologist and technologist know how to use them to advantage.

Chapter
SEVENTEEN

Biologic Effects
of MRI

Many noninvasive medical imaging modalities are currently available such as x-ray imaging, radioisotope scanning, ultrasonography, and, as we have learned in this volume, magnetic resonance imaging. Being noninvasive, each of these modalities is inherently safe. Ultrasonography and MRI prevail in safety considerations because neither employs ionizing radiation. Ionizing radiation can induce malignant disease and genetic mutations, although the risk of such responses is vanishingly low.

Human response to medical ionizing radiation follows a linear-quadratic dose-response relationship such as that shown in Figure 17-1. This is a nonthreshold dose-response relationship, which simply means that no dose of ionizing radiation is considered absolutely safe. Even the smallest dose carries a risk of response, albeit insignificant. At low radiation doses, the increase in response is very low. Only after rather high radiation doses, say 0.25 Gy or above, would the anticipated response be detectable.

Exposure to the energy fields of MRI, both individually and collectively, results in the fundamentally different dose-response relationship shown in Figure 17-2. Such a dose-response relationship is known as a threshold, nonlinear relationship. Regardless of the MRI field, there is a level of dose, D_T, the **threshold dose,** below which no response will be elicited. Below D_T MRI is

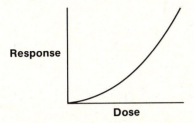

Figure 17-1. The dose-response relationship for medical ionizing radiation is linear-quadratic. It is also nonthreshold, suggesting that even the smallest radiation dose carries a risk, although such risk may be lower than that from other everyday factors.

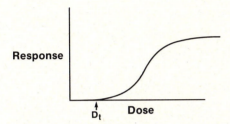

Figure 17-2. The response following exposure to the energy fields of MRI is threshold, nonlinear in form.

safe. D_T is considerably higher than any of the field intensities employed for clinical MRI examination. Above D_T the response to MRI exposure increases slowly at first and then more rapidly until 100% response would be observed.

MRI is relatively new and advancing rapidly, and so all of the radiobiologic questions are not completely answered. However, it does appear that MRI as currently employed is safe for all workers and patients. Experimental observations suggest that D_T for all of the MRI energy fields is considerably higher than the intensities employed for clinical examinations.

MRI COMPONENTS OF CONCERN

Although MRI is considered by all to be safe, radiobiologists will be busy for many years stretching their ability to detect human responses. It is certain that the delayed determination that x-ray exposure can cause cancer and leukemia will not be repeated with MRI, since the energy fields are nonionizing.

The potential health hazards of MRI lie in either the **static magnetic field,** the transient **gradient magnetic fields,** the **RF pulsed electromagnetic fields,** or a combination of these. There is already a wealth of radiobiologic data to show that, individually, such fields at the levels employed for MRI are innocuous. In addition to following a threshold dose-response relationship, these fields exhibit a time-intensity relationship as shown schematically in Figure 17-3. The threshold intensity, D_T, applies to continuous exposure. Above this threshold, shorter exposure times will produce the same response. What is

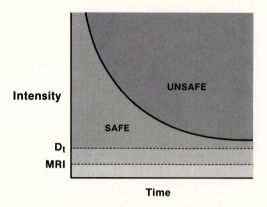

Figure 17-3.   Individually, the MRI energy fields follow this type of time-intensity relationship to produce a human response.

not fully understood is whether in combination these MRI energy fields have adverse health effects.

Before we discuss the known biologic effects of MRI in humans, an examination of each of the MRI fields and their effects on other biologic systems is in order.

Static Magnetic Fields

There is no evidence based on scientific investigation to show that intense magnetic fields produce harmful effects in mammals. Mechanisms have been suggested and each has been subject to considerable investigation, but the result is always the same. The findings are negative.

There are few studies of the effects of long-term exposure to intense static magnetic fields using proper controls and large sample sizes. Some experiments have been designed to detect growth abnormalities, biochemical disruption, and malignant disease induction in rodents at magnetic field strengths up to 5 T. All such observations have been negative. It can be argued for each that the sample size was too small.

Other reports deal with effects of intense magnetic fields on cultured cell lines and suggest that there is no adverse effect on cell growth at magnetic fields up to 7 T. Such experiments consist of conventional culturing of human fibroblasts. Lengthening the exposure time does not produce a positive response. It has been suggested that proton tunneling in DNA molecules may be affected by intense static magnetic fields, which may alter the base pairing and thereby cause point mutations. This has not been observed at either the molecular level or the cell level.

The navigational ability of adult bees and pigeons is considered to be mediated by granules of magnetite deposits in the abdominal region and in the head, respectively, as suggested in Figure 17-4. These magnetic deposits serve as a sort of built-in compass. Experiments have not yet been conducted to determine if these characteristics can be disturbed by intense magnetic fields. It

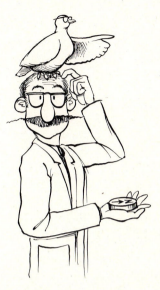

Figure 17-4.   It has been shown that magnetic deposits in the head of the pigeon allow it to know which way is north.

is unimportant anyway because humans do not rely on such an internal compass.

Some speculation exists concerning bioeffects of intense magnetic fields on growth rate, mutation, fertility, and blood cell count in mammals. Growth rate and mutation effects have been reported in animals as well as on yeasts, but the results have been equivocal or not reproducible. Monkeys exposed to a static magnetic field of 7 T for up to 1 hour experienced a transient decrease in heart rate and sinus arrhythmia, whereas a later study failed to demonstrate such effects when the exposure was limited to 15 minutes at 10 T.

The evidence for static magnetic field effects on the developing embryo of pregnant mice exposed at various times during gestation has shown no consistently statistical alterations in the offspring when compared with nonexposed control mice. These studies have employed acceptably large sample sizes and have been repeated with similar negative results.

Russian investigators have reported histologic changes in guinea pigs exposed to field strengths of 2 mT and 700 mT for up to 21 days. They found transient changes in liver, kidney, testes, and lens epithelium. However, such changes were not observed by American investigators when rats were exposed to 1.2 T for 1 month.

A static magnetic field of 0.3 T with continuous exposure up to 66 hours does not affect spermatogenesis in mice. However, it has been found that fertilization was enhanced by exposure of rainbow trout sperm and ova to a static magnetic field of 1 T for 1 hour prior to fertilization.

Transient Magnetic Fields

In MRI the gradient magnetic fields are pulsed and therefore are said to be **transient.** Such transient magnetic fields can induce electric currents, as was discussed in Chapter 2. A transient magnetic field of 3 T/s will result in an electric current density of approximately 3 A/cm^2.

Because some cells and tissues are electric conductors, the transient gradient magnetic fields may induce or interfere with normal conduction pathways. Depending on the intensity of the induced electric current, the normal function of nerve cells and muscle fibers may be affected. The threshold current density of transient magnetic fields depends mainly on the tissue conductivity and the on-time of the field.

Radio Frequency Fields

The most commonly reported effect of exposure of RF fields is an increase in body temperature. This increase is a function of the absorbed energy, which in turn is dependent on various parameters of the exposure system. These parameters include frequency, exposure time, and the mass of the exposed object.

The basic measure of **dose** of RF energy is the **specific absorption rate (SAR),** and it has units of W/kg. It may be expressed as averaged over a whole body or any of its tissues. It may also be expressed in time, averaged over a long time or over a single pulse. SAR is a measure of the power absorbed per unit time per unit mass. **SAR is to MRI what the gray is to ionizing radiation.** The mathematical formulation of SAR is much more difficult, however, and not necessary here.

The expression of **exposure** to RF is in the units of power density, W/m^2. This is equivalent to C/kg for ionizing radiation. Biologic effects of RF, therefore, are associated with the SAR. The SAR, in turn, is related to the RF power density as it varies in time (temporal) and in space (spatial). Maximum permissible exposure limits are expressed as power density and set 100 times lower than levels known to cause a response.

Anatomic abnormalities in the offspring of pregnant animals have been reported when the SAR during whole body exposure exceeded 20 W/kg. The amount of energy absorbed by the animal resulted in a slight rise in body temperature. If the rate of energy absorption exceeded the rate of heat loss, there was an increase in body temperature. When such temperature increases last for long periods, adverse biologic effects can be expected.

Exposure to microwave radiation (frequencies higher than those used in MRI) similarly causes an increase in body temperature. Such exposure has been associated with a decrease in fertility and testicular degeneration in mice, although such reports have not been confirmed by repetitive experiments.

Combined MRI Fields

At present there have been no large-scale or long-term studies in experimental animals with respect to biohazards of the combined fields of MRI. A limited number of short-term studies using clinical MR imagers on animals has been reported with consistently negative results. However, not all such experiments involved exposure to all three MRI fields.

Mutagenic or lethal effects in **Escherichia coli** were not observed when the bacterial cells were exposed to MRI fields typically used even with exposure of up to 5 hours. When human peripheral blood lymphocytes grown in tissue culture were exposed to MRI, no significant differences between exposed and control groups were found with respect to chromosomal lesions or sister chromatid exchanges. Similar cytogenetic studies have been conducted using several mammalian cells (for example, HeLa cells, Chinese hamster cells) with MRI exposure, and all have reported negative results in terms of chromosome aberrations, sisters chromatid exchanges, or DNA synthesis.

The effect of MRI on the early development of an amphibian system has also shown the absence of deleterious bioeffects. These studies were conducted using frog spermatozoa, eggs fertilized during second meiotic division, and embryos during cleavage. All were subjected separately to 30-MHz continuous wave RF in a static magnetic field of 0.7 mT for 20 minutes. These specimens were compared with unexposed groups at similar stages with respect to damage in genetic material, interference with meiotic cell division, and impairment in the development of embryos. No significant differences were observed following such treatment, suggesting that MRI exposure, at the doses used, does not cause detectable adverse effects in the amphibian system.

HUMAN RESPONSES TO MRI

Of the three MRI energy fields, only two, transient magnetic fields and RF fields, have been shown to induce responses in humans, but then only at exceedingly high intensities. There are no known effects from static magnetic fields. Transient magnetic fields are known to induce **magnetic phosphenes**, stimulate **healing in bones**, and cause **cardiac fibrillation.** RF exposure has been implicated in **tissue heating, induction of blood dyscrasia,** and **cataract formation.** Each of these responses is considered to be acute. There are no known long-term effects of MRI fields.

The extent of SAR tolerance in a subject depends on many factors, principally oxygen supply and humidity. Brain, kidney, and liver are examples of high vascularity. The lens of eye and testes have poor vascularity and therefore less oxygen supply. It is therefore suspected that the testes and lens are more susceptible to biological damage by RF energy.

Effects of Transient Magnetic Fields

Magnetic phosphenes are flashes of light that we sometimes perceive with our eyes closed. M.A. D'Arsonval first reported magnetic phosphene induction in 1896, and the introduction of MRI has rekindled research in this area. This phenomenon is caused by electrical stimulation of the sensory receptors of the retina as a result of transient magnetic fields. The threshold for such magnetic field change in humans for induction of magnetic phosphene is approximately

TABLE 17-1. Clinical MRI exposure limits recommended by the U.S. Center for Devices and Radiological Health and the British National Radiological Protection Board

MRI Components of Concern	Recommended Limits	
	U.S.	British
Static magnetic fields	<2.0 T	<2.5 T
Varying magnetic fields	<3.0 T/sec	<20.0 T/sec
Average power absorbed		
whole body	<0.4 W/kg	<0.4 W/kg
averaged over any 1 g of tissue	<2.0 W/kg	<4.0 W/kg

3 T/s at low frequencies. Magnetic phosphene induction has not been observed in the RF region, but only at frequencies less than 100 Hz.

Bone healing is accelerated if a low-frequency coil is positioned over the fracture. The precise mechanism of action is unknown, but it works and it is an accepted adjunctive therapy. Treatments lasting several minutes are given repeatedly during a 2- to 5-week course. Apparently, such bone healing is not stimulated by transient magnetic fields.

Ventricular fibrillation is another potential hazard of electric currents induced by transient magnetic fields. This happens when the current density in cardiac tissue is above approximately 0.5 mA/cm^2 applied for more than 3 seconds. The threshold for such an effect is thought to be approximately 0.1 mA/cm^2. Such disruption of heartbeat can result in a drop in blood pressure. However, ventricular fibrillation ceases and heartbeat returns to normal when the induced electric current is interrupted. This response has not been observed in humans experimentally or clinically except for patients with pacemakers.

Each of these responses that can be induced by changing magnetic fields has a threshold that is an unknown but obviously complex function of frequency, waveform, pulsatile nature, and duration. Presumably, they each follow a time-intensity relationship such as that in Figure 17-3.

Effects of RF Exposure

The hazard of exposure to RF radiation is associated with heating. Thermal effects on tissue are related to frequency and waveform, and the hazard is one of cooking as in a microwave oven. Such effects have been observed in experimental animals but not in humans.

Heating of avascular structures such as the lens of the eye is known to produce cataracts. Such has been demonstrated experimentally in animals and has been observed in humans. Some evidence is available to suggest that ship-bound sailors working near radio antennae were exposed to high-intensity RF and subsequently developed cataracts.

Exposure to intense RF has been shown to result in nonspecific blood changes, principally lymphatic depression. Such was thought to be the case

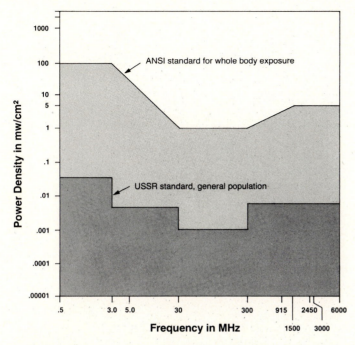

Figure 17-5.   Maximum permissible RF power densities are related to frequency. (Courtesy Holaday Instruments, Inc.)

some years ago in U.S. Embassy personnel who were alleged to have been exposed to RF by sources outside the embassy.

There have been no large-scale epidemiological or other studies in humans with respect to harmful effects of MRI. A well-controlled long-term study requires years of effort on the part of dedicated and experienced researchers using a sufficiently large population of individuals exposed to MRI to show any such effects. A prospective study of patients exposed to clinical MRI at present is lacking, but it may be too early to conduct such a study.

RECOMMENDED GUIDELINES

Reports of the first MRI patients studied date back to only early 1981. During the intervening years, several thousand patients worldwide have been imaged by MRI. The most predictable results of exposure to the MRI components are increase in temperature, physiochemical changes, and induction of electric currents. So far, none of these changes or any such adverse acute effects have been reported in patients undergoing clinical MRI evaluation. However, approximately 5% of all patients experience claustrophobia. Another 10% will sleep during the examination.

In light of the rapid progress in the application of MRI in medical diagnosis, maximum permissible limits of each component field of a clinical MR imager have been recommended by the Center for Devices and Radiologic Health of the United States Department of Health and Human Services and by

TABLE 17-2.   SAR levels from which RF exposure limits are derived

Population	Whole-Body Exposure	Tissue Exposure (1 g)
Occupational	0.4 W/kg	4.0 W/kg
General public	0.08 W/kg	0.8 W/kg

TABLE 17-3.   Recommendations of the International Radiation Protection Association (IRPA) for exposure limits to RF radiation

Frequency Range (MHz)	Power Density Limit Unit (W/m²)	
	Occupational	General Public
0.1–1	100	20
>1–10	100/f	20/f
>10–400	10	2
>400–2K	f/40	f/200
>2K–300K	50	10

f = Frequency.

the British National Radiological Protection Board. These guidelines are shown in Table 17-1.

The United States recommends that the static magnetic field not exceed 2 T; the British limit is 2.5 T. Transient magnetic fields are limited to 3 T/s by the United States and to 20 T/s by Britain. SAR limitations are 0.4 W/kg for both countries. Figure 17-5 compares the 1982 American National Standard Institute (ANSI) standard for whole-body exposure with the limitations employed by the USSR. These standards acknowledge that biologic responses are related not only to the power density but also to the frequency.

In addition, it has been suggested that MR examinations not be given to patients fitted with cardiac pacemakers, persons with large metallic implants, and pregnant women during the entire gestation period, but especially during the first trimester.

In 1983 the International Radiation Protection Association (IRPA) recommended interim guidelines on limits of exposure to RF electromagnetic fields. These guidelines are established for occupationally exposed persons and the general public. The limits are established on the basis of the SAR values shown in Table 17-2. The resulting RF exposure limits are shown in Table 17-3. The basal metabolic rate for humans is approximately 1 W/kg at rest. During exertion the metabolic rate may increase to 15 W/kg.

SUMMARY

A considerable amount of data shows that the energy fields employed in MRI are harmless. At much higher field intensities, positive responses have been reported in biologic targets other than humans. Our understanding of the exposure of humans to the combined fields of MRI is not so complete. Many observations of humans exposed to MRI have consistently resulted in negative findings. Nevertheless, maximum permissible operating intensities have been prescribed.

Chapter
EIGHTEEN

Administering a Magnetic Resonance Imager

The time to begin preparing for the daily operation of an MR imager is 6 months to a year before the scheduled turnover date from the manufacturer. The reasons for this long planning time become clear as soon as one begins to delve into all that needs to be accomplished before the first patient is put into the gantry. A fair amount of research and thought are required in producing a workable clinical environment, as shown in the chart in Figure 18-1.

For the establishment of a properly functioning magnetic resonance imager, the time from conception to operation may take up to 2 years. In Chapter 8 it was pointed out that the first step in this process was selection of the imager. This is to be followed by site selection and design of the facility. Approximately 1 year prior to operation, attention should be focused on personnel, equipment, and administration.

First one must identify all of the necessary ancillary equipment and submit purchase orders. Then a competent staff must be hired and sufficient time allowed for adequate training of these new employees. Staff scheduling must be arranged and scanning protocols established. Service and safety arrangements are necessary.

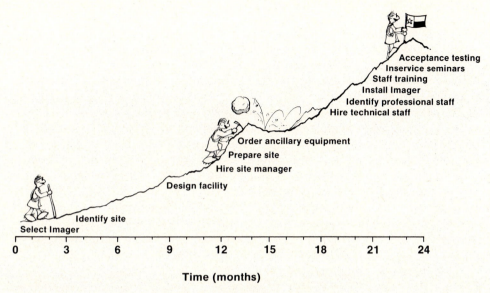

Figure 18-1. The several steps and time sequence for establishing MRI have been likened to climbing a mountain, though the former may take more time.

ANCILLARY EQUIPMENT

Shown in the box below is a list of equipment that is necessary for the proper operation of most MR imagers. This list is offered as a planning guide for initial start-up. **Everything that goes into the magnet room must be nonmagnetic.**

Ancillary equipment necessary for MRI start-up

Fire extinguisher(s)
Gurney(s)
Wheelchair(s)
Intravenous pole(s)
Step stool
O_2 tank (if there is no piped-in O_2)
Wooden chairs
Tools
Respirator (that will work in the magnetic field)
Stethoscope
Plastic bucket, mop
Central vacuum (if there is carpet)

Only recently has nonmagnetic equipment for use with an MR imager become readily available. The primary materials used in such equipment are sturdy plastics, aluminum, wood, and high-grade stainless steel. There are other metals and alloys that are also nonmagnetic, but it is always best to check any large metal object before it enters the imaging room. Small magnets should be readily available for testing any questionable object.

It pays to shop when purchasing nonmagnetic equipment; it appears that the mere word *nonmagnetic* in the description of the equipment allows for a substantial increase in price.

Nonmagnetic gurneys are now available from many x-ray supply companies. Nonmagnetic stretchers are more difficult to find and considerably more expensive but are more versatile and adaptable because they have more options, such as raised head and adjustable height. Wheelchairs are also available from x-ray supply companies, as are intravenous poles and step stools.

Stainless-steel or aluminum oxygen cylinders and respirators are more difficult to locate. The cylinders should be obtainable either from a local gas supply company or from the cryogen supplier. A respirator that works in the magnetic field is primarily plastic with no metal gauges. The fittings should be nonmagnetic brass or aluminum.

Tools can be purchased from the vendor or from companies that provide nonmagnetic supplies for research laboratories containing magnets. Nonmagnetic fire extinguishers should be kept in the area to avoid any unfortunate accidents during an emergency. A local supply company should be consulted for this.

HUMAN RESOURCES

Staffing

Staffing will certainly differ from facility to facility and also between a hospital and an imaging center. The number of staff will depend principally on the demand placed on the magnet by referring physicians and radiologists. Table 18-1 identifies a representative start-up staff for both a hospital and an imaging center. After a few months of operation it may be necessary to increase hours and days of imaging. Fully used MR imagers will eventually operate 18 hours a day, 6 days a week. This will create a great demand on technologists and radiologists to perform complete diagnostic examinations in the most efficient and timely manner possible. It may be necessary to schedule staggered shifts rather quickly after start-up.

What training and experience should be required for operation of the MR imager? At present very few programs are available to train competent technical personnel specifically in MRI. Essentially all that is available are on-the-job training, a few continuing education seminars, and training provided by manufacturers.

Radiologic technologists with extensive experience in CT are an obvious choice to perform as MRI technologists. Such individuals have already demonstrated competence as imaging technologists by completing a minimum 2-year training program and passing the examination of the American Registry of Radiologic Technologists (ARRT). Their experiences in patient care, trans-

Table 18-1. Representative staffing for start-up of an MRI facility

Staff Member	Number		Duties
	Hospital	Clinic	
Radiologist	2	2	Image interpretation
Receptionist/secretary	3	2	Scheduling, filing, typing
Imaging technologist	4	2	MR imager operation
Darkroom technician/aide	2	1	Filming, filing
Radiology nurse	1	0	Patient support

axial anatomy, and computer operation can shorten the learning time required for operating an MR imager. Ultrasound and nuclear medicine technologists are also likely choices. They have an excellent background in sectional anatomy and pathology and are trained in medical imaging.

Any number of other qualified technical personnel could be trained to operate an MR imager. However, registered radiologic technologists with CT experience may prove to be the most effective MRI technologists. They already are familiar with patient positioning, sectional anatomy, and operation of a rather complex console. Becoming comfortable with and understanding the physical principles of MRI are another matter.

For the technical staff to develop the necessary competence not only to operate the MR imager but also to exercise independent judgment about imaging techniques, they should receive appropriate continuing education. Ideally, there would be an opportunity to send the MRI technologists to regional seminars before the magnet is fully operational. It is very important for operators to have a basic understanding of what occurs during MRI if they are to provide adequate physician assistance.

The physical basis for MRI is totally different from that for x-ray imaging. Thought processes equating more dense tissue to white and less dense tissue to black on a radiograph cannot be applied to MRI. MRI is much more complex. Technologists and physicians need to think in terms of signal intensity. **Strong signal intensity results in a bright image, and weak signal intensity results in a dark image.** To complicate matters, MRI signal intensity can be completely reversed depending on the nature of the RF pulse sequence. The technologist and radiologist must understand these imaging parameters.

Scheduling

Experience has shown that 2 to 2½ hours per examination should be allowed initially. Early experiments with RF pulse sequences and patient positioning require considerable time. However, it will not be long before the average examination time is reduced to less than 1 hour. At that time the scheduling of technologists can be somewhat altered. Rapid imaging RF pulse sequences are emerging that may shorten examination times further.

TECHNOLOGIST SCHEDULING. During the initial start-up phase everything will be slow because of such factors as unfamiliarity with operating controls, difficulty in setting up imaging protocols, and selection of appropriate hard copies. Depending on the institution, this will last 1 to 6 months. The technologists should become involved and a part of the final product. The entire department will benefit from this interaction. Time and effort expended initially will pay off later.

PATIENT SCHEDULING. Seldom should it be necessary to repeat a patient examination because it is incomplete. This not only increases the work load but also disrupts the schedule. Nevertheless, reexamination is sometimes required because of inability to complete the examination due to patient motion. The appearance of a questionable area upon review of the images may also require additional imaging.

The magnet should not remain idle because of misinformation or scheduling inefficiency. **All outpatients should be called the day before their scheduled examination** for confirmation of appointment to ensure that they know the time of their appointment and to give instructions and directions to the MRI suite. Time should be taken to answer questions or discuss fears they may have. Such attention will help tremendously in ensuring their arrival on time. One needs to make every effort to avoid the "empty table syndrome."

It is helpful to schedule similar examinations back to back. If possible, separate segments of each day should be scheduled for head, body, and surface coil imaging. This eliminates the need for switching equipment or coils from patient to patient and saves considerable time.

Request Form: No patient should be examined without a properly executed request by a referring physician. Figure 18-2 is a facsimile of a request form for an MRI examination. As much medical information as possible should be provided with the request. In addition to giving standard identification data, the requesting physician should provide pertinent information on the patient's clinical history and specific information as to why the MRI is requested. In particular, the referring physician should be required to determine and state that the patient has no intracranial aneurysm or bypass clips, cardiac pacemaker, artificial limb, metal prosthesis, or metal fragments.

Consent Form: When any hardware or software of the MR imager is not approved by the Food and Drug Administration (FDA), the FDA requires that a consent form be obtained from each patient. If all of the hardware and software are approved or if software or hardware upgrades that are not FDA approved are implemented, it is again necessary to obtain the consent form. Nevertheless, during this early era of MRI it is probably advisable to obtain a consent form from each patient. Figure 18-3 presents such an informed consent form. In addition to providing general information and identification, the form must state that the patient understands the nature of the examination and that all the patient's questions have been answered.

Of particular importance, the patient should be required to respond to the same questions posed to the clinician regarding clips, pacemakers, prostheses, and other metal devices. A basic explanation of MRI should be provided to the

Precessional Saints Memorial Hospital   **MRI Information Request Form**

Date Received_____ By _____ Nursing Extension _____ Date Scheduled_____

Patient Name _____
                          Last   First   Middle Initial

Date of Birth _____ Sex _____   Previous MRI _____
                          M   D   Y

Hospital # [ ][ ][ ][ ][ ][ ][ ][ ][ ][ ][ ]   Region of Interest _____

Patient Location_____   Referring Physician _____

Patient Age_____ Weight _____ Lb.   Height _____ Ft. _____In.

Travel By: Walk   Wheelchair   Stretcher

Does Patient Require: O₂   I.V.   Infusion Pump   Other:

If OP: Home Phone_____ Work _____

Pertinent Clinical Hx: _____
_____
_____
_____

Specific Reason for MRI: _____
_____

Eye make-up must be removed before MRI examination

1. Subject in fair state of health.	Y	N
2. Subject states she is not pregnant.	Y	N
3. Subject is able to give voluntary informed consent, or is accompanied by someone legally responsible to do so.	Y	N
4. Review of medical history with patient indicates absence of:		
— intracranial aneurysm or bypass clips	Y	N
— cardiac pacemaker, neuro/biostimulator	Y	N
— artificial limb/joint prostheses	Y	N
— cardiac valve prostheses	Y	N
— middle ear prostheses	Y	N
— metal fragments, shrapnel, bullet fragments	Y	N
— permanent eyeliner (cosmetic tattooing)	Y	N
— other _____	Y	N

Figure 18-2. A representative MRI request form.

patient. A brief and clearly stated pamphlet would be sufficient. The patient should be made aware that MRI is a benign examination and that there are no adverse side effects. Also included should be a statement noting responsibility of payment.

Before the examination, the procedure should be explained to the pa-

Resonance Regional Medical Center

Your physician has ordered an MRI examination as part of the diagnostic tests for your medical evaluation. This procedure is relatively new and can provide information which will enhance your diagnosis. The procedure is accomplished by using a strong magnetic field, radio-frequency waves and a computer to generate the image. No x-rays or radioactive materials are necessary. Because this technology is new and considered investigational, permission forms are required for record-keeping.

MRI systems have been in use for several years with no harmful side effects reported, except in patients with intracranial metal. Your participation in this study is voluntary and you may withdraw at any time. Because of the nature of the magnetic field, it is necessary to know if you have had certain surgeries or traumas which could have resulted in any metal implants in the body. Please inform the technologist or nurse if you have any of the following (check the appropriate lines):

	No	Yes
1. Cardiac valve prosthesis	☐	☐
2. Cardiac pacemaker or pacer wire implants	☐	☐
3. Intracranial aneurysm or bypass surgery	☐	☐
4. Middle ear prosthesis	☐	☐
5. Neuro or bio-stimulator	☐	☐
6. Joint or limb prosthesis	☐	☐
7. Old shrapnel or welding wounds or accidents	☐	☐
8. Other internal metal	☐	☐

Qualified medical and technical personnel will be in attendance throughout the entire procedure.

There is a procedure charge for the MRI examination for which you are responsible, but if you have insurance you may file for reimbursement.

All data collected in this study is confidential as part of your patient record. if the data is used for research studies or publications, no patient identification will appear. This information will be used only for educational, research, and scientific purposes.

In the event of physical injury incurred during the procedure described to me, Resonance Regional Medical Center is not able to offer financial compensation, nor to absorb the costs of medical treatment. However, necessary facilities, emergency treatment, and professional services will be available to research subjects, just as they are to the community generally.

Signed: _____   Date: _____
                        Patient's Name

Child's Assent _____   Age: _____
                        (If seven or older)

_____   Date: _____
                        Parent / Guardian

_____   Date: _____
                        Witness

Figure 18-3.   A typical informed consent form to be completed by the patient.

tient. The patient should be told that the examination may take as long as an hour and therefore it is important to remain very still and relaxed. The patient should be assured that the examination does not hurt but that loud thumping noises may be heard. Eating and drinking should be avoided for 2 hours before the examination for patient comfort. The patient should be reminded that this is a diagnostic examination and not a treatment.

SCANNING PROTOCOLS

Once the scanner is operational and qualified imaging technologists are on staff, it will be evident that the choices presented for collection of images from a patient are almost endless. Most imagers are fairly versatile and allow for

Table 18-2. **RF pulse sequences that emphasize the principal MRI parameters**

MRI Parameter	RF Pulse Sequence	TR (ms)	TE (ms)	TI (ms)
SD	Spin echo	2000	30–50	
TI	Spin echo	500–1000	30–50	
T1	Inversion recovery	2000	30–50	100–500
T2	Spin echo	1000	50–150	

wide variations in RF pulse sequences. The ultimate goal is to find optimal RF pulse sequences for each patient and for each suspected pathology. To achieve this ideal, the MRI technologist must work closely with the radiologist. It is the primary responsibility of the technologist to learn how to manipulate the console controls in order to optimize each examination.

The number of available RF pulse sequences is enormous. With MRI there is no correct RF pulse sequence for a body part or pathology, but with experience better optimization can be obtained. In general, one will select that RF pulse sequence that will provide the most information in the least time. Normally, two RF pulse sequences are employed:—SD-weighted images will be obtained for anatomy and T2-weighted images for pathology.

MRI is valuable because of the enhanced contrast resolution owing to differences in the basic MRI parameters of SD, T1, and T2. Most pathologic processes cause changes in T1 and T2; therefore, RF pulse sequences in general, are tailored to emphasize such changes. Table 18-2 shows ranges of values for TR, TE, and TI for several RF pulse sequences designed to emphasize a given MRI parameter.

During use of the spin echo RF pulse sequence, increases in T1 tend to reduce signal intensity and increases in T2 tend to increase signal intensity. Therefore, it is rarely sufficient to use a single spin echo for imaging. One usually obtains an early spin echo image and a late spin echo image to avoid having pathology appear isointense with normal tissue.

Because T1 and T2 values for the brain are long and for cerebrospinal fluid (CSF) even longer when compared with those for other body tissues, RF pulse sequences for imaging of the central nervous system (CNS) are usually not appropriate for body imaging. Table 18-3 presents representative scanning protocols that are appropriate for initial imaging. With experience, these protocols can be varied to accommodate suspected pathology. Technologists and radiologists will want to try different RF pulse sequences until one is found that works best for their magnet and patient population. Technologists must be open to change and learn from the experiences of others.

IMAGER MAINTENANCE

An MR imager is a highly complex instrument that requires regularly scheduled preventive maintenance and unscheduled service for repairs as needed. A

Table 18-3. Suggested protocols for start-up imaging

Examination	Image Plane	TE (ms)	TR (ms)
Brain	Transaxial	40/80	2000
Spine	Transaxial	35/70	1000
	Coronal	40/80	800
	Sagittal	40/80	800
Chest	Coronal	30/60	1000
	Transaxial	30/60	1500
Abdomen	Transaxial	30/60	800
	Coronal	25/50	500
Pelvis	Coronal	25/50	800
	Transaxial	30/60	1000
Extremities	Sagittal	40/80	700
	Coronal	40/80	700

minimum of 14 hours per month can be expected for regular cryogen replacement and preventive maintenance. The warranty period for parts and labor for an MR imager should be at least 1 year. Longer service contracts are available but at considerable expense. Warranty service is expected to occur during normal working hours. Extended coverage for service after hours is generally offered at a higher hourly labor rate.

Preventive Maintenance

The sophisticated support systems for the main magnet require the most attention during regularly scheduled preventive maintenance. Failure of any electronic components will seriously affect the quality of the image and can disrupt imaging entirely. The magnet must be constantly fine tuned to keep the quality of the MR signal high to produce images with maximum signal and minimum noise. It may be necessary to have a service engineer on site several days each week to maintain optimum operation. Actual monthly operating hours with an MR imager will be less than expected owing to the preventive maintenance required. This reduction in imaging time will be further accentuated if service is performed during normal working hours.

Several support systems for the magnet may include items that require regular preventive maintenance as specified by the manufacturer. These systems may include a chilled water system, a Halon system, oxygen alarms, compressed air and pumps, and air-conditioning systems. A mobile MRI is equipped with generators that will require frequent service.

Many of these items have components that are not normal off-the-shelf hardware store items and may have a long lead time for replacement. Therefore, it may be necessary to have some components available for replacement at the site to preclude weeks of downtime resulting from equipment failure and parts delivery.

Before operation of an MR imager, the person responsible for service and preventive maintenance on the system and support systems must be identified. That individual then should be charged with scheduling such maintenance and deciding what backup parts and systems should be available on site.

Regular preventive maintenance on the MR system will include diagnostics on the software and checks of the RF subsystem. Changes in RF frequency do occur. Each system normally has a 10- to 20-Hz drift each day. The gradient sensitivity and offset can drift, and readjustment of the free induction decay (FID) may be necessary to maintain image quality. Cryogen levels should be monitored daily, and any differences in cryogen boil-off should be noted for possible problems. For safety procedure checks, the emergency shutdown and quench buttons should be verified as operational.

Before the imager is purchased, an estimate of maintenance costs after the warranty period has ended will be helpful. Negotiations for service should be done as the system is purchased so that a realistic picture of operating expenditures will be available in the planning stages. Service contracts for MRI systems are more expensive than those for any other imaging system. Costs may exceed $150,000 per year.

Repairs

The components that require the most attention are the electronics. Once the magnet is energized, it will not require service except for the superconducting magnet, which requires cryogen replacement. Unless a quench occurs, the magnet should not require repair. Nevertheless, the electronic components of the MR system are the primary elements of the repair and service process. Small glitches in the software programs can usually be handled by rebooting the system or by service advice given over the telephone. Such glitches can usually be overcome in 30 minutes. The system will experience the normal problems with disk and tape drives that exist with any other computer-assisted technology.

Repairs for intermediate-level problems are usually not completed in less than 4-hours. Elusive repairs to correct a loss of image quality can become a marathon, lasting 12 to 48 hours. Obviously, these marathons should not take place during normal working hours, or the patient load would fall to an unacceptable level. There must be considerable trade-offs between the cost of service after hours, revenue generated by the imager, and the completion of the patient schedule.

Because of the sensitivity of an MR imager and the complex problems associated with repair and service, several items are necessary to monitor the service provided. The following items will provide some controls for the cost of repairs.

LENGTH OF TIME REQUIRED FOR REPAIR.   All the time spent for repairs should be due to failure of the equipment. Service personnel should not add time to the service report for such things as filling out the service report. All times should be logged in and out by the service personnel.

REPAIR COMPLETED, PROBLEM UNSOLVED.   Many hours may be spent trying to isolate the event that causes the problem. It is not uncommon to put the imager out of service several times to correct the same repair. There should be an awareness of how long this is happening, and expert repair help should be requested.

TRAINING AND COMPETENCE OF SERVICE PERSONNEL.   Frequently more than one service engineer is required to correct a problem. If additional engineers are on site for training or experience and are not productive, there should be no charge for the additional personnel.

COMMUNICATION WITH HEADQUARTERS FOR EXTENDED SERVICE PROBLEMS.   Some persistent problems require that assistance from the factory be available for resolution.

RESPONSE TIME TO REPORTED SERVICE PROBLEMS.   Time for repair of problems should not include the travel time of service personnel to the facility. It is wise to negotiate for a minimum response time for a service engineer to respond to requests for assistance. If service is required over the weekends, this item should be addressed during the purchase negotiations.

AVAILABILITY OF PARTS LOCALLY.   Parts for the imager should be available locally. Repair budgets should be increased significantly after the warranty period to include replacement components. Knowledge of the magnet and its components is mandatory for the MRI administrator or technologist to control repair costs.

Cryogen Replacement

The most popular type of magnet, the superconducting magnet, requires cryogenic gases for cooling. The principle of the superconducting magnet is to create an environment that does not require a continuous electrical energy source. The 15 or more miles of windings in the core of a superconducting magnet must be cooled to less than 9.5 K, a mere $-260°$ C. This is accomplished through the construction of the sophisticated giant Thermos bottle that was described in Chapter 7.

As long as the windings of the main magnet remain less than 9.5 K, the magnetic field will be sustained at a constant field strength. Cryogen must be replaced on a regular schedule, and this is a technical problem that must be considered before operation. Abrupt loss of cryogens will result in a magnet quench that can be disastrous.

Liquid nitrogen is a fairly stable cryogen with which to work because it has a boiling point of 77 K. Liquid helium is not so stable because its boiling point is 4.2 K. The difference between the operating temperature of the magnet and the boiling point of helium is only about 5 K.

Once the initial warranty period is over, it is necessary to obtain a contract with a cryogen supply company. A **reliable** cryogen supply company is extremely important.

Cryogen replacement is a critical operation. It must be done by knowledgeable, fully trained personnel. It is usually best to contract with companies that specialize in cryogen replacement. Regardless of who does the replacement, proper safety procedures must be followed. Safety glasses must be worn for eye protection and heavy gloves for hand protection. All connective tubing and parts must be precooled to avoid the introduction of heat into either the cryogen transport dewars or the magnet itself.

Nitrogen usually must be replaced weekly, and helium replacement is required every 3 to 4 weeks. These liquids vaporize during filling of the magnet and during transport. Cryogens cannot be stored for more than several days in the transport dewars or else the dewars may be empty when the magnet is ready for filling. The supplier must adhere to accurate cryogen delivery schedules after proper planning on the part of the MRI facility. Emergency deliveries of cryogens can triple the cost, especially for helium.

Helium gas is obtained commercially from certain deposits of natural gas in Texas, Kansas, and New Mexico, where it occurs in concentrations up to 7%. Helium is separated by a process of freezing out the less volatile components, leaving the helium gas that must then be liquefied. All United States production of helium is under the control of the U.S. Bureau of Mines.

Spontaneous boil-off of cryogens consumes approximately 1 to 2% of the helium and 5 to 7% of the nitrogen per day on a stationary magnet. Cryogen consumption for a mobile magnet can be considerably higher, depending on whether the magnet is moved frequently or is operated in a stationary location. If the magnet is moved frequently and must be ramped up and down for moving, an additional 1% will be used during the ramping. Critical cryogen levels are reached at approximately 50% of the total volume. Below this level a quench is possible.

Magnet Quench

Helium is an important choice for a cryogen in magnets because of its chemical inactivity and its low density. However, this presents special problems if the liquid helium begins to warm or is exposed to room temperature. Charles's Law states that "at constant pressure, the volume of a given mass of gas is directly proportional to the absolute temperature." The importance of this law is apparent if the magnet should quench. A quench occurs when the temperature of the liquid gases—nitrogen and helium—exceeds their respective boiling points. The liquid gases vaporize, causing the main magnet windings to rise in temperature and become electrically resistive. This results in more heat, which results in more liquid boil-off. The magnet windings cannot sustain the high current in the resistive phase and can be severely damaged. If this occurs, the magnetic field intensity will drop rapidly to zero, and the imager ceases to function.

It is possible during a quench for 100 to 150 L of helium and nitrogen to be vaporized in less than 1 minute. This will produce approximately 4000 cubic feet of gas at room temperature and normal pressure. This can quickly displace all the oxygen in the room and present an emergency safety hazard. For this reason, it is recommended that every superconducting magnet be equipped in the control room with an oxygen monitor that will sound an alarm if the oxygen level in the imaging room drops below 140 ppm. Normal levels of oxygen in air are 150 ppm (20%) by volume. This assumes even greater importance if the design of the magnet room does not allow the technologists to view the cryogen port directly. However, most superconducting magnets are vented through a cryogen vaporization duct to the outside of the facility to prevent an undue safety hazard to personnel and patients.

Should a quench occur, the magnet will quickly lose its magnetic field and become inoperable. The magnet must then be recooled and restarted, which can take a considerable time, assuming the magnet has not been damaged from the overheating. Quenching is a very expensive and hazardous event and must be avoided.

QUALITY ASSURANCE

It is important to evaluate the image on a daily basis to maintain image quality. This is best accomplished by using the first half an hour of the day for quality assurance. A standard reference measurement on an MR phantom should be done daily and the images and data saved over at least a month's time to evaluate subtle changes in image quality and signal-to-noise ratio. A reduction in the signal-to-noise ratio may be the first indication of a problem. Phantom images can be used to identify and evaluate artifacts that occur. Artifacts that are attributed to the inhomogeneity of a living system may be in error and should be cross-referenced to a phantom image for identification.

Several MRI quality assurance phantoms have been developed by medical physicists, a few of which are shown in Figure 18-4. The American Association of Physicists in Medicine (AAPM) has a large compendium of such phantoms available upon request. The box below lists the important image characteristics to be evaluated by such phantoms.

Image characteristics to be evaluated with MRI quality assurance phantoms

Image Characteristic	Phantom Configuration
Noise	Uniform liquid bath
Uniformity	Measure of signal throughout uniform liquid bath
Spatial resolution	Hole pattern or bar pattern
Contrast resolution	Hole pattern in various thicknesses of plastic
Linearity	Step wedge or various paramagnetic samples
Sensitivity profile	Ramped wedge or rod
Slice contiguity	Ramp or helix

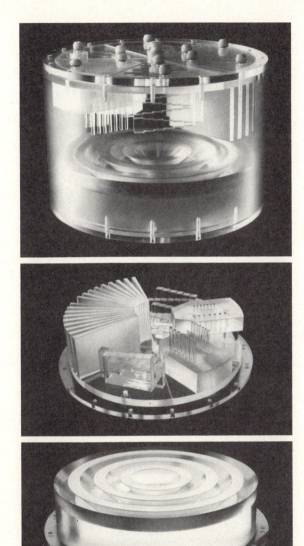

Figure 18-4.   Examples of MRI quality assurance phantoms. (Courtesy Hy Glasser, Nuclear Associates, Inc.)

Keeping the signal-to-noise ratio at a level that produces excellent diagnostic images should be a closely monitored procedure. Even with magnetic and RF shielding, small subcomponents of the support systems can introduce interference that causes image degradation.

An example of a small subcomponent that can create interference is a water valve in the chilled water system opening and sticking during regular operations. This interference can alter the images, making it appear as if the patient is moving during data acquisition. Also, any introduction of additional electrical systems that are interfaced with the computer can "cross-talk" with the wiring beneath the computer floor and affect image quality.

SAFETY

Access to the magnet room must be strictly controlled because of potential adverse effects of both the magnet on visitors and visitors on the magnet. Signs cautioning entrance to the magnet room must be prominently displayed in many areas in addition to the entrance door. An example of such warning signs is shown in Figure 18-5. Because most people read and ignore such signs, additional measures must be taken to control entrance to the MRI room. This is particularly important with permanent and superconducting magnets because their magnetic field cannot be interrupted or turned off.

Visitors' Effect on Magnet

When the MR imager first becomes energized, in-service training sessions for many departments in the hospital or clinic must be conducted. There will be much curiosity and many rumors about the magnet. Questions such as "Can it pull the fillings out of your teeth?" or "Can it cause one to become disoriented?" or "Does it cause sterility?" will be heard. The departments that require the most attention to this regard are building services, public relations, and personnel.

In-service training sessions with the supervisors of the building services department and with the employees performing the work are vital to the safety of the imager. For example, one hospital had a central vacuum installed in the area because the magnet room was carpeted. Within a week of an in-service session, a janitorial employee decided the central vacuum was too troublesome and entered the magnet room with a conventional vacuum cleaner. Fortunately, only a chip was knocked off the cover of the magnet cowling, which is where the vacuum cleaner struck when it was pulled out of the janitor's hands. Needless to say, at that hospital no one in building services ever had to be told again not to take anything magnetic into the room.

The public relations department must be made aware of the nature of the MR imager because its members will be touring the facility with visitors. Another reported incident, much more benign in nature, occurred after a magnet was first brought up to field. There was a group of medical and administrative dignitaries visiting from a nearby city who were in the preliminary stages of planning for MRI. Signs were posted prominently as to what should and

WARNING
MAGNETIC FIELD

THE FIELD OF THIS MAGNET ATTRACTS OBJECTS CONTAINING IRON, STEEL, NICKEL OR COBALT. SUCH OBJECTS MUST <u>NOT</u> BE BROUGHT INTO THIS AREA. <u>LARGE</u> OBJECTS CANNOT BE RESTRAINED.

PERSONS WITH IMPLANTS OR PROSTHETIC DEVICES SHOULD <u>NOT</u> ENTER THIS AREA. PACEMAKERS MAY BE DISABLED.

DATA ON CREDIT CARDS AND MAGNETIC STORAGE MEDIA CAN BE ERASED. WATCHES, CAMERAS, AND INSTRUMENTS CAN BE DAMAGED.

Figure 18-5. Warning sign for the entrance to the MRI suite.

Personal effects that should be removed from visitors and patients before entering the 0.5-mT exclusion area

Analog watches
Tape recorders
Magnetized credit cards
Calculators
Jewelry
Shoes with metal supports
Wigs
Hairpins, barrettes
Dentures (when the head or cervical spine is being imaged)

should not enter the magnet room. One visitor was warned by an employee that he should not wear his analog watch into the magnetic field. The man expressed little concern because it was a gold watch. The employee responded that although gold is nonmagnetic, the watch's gears and springs are not made of gold.

As was stated earlier, MRI requires a whole different thought process. If care and constant monitoring are not practiced, the potential for hazard is always present. The box on page 351 lists personal belongings that should be removed from visitors or patients before they enter the exclusion area.

Magnetic Effects on Visitors

The magnetic fringe field may have potentially harmful effects on some visitors. The fringe field of a superconducting MR imager should be considered hazardous. The following box lists those persons who should not be allowed access to the imaging room or within the 0.5-mT exclusion area. Any patient, employee, or family member entering the magnet room should be properly screened.

People who should not be allowed within the 0.5-mT exclusion area

Patients with pacemakers
Patients with intracranial aneurysm clips
Persons subject to uncontrollable seizures

PATIENT HAZARDS

Scheduling personnel must carefully screen patients. Although MRI is generally considered harmless, certain patients should not be imaged because of possible adverse reactions to the examination. It is not always easy to identify those patients who should be excluded because the criteria for exclusion are not obvious even to those familiar with MRI. Certain occupational groups, surgical patients, and pregnant women should not be imaged. The responsibility usually rests with the technologist to recognize the potentially unacceptable patient.

Occupational Groups

Members of several occupational groups should be viewed with suspicion before MRI is done because they may have foreign metallic objects in the body. Often the presence of such objects is unknown. There is a risk for patients who work with metal on a regular basis. Welders, machinists, and auto mechanics come into contact with metal shavings and filings. Most people who work in such a capacity should take protective measures such as wearing safety glasses and other protective apparel. They should be able to give a negative history of possible injury. Exclusion of patients having intraorbital metal is not uncommon. This practice prevents injury caused by magnetic metal torquing in the magnetic field, as has been reported.

Patients who have metal fragments in their bodies may present with no prior history of foreign body injury. Usually these fragments are fixed in subcutaneous tissue, but the possibility of a hazard always exists. Another suspicious group is military veterans. If any doubt exists, stereo orbit radiographs of patients with previous foreign body injury involving metal to the orbits should be routinely obtained.

Surgical Clips and Prostheses

Numerous neurosurgical clips and implants have been tested, and some have been found to be magnetic. It is impossible to recognize their type on any radiograph. Even if all neurosurgical clips were changed to nonmagnetic materials today, it would be impossible to know in the future whether a patient had one of the old magnetic aneurysm clips or a new nonmagnetic one. The patient with neurosurgical clips is simply not imaged because of the risk.

Middle ear prostheses are not considered hazardous to patients but may somewhat compromise the image quality. Many but not all middle ear prostheses have been tested to be nonmagnetic. Some minor image degradation in the area of the implant or prosthesis may occur.

Surgical clips and sutures in the abdomen are a bit more of a problem. There is no contraindication to the use of MRI in the patient with surgical clips in the abdomen. On occasion significant artifacts indicating magnetic metal clips will appear. Trial and error is the only way to determine if abdominal surgical clips will produce artifacts that are objectionable.

Joint prostheses are primarily constructed of stainless steel and do not cause a problem unless the area of interest is directly next to the prosthesis. For example, it is possible to image the lumbar spine of a patient with bilateral hip prostheses. However, it is usually not possible to obtain a complete diagnostic examination of the pelvis.

Pregnant Women

There are no data currently available to suggest that any harmful effects will occur to a pregnant woman. Pregnancy is not a contraindication to MRI. However, it is generally believed that until more research data are available, pregnant women should not be imaged other than in exceptional situations.

SUMMARY

MRI is so new that considerable time and planning are required to establish a new facility. The problems of equipment selection, siting, and facility design are enormous. Adequate attention is imperative to ensure that all material and ancillary equipment that enter the magnet room are nonmagnetic. Proper planning for staff and patients is essential. Included in such planning are preparation of scheduling forms and provision of informative brochures.

Maintenance of an MR imager is no trivial task. Adequate financial resources and time must be allocated to maintenance, including cryogen replacement. A routine program of quality assurance should be instituted with proper phantom design to ensure that image quality is maintained at a high level. Procedures must be established to control entry to the magnet room. Visitors can adversely affect the magnet, and the magnet can adversely affect visitors. Patient screening is essential.

APPENDIX
A

The Bloch Equations

Within a few weeks after his announcement in 1946 of the discovery of "nuclear induction," which has come to be known as nuclear magnetic resonance (NMR)*, Felix Bloch published a set of equations that describe NMR. The most remarkable feature of this set of three coupled differential equations is Bloch's clarity of exposition. In addition to providing a description of the NMR experiments, the Bloch equations are applicable to many other areas of physics. Scientists compare the power of these equations with that of the Maxwell equations, which relate electric and magnetic fields to electric charges and currents and form the basis for the theory of electromagnetic waves.

Even though NMR scientists in physics, chemistry, and engineering substantially alter the mathematical notation of the equations, Bloch's equation set, which predicts the behavior of spin systems in a magnetic field, is nearly infallible, no matter the form of the equations. Despite the complicated appearance of the Bloch equations, an intense study session can provide excellent insight into the behavior of spins in magnetic resonance imaging. Familiarity with spin behavior is critical to understanding the significance of magnetic resonance measurement parameters. This tutorial appendix provides a simplistic development of the Bloch equations.

*The Bloch announcement from Stanford University was one of two. A simultaneous discovery was made by Edward Purcell at Harvard University. The two men subsequently shared the 1952 Nobel prize in physics.

First, the reader should consider several basic precepts. Nuclear magnetization is often described as a vector in three-dimensional Cartesian space with components M_x, M_y, and M_z. By convention, the Cartesian coordinate system is oriented with the Z axis parallel to the direction of the applied field (B_o); the X and Y axes are mutually perpendicular to each other and to the Z axis. The laws of thermodynamics set the maximum nuclear magnetization at a value M_o, and its magnitude $(M_x^2 + M_y^2 + M_z^2)^{1/2}$ can never exceed M_o.

Bloch postulated two relaxation times, transverse and longitudinal, associated T1 with M_z and T2 with M_x and M_y, and gave them the symbols T1 and T2. T1 and T2 are time constants for a first-order kinetics process, which can be incorporated into a set of coupled differential equations as follows:

$$\frac{d\,M_x}{dt} = \frac{M_x}{T2} \tag{1a}$$

$$\frac{d\,M_y}{dt} = \frac{M_y}{T2} \tag{1b}$$

$$\frac{d\,M_z}{dt} = \frac{(M_z - M_o)}{T1} \tag{1c}$$

The first two equations state that the transverse components of the nuclear magnetization decay with the time constant T2. The third equation states that the longitudinal component builds up to the value M_o with a time constant T1.

Let us look at some interpretations and applications of equations (1a), (1b), and (1c). If we consider a spin system at equilibrium created by placing a sample in a field B_o for a time t (long as compared to T1 and T2), the following definition applies:

$$\frac{d\,M_x}{dt} = \frac{d\,M_y}{dt} = \frac{d\,M_z}{dt} = 0 \tag{2}$$

That is, the components of the nuclear magnetization do not change with time when the spin system is at equilibrium.

On the other hand, suppose by the intervention of an external force, or pertubation, the net magnetization M_o is transformed from the Z axis to the Y axis, as shown in Figure A-1. The time history predicted by equations (1a), (1b), and (1c) can be used to interpret the Bloch equations. Plots are shown in Figure A-2.

The graphs in Figure A-2 have been generated by stepwise solution of equations (1a), (1b), and (1c) with $M_y = M_o$, T2 = 0.1 s, and T1 = 0.5 s. We find that M_y decreases with time constant T2 and approaches zero after several T2 periods. M_x was initially zero and remains at that value. M_z, also initially zero, increases with time until, after several T1 periods, it becomes essentially M_o. As developed in this tutorial, equations 1a, 1b, and 1c are the mathematical statement of the T1 and T2 relationships for the on-resonance rotating frame of reference.

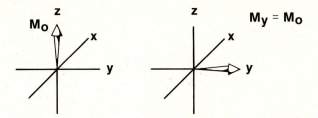

Figure A-1.

Note: Numerical integration is a commonly employed digital computing technique. The name is formidable; the technique need not be. For illustrations in the appendix, we assume a small time change; calculate the difference in the value of M_x, M_y, and M_z that occurs in the time interval; correct the M_x, M_y, or M_z values; and repeat the operation. The NMR enthusiast can accomplish several such steps on a hand-held computer and then estimate the curves found here.

At this point, it is appropriate to remember that T1 must always be equal to or greater than T2. If this restriction is violated, the magnitude of the M_o vector can easily exceed the thermodynamic M_o limit. Indeed, there is no known substance with T2 greater than T1.

Two factors cause us to elaborate on equations (1a), (1b), and (1c). First, there is no method for observing M_z directly, a fundamental truth guaranteed by quantum mechanics. Second, we have not yet discussed a physical means of perturbing equilibrated spin systems. Introducing an RF field in the X-Y plane solves both these limitations. An RF field is electromagnetic in description and can be shown to apply a secondary magnetic field, B_1, along the X axis of our coordinate system. The effect of B_1 is to rotate the vector M_o about the X axis at a rate γB_1, where γ equals the gyromagnetic ratio of the nucleus under observation. Incorporation of this effect changes equations 1a, 1b, and 1c into equations (3a), (3b), and (3c).

$$\frac{d\,M_x}{dt} = \frac{M_x}{T2} \tag{3a}$$

$$\frac{d\,M_y}{dt} = \frac{M_y}{T2} + \gamma\,B_1M_z \tag{3b}$$

$$\frac{d\,M_z}{dt} = \frac{(M_z - M_o)}{T1} - \gamma\,B_1M_y \tag{3c}$$

Equations (3a), (3b), and (3c) are simply a mathematical statement that any vector in the Y-Z plane is rotated by B_1 to a new location. Figure A-3 shows the effect of γB_1 on a spin system that is initially at equilibrium.

The RF field B_1 creates a motion of M_o around the X axis. The trajectory of M_o can be interrupted at will by turning off the RF oscillator. In this case,

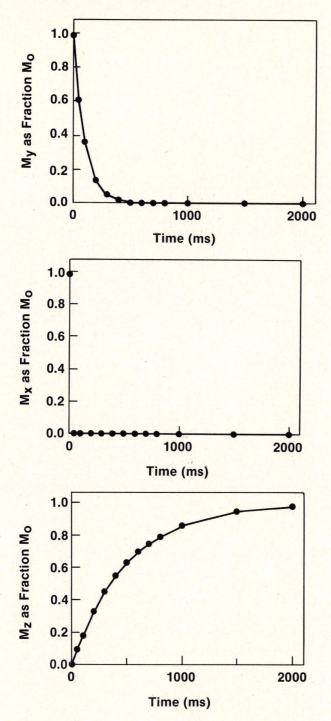

Figure A-2.

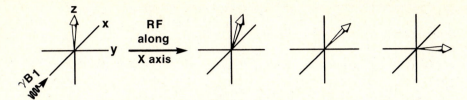

Figure A-3.

equations (3a), (3b), and (3c) simplify to equations (1a), (1b), and (1c), with the components M_x, M_y, and M_z being determined by the time at which the RF field was turned off, after which the behavior shown in Figure A-2 results.

Until now, discussion has been about the on-resonance rotating frame. The off-resonance rotating frame requires another modification of the equations. The terms to be included are ω, the frequency of the rotating frame, and ω_o, the resonance frequency, or γB_o. A difference $(\omega - \omega_o)$ corresponding to 1,000 Hz means the magnetization rotates 1,000 times per second. Mathematically, rotating magnetization in the X-Y plane is incorporated by decreasing M_x and increasing M_y with respect to time, as shown in equations (4a), (4b), and (4c). A comparable form exists for rotation in the Y-Z plane. The Bloch equations in the form of equations (4a), (4b), and (4c), which incorporate both of these features, are very reliable descriptors of the magnetization vectors in a sample during an NMR observation.

$$\frac{d M_x}{dt} = - \frac{M_x}{T2} + (\omega - \omega_o) M_y \tag{4a}$$

$$\frac{d M_y}{dt} = - \frac{M_y}{T2} - (\omega - \omega_o) M_y + \gamma B_1 M_z \tag{4b}$$

$$\frac{d M_z}{dt} = - \frac{(M_z - M_o)}{T1} - \gamma B_1 M_y \tag{4c}$$

The offset terms appear in M_x and M_y only. Numerical integration leads to the time history shown in Figure A-4.

In this case, the detected signal is a damped sine wave for M_x and a damped cosine wave for M_y. This is indeed the observed quadrature NMR signal.

The parameters M_x, M_y, and M_z are all effected by an RF pulse, and these give rise to three plots analogous to those in Figure A-4. Iteration will show that B_o magnetization varies with time and is effected by repeated excitation. The solution of these three equations by computer, and a plot of the results versus time, permits the NMR user to visualize all of the events during an NMR observation either spectroscopically or by imaging.

What faults exist in this analysis of NMR? One drawback is the assumption of a perfectly homogeneous magnetic field. In an inhomogeneous magnetic field, each individual nucleus will have a unique offset frequency

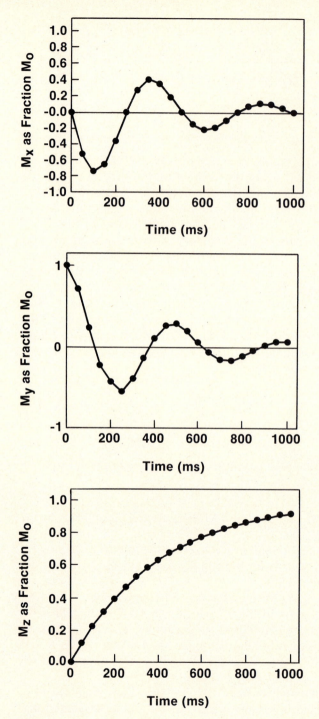

Figure A-4.

($\omega - \omega_o$). The NMR signal behavior observed for this sample is the summed behavior of the various nuclei. This process, called forming the **ensemble average,** provides the intellectual bridge between the behavior of an isolated spin system and multiple spin systems found in imaging applications. We will not show the ensemble averaging procedure here but simply note that it can and does provide a cogent explanation for the spin echo and image formation by gradient modulation. A second omission is that the Bloch equations make no provision for the spin-spin coupling interaction that is always present in spectroscopy.

In conclusion, the versatile Bloch equations of nuclear induction (how spin systems behave in a magnetic field) lend themselves to modification and approximations suitable for interpreting magnetic resonance observations. A basic understanding of these equations is essential before the novice can become an expert in MRI interpretation.

Glossary of MRI Terms*

Absolute zero: temperature of which material has no thermal energy and metals lose electrical resistance (O K, $-273.26°$ C, $459.69°$ F).

Acquisition: process of detecting and storing NMR signals.

Acquisition time: time required for acquisition of the NMR signals. Distinct from reconstruction time.

Air core magnet: electromagnet, either resistive or superconducting, in which the conductor windings provide the magnetic field without flux enhancement by ferromagnetic materials.

Analog-to-digital converter (ADC): part of the computer system that converts ordinary (analog) voltages, such as the detected NMR signal, into digital numerical form.

Angular frequency (ω): frequency of oscillation or rotation commonly designated by the Greek letter ω: $\omega = 2f$, where f is frequency (MHz).

Angular momentum: vector quantity given by the product of the momentum of a particle and its position. In the absence of external forces, the angular momentum remains constant, with the result that any rotating body

*The glossary is adapted from publications by the American College of Radiology, Diasonics, General Electric Company, Phillips Medical Systems, Picker International, Inc., and Siemens Medical Systems.

tends to maintain the same axis of rotation. When a torque is applied to a rotating body, the resulting change in angular momentum results in precession.

Antenna: device to send or receive electromagnetic radiation in the RF region of the spectrum.

Array process: optional component of computer system specially designed to speed up numerical calculations.

Artifacts: false features of an image caused by patient instability or equipment deficiencies.

B_0: conventional symbol for the main magnetic field in an MRI system. Measured in tesla (T).

B_1: conventional symbol for the RF magnetic induction field used in an MRI system. It is useful to consider it as composed of two oppositely rotating vectors, usually in a plane transverse to B_0. At the Larmor frequency, the vector rotating in the same direction as the precessing spins will interact strongly with the spins.

Bloch equations: equations of motion for the macroscopic net magnetization vector. They include the effects of precession about the magnetic field (static and radio frequency) and the T1 and T2 relaxation times.

Boil-off: cryogens returning to the gaseous from the liquid state and discharging from the imager.

Boltzmann distribution: system of particles in thermal equilibrium that exchange energy in collisions. For example, in MRI at room temperature, the difference in number of spins aligned with and against the Boltzmann field is about one part in a million; the small excess of nuclei in the lower-energy state is the basis of the net magnetization and the resonance phenomenon.

Carr-Purcell (CP) sequence: sequence of a 90° RF pulse followed by repeated 180° RF pulses to produce a train of spin echoes.

Carr-Purcell-Meiboom-Gill (CPMG) sequence: modification of Carr-Purcell RF pulse sequence with 90° phase shift in the rotating frame of reference between the 90° pulse and the subsequent 180° pulses to reduce accumulating effects of imperfections in the 180° pulses.

Chemical shift: change in the Larmor frequency of a given nucleus when bound in different sites in a molecule, owing to the magnetic shielding effects of the electron orbitals.

Coherence: maintenance of a constant-phase relationship between rotating or oscillating waves or objects. Loss of phase coherence of the spins results in a decrease in the transverse magnetization and hence a decrease in the NMR signal.

Coil: single or multiple loops of wire designed either to produce a magnetic field from current flowing through the wire or to detect a changing magnetic field by voltage induced in the wire.

Computer: electronic hardware for controlling the RF and gradient pulses and processing the NMR signals to produce an image.

Contrast: relative difference of the MRI signal intensities and the associated image brightness in adjacent regions.

Contrast resolution: ability of an imaging process to distinguish adjacent soft tissues from one another. This is the principal advantage of MRI.

Crossed-coil: pair of coils arranged with their magnetic fields at right angles to each other so as to minimize their mutual electromagnetic interaction.

Cryogen: atmospheric gases such as nitrogen and helium that have been cooled sufficiently to condense into a liquid.

Cryostat: apparatus for maintaining a constant low temperature. Requires vacuum chambers to help with thermal isolation.

dB/dt: rate of change of the magnetic field with time. Because changing magnetic fields can induce electrical fields, this is one area of potential concern for safety limits.

Demodulator: another term for detector, by analogy to broadcast radio receivers.

Detector: portion of the receiver that demodulates the RF NMR signal and converts it to a lower-frequency signal. Most detectors now used are phase sensitive and also give phase information about the RF signal.

Diamagnetic: type of substance that will slightly decrease a magnetic field when placed within it.

Diffusion: process by which molecules or other particles intermingle and migrate because of their random thermal motion.

Digital-to-analog converter (DAC): part of the computer system that converts digital numbers into ordinary analog voltages or currents.

Echo planar imaging: technique in which a complete planar image is obtained from one selective excitation pulse. The spin echo is observed while periodically switching the Y-gradient in the presence of a static X-gradient magnetic field.

Echo time: see *TE echo time.*

Eddy currents: electric currents induced in a conductor by a changing magnetic field or by motion of the conductor through a magnetic field.

Excitation: putting energy into the spin system by way of an RF pulse.

Exclusion time: part of the imaging suite and surrounding areas from which people must be restricted because of possible magnetic field hazards.

Faraday shield: electrical conductor interposed between MR imager and the environment to block out ambient electromagnetic radiation.

Fast Fourier transform (FFT): efficient computational method of performing a Fourier transform.

Ferromagnetic: substance, such as iron, that has a large positive magnetic susceptibility.

Filling factor: measure of the geometric relationship of the RF coil and the body. It affects the efficiency of irradiating the body and detecting MRI signals, thereby affecting the signal-to-noise ratio. Achieving a high filling factor requires fitting the coil closely to the body.

Filtered back projection: mathematical technique used in reconstruction from projections to create images from a set of multiple projection profiles.

Flip angle: amount of rotation of the net magnetization vector produced by an RF pulse, with respect to the direction of the static magnetic field B_o.

Fourier transform (FT): mathematical procedure to separate the frequency components of a signal from its amplitudes as a function of time. The Fourier transform is used to generate the spectrum from the FID and is essential to most imaging techniques.

Fourier transform imaging: MRI techniques in which at least one dimension is phase encoded by applying variable gradient pulses along that dimension. The Fourier transform is then used to reconstruct an image from the set of encoded MRI signals.

Free induction decay (FID): if transverse magnetization (M_{xy}) of the spins is produced, a transient NMR signal will result that will decay with a characteristic time constant T2 (or T2*); this decaying signal is the FID.

Frequency (f): number of repetitions of a periodic process per unit time. For RF electromagnetic radiation applied to MRI, the range is from 10 MHz to 100 MHz.

Fringe field: Stray magnetic field that exists outside the imager.

Gauss (G): unit of magnetic flux density in the older CGS system. The currently preferred (SI) unit is the tesla (T) (1T = 10,000 G).

Golay coil: coil used to create gradient magnetic field, perpendicular to the main magnetic field.

Gradient: amount and direction of the rate of change in space of some quantity, such as magnetic field strength.

Gradient coils: current-carrying coils designed to produce a desired gradient magnetic field. Proper design of the size and configuration of the coils is necessary to produce a controlled and uniform gradient.

Gradient magnetic field: magnetic field that changes in strength in a given direction (T/m).

Gradient pulse: briefly applied gradient magnetic field.

G_x, G_y, G_z: conventional symbols for gradient magnetic field. Used with subscripts to denote spatial direction along which the field changes.

Gyromagnetic ratio (γ): ratio of the magnetic moment to the angular momentum of a particle. This is a constant for a given nucleus (MHz/T).

Hardware: electrical and mechanical components of a computer.

Helmholtz coil: pair of current-carrying coils used to create uniform magnetic field in the space between them.

Hertz (Hz): standard (SI) unit of frequency; equal to the old unit cycles per second.

Homogeneity: uniformity in MRI. The homogeneity of the static magnetic field is an important characteristic of the quality of the magnet. Homogeneity requirements for MRI are generally lower than the homogeneity requirements for NMR spectroscopy.

Image acquisition time: time required to receive all of the NMR signals necessary to produce an MR image. The additional image reconstruction time will also be important to determine how quickly the image can be viewed.

Inductance: measure of the magnetic coupling between two current-carrying loops reflecting their spatial relationship. One of the principal determinants of the resonance frequency of an RF circuit.

Inhomogeneity: degree of lack of homogeneity—for example, the fractional deviation of the local magnetic field from the average value of the field.

Inversion: nonequilibrium state in which the net magnetization vector is oriented opposite to the Boltzmann magnetic field.

Inversion recovery (IR): RF pulse sequence for MRI wherein the net magnetization is inverted and returns to equilibrium with the emission of an NMR signal.

Inversion time (TI): time between the 180° RF inversion pulse and the subsequent 90° RF pulse to bring net magnetization onto the X-Y plane.

Iron core magnet: usually a resistive electromagnet in which the conductor is wound on an iron core to enhance the magnetic field.

Larmor equation: $\omega = \gamma B$ states that the frequency of precession of the nuclear magnetic moment is proportional to the magnetic field.

Larmor frequency (ω): frequency at which magnetic resonance can be excited; given by the Larmor equation. For hydrogen nuclei, the Larmor frequency is 42.6 MHz/T.

Lattice: magnetic environment with which nuclei exchange energy in longitudinal relaxation.

Longitudinal magnetization (M_z): component of the net magnetization vector along the static magnetic field.

Longitudinal relaxation: return of longitudinal magnetization to its equilibrium value after excitation; requires exchange of energy between the nuclear spins and the lattice.

Longitudinal relaxation time: see *T1*.

M: conventional symbol for net magnetization vector.

M_o: equilibrium value of the net magnetization vector directed along the static magnetic field.

Magnetic dipole: north and south magnetic poles separated by a finite distance.

Magnetic induction (B): also called magnetic flux density and magnetic field intensity. It is the net magnetic effect from an externally applied magnetic field and the resulting magnetization. Measured in tesla (T).

Magnetic moment: measure of the net magnetic properties of an object or particle.

Magnetic resonance imaging: creation of images of patients by use of the nuclear magnetic resonance phenomenon. Image brightness in a given region is usually dependent on the spin density and the relaxation times.

Magnetic susceptibility: measure of the ability of a substance to become magnetized.

Maxwell coil: particular kind of gradient coil, commonly used to create gradient magnetic fields along the direction of the main magnetic field.

Megahertz (MHz): unit of frequency, equal to 1 million hertz.

M_{xy}: see *Transverse magnetization* (M_{xy}).

M_z: see *Longitudinal magnetization* (M_z).

Net magnetization vector: net magnetic moment per unit volume of a sample in a given region; considered the integrated effect of all the individual microscopic nuclear magnetic moments. The magnetic polarization of a material produced by a magnetic field.

Nuclear magnetic resonance (NMR): absorption or emission of electromagnetic energy by nuclei in a static magnetic field, after excitation by a suitable RF magnetic field. The peak resonance frequency is proportional to the magnetic field and is given by the Larmor equation.

Nuclear magnetic resonance signal: electromagnetic signal in the RF range produced by the precession of the transverse magnetization (M_{xy}) of the nuclear spins.

Nuclear spin quantum number: property of all nuclei related to the largest measurable component of the nuclear angular momentum.

Paramagnetic: type of substance with a small but positive magnetic susceptibility. The addition of a small amount of paramagnetic substance may greatly reduce the relaxation times of a substance. Paramagnetic substances are considered promising for use as contrast agents in MRI.

Partial saturation (PS): excitation technique applying repeated 90° RF pulses at times on the order of or shorter than T1. Although partial saturation is also commonly referred to as saturation recovery, the latter term should properly be reserved for the particular case of partial saturation when the 90° RF pulses are far enough apart in time that the return of nuclear spins to equilibrium is complete.

Permanent magnet: magnet whose magnetic field originates from permanently magnetized material.

Permeability: tendency of a substance to concentrate the imaginary lines of the magnetic field.

Phantom: artificial object of known dimensions and properties used to test aspects of an MR imager.

Phase: in a periodic function such as rotational or harmonic motion, the position relative to a particular part of the cycle.

Pixel: acronym for a picture element; the smallest discrete part of a digital image display.

Planar imaging: imaging technique in which image of a plane is built up from signals received from the whole plane.

Precession: comparatively slow gyration of the axis of a spinning body so as to trace out a cone, caused by the application of a torque tending to change the direction of the rotation axis.

Probe: portion of an MR imager comprising the patient container and the RF coils, with some associated electronics.

Projection reconstruction: see *Reconstruction from projections.*

Proton density: see *Spin density.*

Pulse, 90°: RF pulse designed to rotate the net magnetization vector 90° to the main magnetic field. If the spins are initially aligned with the magnetic field, this pulse will produce transverse magnetization and an FID.

Pulse, 180°: RF pulse designed to rotate the net magnetization vector 180°. If the spins are initially aligned with the magnetic field, this pulse will produce inversion. If the spins are initially in the X-Y plane, a spin echo will result.

Pulse length: time duration of an RF pulse. For an RF pulse near the Larmor frequency, the longer the pulse length, the greater the angle of rotation of the net magnetization vector will be.

Pulse NMR: NMR techniques that use RF pulses and Fourier transformation of the NMR signal; have largely replaced older continuous-wave techniques.

Pulse programmer: part of the computer system that controls the timing, duration, and amplitude of the RF and gradient pulses.

Pulse sequences: set of RF or gradient magnetic field pulses and time spacings between these pulses.

Quadrature detector: phase-sensitive detector or demodulator that detects the components of the NMR signal in phase with a reference oscillation and 90° out of phase with the reference oscillator.

Quality factor (Q): applies to any electrical circuit component; most often the coil Q is limiting. Inversely related to the fraction of energy in an oscillating system lost in one oscillation cycle. The Q of a coil will depend on whether it is unloaded (no patient) or loaded (patient).

Quantum mechanics: physics of very small objects, based on the concept that all physical quantities can exist only as discrete units.

Quenching: loss of superconductivity of the current-carrying coil that may occur unexpectedly in a superconducting magnet. As the magnet becomes resistive, heat will be released that can result in rapid evaporation of liquid helium in the cryostat.

Radio frequency (RF): electromagnetic radiation just lower in energy than infrared. The RF used in MRI is commonly in the 10- to 100-MHz range.

Receiver: portion of the MR imager that detects and amplifies RF signals picked up by the receiving coil. Includes a preamplifier, amplifier, and demodulator.

Receiver coil: coil of the RF receiver; detects the NMR signal.

Reconstruction from projections: MRI technique in which a set of projection profiles of the body is obtained by observing NMR signals in the presence of a suitable corresponding set of gradient magnetic fields. Images can then be reconstructed using techniques analogous to those used in computed tomography, such as filtered back-projection.

Relaxation time: after excitation, the nuclear spins will tend to return to their equilibrium position, in accordance with these time constants.

Rephasing gradient: gradient magnetic field applied briefly after a selective excitation pulse, in the opposite direction to the gradient used for the selective excitation. The result of the gradient reversal is a rephasing of the spins, forming a spin echo.

Repetition time: see *TR repetition time.*

Resistive magnet: magnet whose magnetic field originates from current flowing through an ordinary electrical conductor.

Resonance: large-amplitude vibration in a mechanical or electrical system caused by a relatively small periodic stimulus with a frequency at or close to a natural frequency of the system.

Resonant frequency (RF): frequency at which resonance phenomenon occurs; given by the Larmor equation for NMR.

RF coil: used for transmitting RF pulses and or receiving NMR signals.

RF enclosure: see *Faraday shield.*

RF pulse: brief burst of RF electromagnetic energy delivered to patient by RF transmitter. If the RF frequency is at the Larmor frequency, the result is rotation of the net magnetization vector and phase coherence of the nuclear spins.

Rotating frame of reference: frame of reference, with corresponding coordinate systems, that is rotating about the axis of the static magnetic field B_o at a frequency equal to that of the applied RF magnetic field, B_1.

Saddle coil: RF coil configuration design commonly used when the static magnetic field is coaxial with the axis of the coil along the long axis of the body.

Saturation: nonequilibrium state in MRI in which equal numbers of spins are aligned against and with the B_o magnetic field so that there is no net magnetization.

Saturation recovery (SR): particular type of partial saturation pulse sequence in which the preceding pulses leave the spins in a state of saturation so that recovery to equilibrium is complete by the time of the next pulse.

Security zone: part of the imaging suite where ferromagnetic objects are intercepted so they do not enter the imaging room. Usually incorporates a metal detector.

Selective excitation: controlling the frquency spectrum of an irradiating RF pulse while imposing a gradient magnetic field on nuclear spins, such that only a desired region will have a suitable resonant frequency to be excited. Commonly used to select a plane for excitation and imaging.

Sensitive plane: technique of selecting a plane for imaging by using an oscillating gradient magnetic field and filtering out the corresponding time-dependent part of the NMR signal.

Sensitive point: technique of selecting a point for imaging by applying three orthogonal, oscillating gradient magnetic fields such that the local magnetic field is time dependent everywhere, except at the desired point, and then filtering out the corresponding time-dependent portion of the NMR signal.

Sensitive volume: region of the object from which NMR signal will predominantly be acquired because of strong magnetic field inhomogeneity elsewhere. Effect can be enhanced by use of a shaped RF field that is strongest in the sensitive volume.

Sequential line imaging: MRI techniques in which the image is built up from successive lines through the object.

Sequential plane imaging: MRI techniques in which the image is built from successive planes in the object.

Shim coils: coils carrying a relatively small current that are used to provide auxiliary magnetic fields to compensate for inhomogeneities in the main magnetic field.

Shimming: correction of inhomogeneity of the main magnetic field of an MR imager owing to imperfections in the magnet or to the presence of external ferromagnetic objects. May involve changing the configuration of the magnet, activating shim coils, or adding small pieces of steel.

Signal averaging: method of improving SNR by averaging several FIDs or spin echoes.

Signal-to-noise ratio (SNR or S/N): used to describe the relative contributions to a detected signal of the true signal and random superimposed signals or noise. The SNR can be improved by averaging several NMR signals, by sampling larger volumes, or by increasing the strength of the B_o magnetic field.

SI unit: universally accepted unit as defined by The General Conference on Weights and Measures. From the French Systeme Internationale.

Software: set of instructions, or programs, that controls the activities of the computer. Programs may be written in machine language, assembly language, or higher-level languages such as Fortran or BASIC.

Solenoid coil: coil of wire wound in the form of a long cylinder. When a current is passed through the coil, a magnetic field is produced along the axis of the coil.

Spatial resolution: ability of an imaging process to distinguish small adjacent high-contrast structures in the object.

Spectrum: array of the intensity of the components of the NMR signal according to frequency.

Spin: intrinsic angular momentum of an elementary particle, or system of particles such as a nucleus, that is responsible for the magnetic moment.

Spin density (SD): density of resonating nuclear spins in a given region; one of the principal determinants of the strength of the NMR signal from that region.

Spin echo: reappearance of an NMR signal after the FID has disappeared. The result of the effective reversal of the dephasing of the nuclear spins.

Spin echo imaging: any one of many MRI techniques in which the spin echo NMR signal rather than the FID is used.

Spin-lattice relaxation time: see *T1*.

Spin-spin relaxation time: see *T2*.

Spin warp imaging: form of Fourier transform imaging in which phase-encoding gradient pulses are applied for a constant duration but with varying amplitude. This is distinct from the original Fourier transform imaging methods in which phase encoding is performed by applying gradient pulses of constant amplitude but varying duration.

Steady-state free precession (SSFP): method of NMR excitation in which strings of RF pulses are applied rapidly and repeatedly with interpulse intervals short compared to those of both T1 and T2.

Superconducting magnet: magnet whose magnetic field originates from current flowing through a superconductor. Such a magnet must be enclosed in a cryostat.

Superconductor: substance whose electrical resistance essentially disappears at temperatures near absolute zero. A commonly used superconductor in MR imagers is niobium-titanium, embedded in a copper matrix.

Surface Coil: simple, flat RF receiver coil placed over a region of interest. It will have an effective selectivity for a volume approximately equal to the coil circumference and one radius deep from the coil center.

T1: spin lattice or longitudinal relaxation time; the characteristic time constant for spins to tend to align themselves with the external magnetic field.

T2: spin-spin or transverse relaxation time; the characteristic time constant for loss of phase coherence among spins oriented at an angle to the main magnetic field owing to interactions between the spins. T2 never exceeds T1.

T2*: characteristic time constant for loss of phase coherence among spins oriented at an angle to the main magnetic field owing to a combination of magnetic field inhomogeneities and spin-spin relaxation. T2* is always much shorter than T2.

Tailored pulse: shaped RF pulse whose magnitude is varied with time in a predetermined manner. Affects the frequency components of an RF pulse in a manner determined by the Fourier transform of the pulse.

TE echo time: time between middle of 90° RF pulse and middle of spin echo.

Tesla (T): preferred (SI) unit of magnetic flux density or magnetic field intensity. One tesla is equal to 10,000 gauss, the older (CSG) unit. One tesla also equals one newton/amp-m.

Thermal equilibrium: state in which all parts of a system are at the same effective temperature. When the relative alignment of the spins with the magnetic field is determined solely by the thermal energy of the system.

TI inversion time: time after middle of inverting RF pulse to middle of 90° pulse to detect amount of longitudinal magnetization.

Time reversal: technique of producing a spin echo by subjecting excited spins to a gradient magnetic field and then reversing the direction of the gradient field.

Torque: force that causes or tends to cause a body to rotate. It is a vector quantity given by the product of the force and the position vector where the force is applied.

Transmitter: portion of the MR imager that produces RF current and delivers it to the transmitting coil.

Transverse magnetization (M_{xy}): component of the net magnetization vector at right angles to the main magnetic field, B_o.

TR repetition time: period between the beginning of a pulse sequence and the beginning of the succeeding and identical pulse sequence.

Tuning: process of adjusting the resonant frequency of the RF circuit to the Larmor frequency. More generally, the process of adjusting the components of the spectrometer for optimal NMR signal strength.

Tunnel: opening into MR imager for patient. Sometimes called the patient aperture.

Two-dimensional fourier transform imaging (2DFT): form of sequential plane imaging using Fourier transform imaging.

Vector: quantity having both magnitude and direction, frequently represented by an arrow whose length is proportional to the magnitude and with an arrowhead at one end to indicate the direction.

Volume imaging: imaging techniques in which NMR signals are gathered from the whole object volume to be imaged at once.

Voxel: volume element; the element of three-dimensional space corresponding to a pixel for a given slice thickness.

Zeugmatography: term for MRI coined from Greek roots suggesting the role of the gradient magnetic field in joining the RF magnetic field to a desired local spatial region through nuclear magnetic resonance.

Index